INTERNATIONAL REVIEW OF

Neurobiology

VOLUME 8

Contributors To This Volume

Denise Albe-Fessard

Raymond A. Beck

David Bowsher

Günter G. Brune

Leonide Goldstein

Paul A. J. Janssen

James L. McGaugh

Lewis F. Petrinovich

Ch. Stumpf

Lowell E. White, Jr.

INTERNATIONAL REVIEW OF

Neurobiology

Edited by CARL C. PFEIFFER
New Jersey Psychiatric Institute
Princeton, New Jersey

JOHN R. SMYTHIES
Department of Psychological Medicine
University of Edinburgh, Edinburgh, Scotland

VOLUME 8

1965

ACADEMIC PRESS • New York and London

ACADEMIC PRESS INC.
111 Fifth Avenue, New York, New York 10003

United Kingdom Edition published by
ACADEMIC PRESS INC. (LONDON) LTD.
Berkeley Square House, London W.1

Library of Congress Catalog Card Number: 59-13822

PRINTED IN THE UNITED STATES OF AMERICA

To

F. Georgi

CONTRIBUTORS

Numbers in parentheses indicate the pages on which the authors' contributions begin.

DENISE ALBE-FESSARD (35), *Faculty of Science, Laboratoire de Physiologie des Centres Nerveux, Paris, France*

RAYMOND A. BECK (265), *Section on Neuropharmacology, Bureau of Research in Neurology and Psychiatry, New Jersey Neuropsychiatric Institute, Princeton, New Jersey*

DAVID BOWSHER (35), *Department of Anatomy, University of Liverpool, Liverpool, England, and Centre d'Etudes de Physiologie Nerveuse, University of Paris, Paris, France*

GÜNTER G. BRUNE (197), *Neurologische Universitätsklinik und -Poliklinik, Hamburg, Germany*

LEONIDE GOLDSTEIN (265), *Section on Neuropharmacology, Bureau of Research in Neurology and Psychiatry, New Jersey Neuropsychiatric Institute, Princeton, New Jersey*

PAUL A. J. JANSSEN (221), *Janssen Pharmaceutica, Research Laboratoria, Beerse, Belgium*

JAMES L. MCGAUGH (139), *Department of Psychobiology, University of California, Irvine, California*

LEWIS F. PETRINOVICH (139), *Department of Psychology, State University of New York, Stony Brook, Long Island, New York*

CH. STUMPF (77), *Department of Pharmacology, Emory University, Atlanta, Georgia, and Institute of Pharmacology, University of Vienna, Vienna, Austria*

LOWELL E. WHITE, JR. (1), *Division of Neurosurgery, University of Washington School of Medicine, Seattle, Washington*

PREFACE

The major aim of this review is to provide a forum in which the latest progress in the many major and different sciences that make up neurobiology can be presented for the edification not only of scientists working in the same science but also of those working in other disciplines.

The usual order for the classification of knowledge in medical science is used in this volume, namely a progression from anatomy and histology through chemistry and physiology to the clinical application of anatomical, physiological, pharmacological, and psychological knowledge. This represents the orderly progression which will ultimately determine success in the general field of neurobiology when the total goal is the better understanding and treatment of all mental disorders. As in the past, particular emphasis has been given to the recent development of basic concepts which are of fundamental importance, and also to those which are likely to further our understanding of neuronal functions and mental diseases. In the past the neurobiological sciences have been most important in progress toward these ends.

These reviews and summaries ordinarily are by invitation, with an annual deadline for receipt of manuscripts by October 1. The editors, however, will be happy to review unsolicited manuscripts if submitted in complete or outline form.

CARL C. PFEIFFER
JOHN R. SMYTHIES

July 1965

CONTENTS

Biogenic Amines in Mental Illness

GÜNTER G. BRUNE

The Evolution of the Butyrophenones, Haloperidol and Trifluperidol, from Meperidine-Like 4-Phenylpiperidines

PAUL A. J. JANSSEN

Amplitude Analysis of the Electroencephalogram (Review of the Information Obtained with the Integrative Method)

LEONIDE GOLDSTEIN AND RAYMOND A. BECK

A MORPHOLOGIC CONCEPT OF THE LIMBIC LOBE

By Lowell E. White, Jr.

Division of Neurosurgery, University of Washington School of Medicine, Seattle, Washington

I. Introduction

The surprising response of the chimpanzee "Becky" following the amputation of her frontal lobes (Jacobson, 1935; Walker, 1944; Fulton, 1951) and the foresighted surgical therapy on the frontal lobe for psychiatric disease (Moniz, 1936; Freeman and Watts, 1950) opened a new era in the quest for knowledge concerning the behavior of man. These epic observations, when considered in the light of the provocative morphologic "emotional mechanism" postulated by Papez (1937), have led to an era of investigation centered around the vegetative activities of the limbic cortex of the brain. These observations have been formulated by many into theories of "emotion" and control of visceral function, imparting to Broca's grand limbic lobe a possible homeostatic function (Pool, 1954; MacLean, 1954; Pribram and Kruger, 1954). Although still shrouded in mystery, recent years have recorded the rebirth of the limbic lobe and an elevation of status approaching that of the basic five senses. In many circles it carries the connotation of "a limbic system."

To the anatomist this suggestion represents a play on words, disrupting an already confusing area of anatomy by many functional terms and amplifying the already cluttered and redundant nomenclature of this poorly differentiated cortex. To the physiologist it offers an area of speculation because of its relative anatomic simplicity and varied evoked responses. To the behavioral psychologist it represents a nonspecific area of basic function, injury to which produces various changes related to volume destroyed, but with little in the way of discrete localization. To the clinician it represents a new vista for the possible understanding of abnormal mental function in psychosomatic and psychiatric diseases.

The description of the limbic lobe by Broca in 1878 stressed the circumferential nature of this part of the brain, emphasizing its location as a border for the cerebral hemisphere. He observed that this border was joined together ventrally by the olfactory portion of the hemispheres to which in 1837 Sir Richard Owen had referred, in relation to its major input, as a rhinencephalon. Rapidly the term rhinencephalon was amplified to include all the border lobe of the brain and was adopted by many authors, particularly those writing in the French language (Gardner, 1881; Elliot Smith, 1910b). This use of the term was generally accepted by human anatomists above the objections of noted comparative anatomists of the day. Thus, anatomists brought to the present era a functional connotation to their nomenclature which has led to considerable objection on the part of recent investigators who have suggested such terms as "visceral brain" (Pool, 1954) and integrated "limbic system" (MacLean, 1954). Does this represent an improvement or simply add to the confusion? Was Broca correct in looking upon this area as a border for the spherical hemisphere? Is this cortex rudimentary in nature or simply old? A careful look at and review of the known morphology of this area in the light of history and recent knowledge may help to clarify this problem and create a unified approach to the nomenclature employed.

The intent of this paper is not to be all inclusive but rather selective in the use of information in essay form. Information will be taken from three sources to arrive, in this author's opinion, at a historically sound, ontogenetically descriptive and phylogenetically consistent morphologic concept compatible with present day usage and adaptable to all fields of neurobiologic endeavor.

II. Terminology

A. Limbic Lobe vs. Rhinencephalon

The purely descriptive term for this area (limbic lobe) of the brain cannot be credited to Broca, for the truly bordering nature of this portion of the brain was recognized by older anatomists. Thomas Willis as early as 1664 pictured this area of the brain and referred to it as the limbus. Later authors (e.g., Solly, 1848; Todd, 1839) although not stressing the Latin term considered its prominence as a primary convolution containing within it the major superior commissure of the hemisphere (the cingulum of later writing). The Latin word *commissura* means a joining together. Early anatomists used the term for any tract of fibers within the brain or spinal cord connecting two points, either ipsilateral or contralateral. Modern usage limits the term to fiber tracts joining right and left sides of the brain or spinal cord.

The commonly applied term for the limbic lobe prior to the work of Broca was used by Foville (1844) (the circonvolution de l'ourlet) and later called the falciform lobe by Schwalbe (1881). Likewise, Broca cannot truly be given the dubious distinction of coining the term rhinencephalon. Apparently both St. Hilaire and Robin in the eighteenth century (Elliot Smith, 1901) used the term to describe uniocular monsters without reference to the brain—a term maintained in the first index volumes of the Army Medical Library of the United States. On independent grounds Sir Richard Owen applied the term between the years 1840 and 1868 to the olfactory bulb and peduncle, establishing a precedent for its use as a descriptive term for a given area of the brain (Owen, 1868; Huxley, 1894). With Broca's careful comparative study of the cerebral convolutions in 1878 he likened this border area of the hemispheres to a tennis racket with the handle represented by the olfactory bulb and peduncle and the racket proper by the cortex circumscribing the medial border of the hemisphere (Fig. 1). He described this area as a continuing band of cortex which he referred to again in Latin as limbic cortex and applied the term grand limbic lobe. He ascribed to this area a possible function—olfaction—but did not use the term rhinencephalon. But, the term having previously been used in relation to olfaction was rapidly adopted by others. Many noted anatomists objected to this, and in rebuttal Sir William Turner (1890) extended the original use of the term by his countryman, Sir Richard Owen, to include not only the olfactory bulb and peduncle but the cortex to which the olfactory tracts were felt

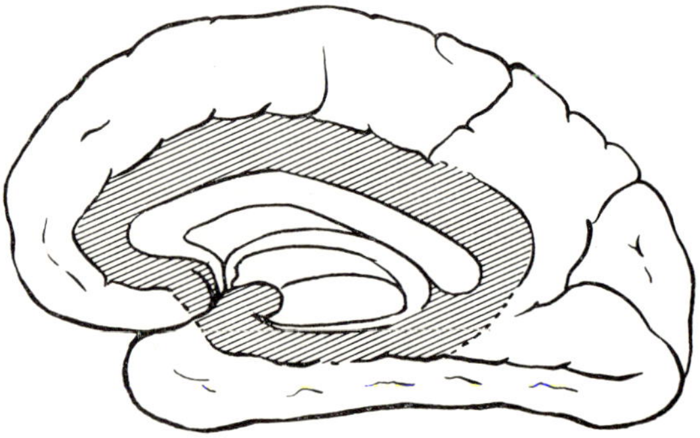

FIG. 1. The crosshatched area represents a diagrammatic overlay of the limbic lobe on the medial surface of the human brain.

primarily to project (olfactory tubercle, the anterior perforate area, and piriform lobe) and used the term rhinencephalon in contradistinction to the rest of the hemisphere which he referred to as pallium. Numerous anatomists of the day including such names as Wilhelm His, David Ferrier, G. P. Putnam, Heinrich Obensteiner, Alex Hill, and G. Elliot Smith objected to the use of the all-inclusive term, rhinencephalon, on comparative anatomic grounds. Furthermore, Wilhelm His in 1895 did not include this definition of the term in the *Basel, Nomina Anatomica,* but rather adopted the description of Sir William Turner which included only the cortex of the base of the brain.

B. PALLIUM

The term pallium was an embryologic term applied to the thin upper portion of the developing hemisphere by Reichert in 1859 in contradistinction to the development of the basal ganglia and their overlying cortex which he termed "stamlappen." In 1901 Elliot

Smith, struck by the confusing use of the term rhinencephalon in one sense for the olfactory lobe of Turner and in the other for the limbic lobe of Broca, and strongly objecting to the structures included in the limbic lobe of Broca (Elliot Smith, 1896d), drew attention to the above concept of pallium by the embryologist and on phylogenetic grounds suggested that in the developed cerebral hemisphere three major subdivisions existed: the older cortex of the medial hemisphere exemplified by the hippocampus; the basal

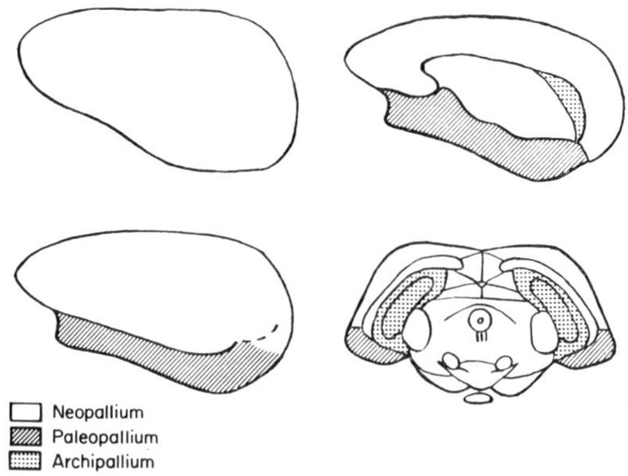

FIG. 2. A diagrammatic representation of the three major divisions of the cerebral cortex depicted on dorsal, medial, lateral, and coronal section views of the rat brain.

cortex associated with the major ganglia of the base; and the newer cortex encompassing the majority of the hemisphere. To the thin pallium he applied the term neopallium. Owing to translation difficulties old brain was considered as archipallium by others which Elliot Smith (1910a) disclaimed and objected to. Apparently to clarify this paleopallium was utilized to separate the cortex commonly thought of as olfactory in nature and associated with basal structures from the other two pallial divisions (Fig. 2).

Not only was the application of terminology difficult during this era, but it was complicated by a lack of acceptance of phylogenetic concepts concerning the development of the medial hemisphere propounded by Owen (1837, 1868). These observations were important to the precepts of Darwin and well known to the populace of the day as well as to the learned Linnean Society, where heated discussions were apparently common on these matters among Owen, Flowers, and Huxley (Elliot Smith, 1910b; Kingsley, 1863). These concepts were of basic importance to the understanding of brain development and their relation to human anatomy. The discussions centered around the morphology of the limbic lobe and particularly the hippocampus and the transverse commissures. Some insight into the strong feeling encountered between these naturalists was recorded by the clergyman Charles Kingsley and well summarized in many passages of his version of the old Greek story, "Water Babies" which he wrote to "my youngest son . . . and all other good little boys" in 1863.

C. Hippocampus

Aside from the over-all concepts of the origin and connections of the medial aspect of the cerebral hemispheres, descriptive anatomists had difficulty in not only setting uniform limits on the structures encompassed by morphologic terms but coined many original terms for previously documented structures. This practice was aptly described by Alex Hill in 1893: "Galen converted illustrations into cognomens for most of the bones, muscles and other parts of the body, but the anatomists of the 17th and 18th centuries, when writing of the parts of the brain, considered it as immaterial whether or not they used the same symbol or illustration as their predecessors . . . if a new illustration occurred to them . . . , by all means let posterity make use of it!" Thus, in 1893, Hill recorded seventeen commonly used synonyms for the hippocampus of Arantius first described in 1587 (and likewise called by him *Bombyx*). Tilney reviewed this multiplicity of terms in 1938 and again reiterated that the term hippocampus was adopted in Basel in 1895 as a part of the *Nomina Anatomica* and represents the most acceptable name, although it may be somewhat confusing on descriptive grounds (Lewis, 1923).

D. Fornicate Gyrus

The remaining cortical components of the limbic lobe do not carry as profound a history as those of the archipallium (Ecker, 1873). The gyri of early nomenclature were usually considered simply as primary or secondary convolutions or folds (Solly, 1848). Arnold (1851) who prepared his anatomical handbook in 1844 referred to the superior longitudinal commissure (cingulum) as a peripheral counterpart of Vesalius' fornix, naming the overlying gyrus of the hemisphere the fornicate gyrus, extending from the subcallosal septal area to the subsplenial hippocampal area. This nomenclature was officially adopted in Basel as the proper name for the primary gyrus of the medial hemisphere eliminating the term convolution de l'ourlet of Foville (1844) and the callosal gyrus of Huxley (1864). The need for a further subdivision of the convolution was necessary. Although the term cingulum had been utilized before the work of Beevor (1891) (Ecker, 1873; Obersteiner and Hill, 1890; Edinger, 1891), thereafter the term cingulate gyrus was commonly used in textbooks, the fornicate gyrus being divided into two main components: (1) the cingulate gyrus related to the corpus callosum and (2) the hippocampal gyrus related to the hippocampus (Elliot Smith, 1903b). The central continuation of the cingulate gyrus cephalad around the genu of the corpus callosum was referred to by Vicq d'Azyr as the peduncle of the corpus callosum, and later the subcallosal gyrus by Zuckerkandl (1887). The relationship of this later gyrus to the precommissural area was recognized by Huxley (1864) and referred to as the septal area which was continuous with the diagonal band of Broca. These two structures form the connecting link between the subcallosal portion of the gyrus fornicatus and the uncus portion of the hippocampal gyrus on the ventromedial surface of the hemisphere—creating the completed ring of the limbic lobe. The following subdivisions of the fornicate gyrus were thus adopted in Basel (His, 1895) as the basic anatomical subdivisions of the fornicate gyrus of Arnold: the subcallosal gyrus, cingulate gyrus, and hippocampal gyrus.

E. Telencephalon Medium

In acallosal animals the concept of the central telencephalic segment or telencephalon medium (telencephalon impar) was accepted. Although this area is present in higher mammals it is much more obvious in lower forms. The relation of this area to the midline septum pellucidum was suggested by Huxley (1864) who first referred to its discrete nuclear area in mammals as the septal area. Other authors stressed in lower forms the relationship of this midline nuclear mass to the olfactory lobe and referred to this cerebral area as paraolfactory (Johnston, 1913). Others stressed its cephalad position in relation to the anterior neuropore and the lamina terminalis—the paraterminal body of Elliot Smith (1896b,c, 1910b). Recent studies by Andy and Stephan (1962, 1963) and Stephan and Andy (1964) show that phylogenetic growth of the septal area occurs in keeping with the growth of the remainder of the related limbic lobe structures. These later observations indicate that this telencephalic element must functionally remain an important cerebral structure apparently not solely related to olfactory function.

F. Longitudinal Fiber Tracts

The major connecting fibers between the hippocampus and the telencephalon medium were described and pictured by Vesalius in 1543 as the fornix, a name surviving undistorted to date. With this prominent name other tracts were named around the fornix, the original superior longitudinal commissure being referred to by Arnold (1851) as the fornix peripherus and only later as the cingulum.

The projection of the various portions of the fornix excited extreme interest. In 1845 Arnold (Arnold, 1851; Elliot Smith, 1896e) in order to establish a distinction between the fornix peripherus and the true fornix of Vesalius referred to the latter as the fornix internus. In 1869 Stieda described fibers in the mouse on each side of the septum joining the fornix from the hippocampus as well as fibers from the cortex above the corpus callosum in which the fornix peripherus was located. In 1872 Forel called attention to the crossing psalterium fornix fibers which he described as connecting the two hippocampi and likewise the longitudinally running fornix fibers. He referred to these, respectively, as the fornix transversus and the fornix longus. In 1882 Ganser again described the longitudinal fibers of the septum perforating the corpus callosum from the fornicate gyrus, a fact previously noted by Meynert (1884) and Huguenin (1879), and referred to these fibers as the fornix longus. Von Koelliker in 1894 suggested the name fornix superior for these perforant fibers (of Ganser) to separate them from those fibers obviously emanating from the area of the hippocampus. Huxley (1864) had previously described the pre- and postcommissural nature of these longitudinal fornix fibers within the septal area and Elliot Smith (1898), upon reviewing the situation, divided the longitudinal fornix into a dorsal portion receiving the perforant system (the fornix superior) and a ventral portion receiving its fibers directly from the hippocampus and related structures.

The other major projection system of the limbic lobe from telencephalon medium is well documented in lower forms (Ariëns

Kappers *et al.*, 1936) and has caused little historical concern—the medial forebrain bundle. Its importance as a major association bundle of the forebrain has recently been emphasized by Herrick (1948).

III. Phylogenetic Development

The study of the comparative neuroanatomic makeup of the various phyla has added immensely to our knowledge of the development of the cerebral hemispheres. This is compared in numerous papers and summarized in the epic work of Sir Richard Owen (1868) and Ariëns Kappers *et al.* (1936).

A. A Promammalian Hemisphere

The development of the vertebrate hemispheres from their rudimentary beginning in the Silurian era to the mammalian brain we know today was an orderly process. This differentiation was probably influenced greatly by the alterations in oxygen tension created by a terrestrial existence. The significance of these changes has been outlined by Herrick (1920), and the significance of the everted hemispheres of ganoid and teleost brains to this orderly evolution has been stressed by Holmgren (1922). The earliest portion of the developing cerebral vesicle is represented by the vertebrate olfactory bulb and the rudimentary development of the primitive hemispheric vesicle. The exact makeup of the promammalian hemisphere is not known for, as is true throughout the phyla, the need for change is depicted by extinction and survival only of the changed and fittest. Elliot Smith in 1910 proposed a diagram for a promammalian brain (Fig. 3) made up of two vesicles, their development centered about a paired central structure which he referred to as the paraterminal body (telencephalon medium). This area was previously referred to by Huxley (1864) as the septal area and by Zuckerkandl (1887) as the subcallosal gyrus, and later by Johnston (1913) as the paraolfactory area.

The differentiation of the cephalad end of the neural tube allowed additional areas of integration for the neural tube (Herrick, 1920). This not only established the receptive areas for the two most powerful distance-receptive senses—sight and smell—but allowed the unimpeded growth of neural nets not specifically related to functional input and output, but rather "associational" in nature. This theory largely propounded throughout the writings of Herrick (1926, 1948, 1956) has come to be, in morphologic circles, relatively uniform in its acceptance. The initial cerebral growth is largely represented by limbic lobe development (von Bonin and Bailey, 1961) and closely related to the deep ganglionic masses of the striatum that reach their peak prominence in birds.

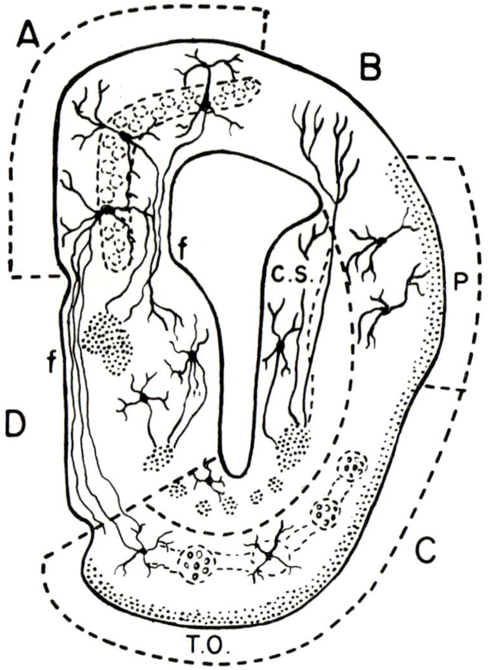

FIG. 3. A coronal section of half of the telencephalon of a possible promammalian brain as modified from Elliot Smith (1910b). Abbreviations: A, archipallium; B, neopallium; C, paleopallium; D, telencephalon medium; c.s., corpus striatum; f, fornix; p, piriform cortex; T.O., olfactory tubercle.

In the primitive promammalian brain the neocortex is relegated to a very insignificant role in the lateral portion of the developing vesicle. Rostrally is located the paired septal area in the region of the terminal plate, dorsally and caudally the hippocampus, and ventrally the piriform cortex and the olfactory tubercle. Fiber association between the two hemispheres occurs within the area of the terminal plate with fibers passing through the primitive septal area. Originally the most prominent of these crossing fibers connect the olfactory tubercles, the piriform cortices, and the hippocampi, but as will be emphasized later, subsequent neocortical interconnecting fibers continue to traverse this area leading to a major distortion of the developing limbic cortex by the corpus callosum.

B. The Commissures

The fundamental plan of the vertebrate brain was the subject of much debate. The source of the major transverse commissures was first propounded in 1837 by Sir Richard Owen and later conclusively established by John Symington in 1892. This observation led to the appreciation of the significance of the corpus callosum as a higher mammalian structure absent in lower mammals such as marsupials and monotremes.

The basic mammalian hemisphere largely represented by the limbic lobe is illustrated in the following drawing of the medial surface of a marsupial brain (Fig. 4). The relationship of the medial rim of tissue to the large foramen of Monro is evident. In this precallosal brain the limbic lobe forms the true boundary of the foramen of Monro and the neocortex is relegated to a lateral position maintaining the same relationship as in the hypothetical promammalian hemisphere (Fig. 3).

The significance of these findings and the true limbic nature of the hippocampus, piriform cortex, and the septal area with its connecting lateral link, the diagonal band of Broca, were described and discussed by Elliot Smith in 1896 (Elliot Smith, 1896a,b,d,e). He in turn referred to this area as the true limbic lobe bordering the foramen of Monro and considered the fornicate gyrus as a further perilimbic neocortical development.

Elliot Smith (1895b, 1903a) laid the groundwork for our understanding of the phylogenetic development of the major cerebral commissures which led directly to the understanding of the somewhat dystrophic and distorted elements (indusium griseum) of the limbic lobe of higher mammals. In early callosal animals the corpus callosum is just forming rostral to the hippocampal commissure which becomes displaced from its usual position in relation to the anterior commissure. There is little distortion of the major bulk of the hippocampus although the portion immediately overlying the corpus callosum is dystrophic with a well-formed, subcallosal, hippocampal extension joining the septal area.

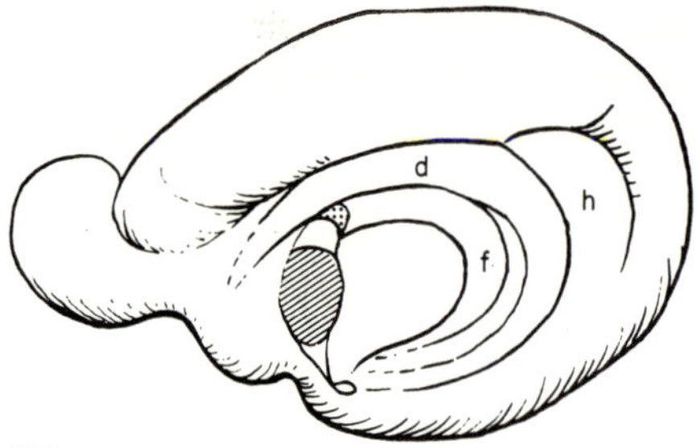

FIG. 4. The medial surface of a marsupial cerebral hemisphere which illustrates the relationship of the anterior and hippocampal commissures, and the absence of the corpus callosum. Abbreviations: f, fornix; d, dentate fascia; h, hippocampus.

As the phylogenetic scale is ascended the corpus callosum increases in size, extending caudad and creating the dorsal flexure in the remaining dorsal hippocampus (Fig. 5). This latter configuration is illustrated by both rodents and carnivores. With the larger corpus callosum the overlying hippocampus becomes more dystrophic and takes on the typical appearance of the indusium griseum with its contained longitudinal hippocampus and dentate

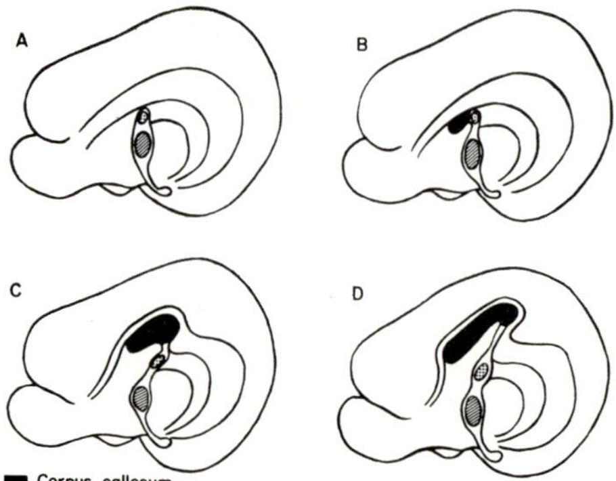

FIG. 5. Diagram of the phylogenetic development of the corpus callosum. This is illustrated on the medial surface of a marsupial hemisphere (see Fig. 4) in order to demonstrate the progressive distortion of the older commissures of the lamina terminalis and the components of the hippocampal formation by the (A–D) progressive development of the corpus callosum.

fascia fiber system, the medial longitudinal striae (Elliot Smith, 1897). With further growth of the corpus callosum the dorsal flexure area becomes somewhat dystrophic and straightened, becoming the fasciola cinerea and the gyrus fasciolaris of primate neuroanatomy. They represent the dorsal continuation of the dentate fascia and hippocampus extending retrosplenially to join the indusium.

C. The Fornix

The prominent fornix projection system of the limbic lobe with the septum remains unchanged by the development of the major cerebral commissures within the septal area (telencephalon medium). Therefore, in the primate the fornix projects from the hippocampus and extends beneath the corpus callosum where it is joined by callosal perforant fibers from the cortex above the corpus callosum. Rostrally the fornix continues to form the border of the foramen of Monro which it skirts to penetrate directly into the septal area. Those fibers that do not end in the septal area continue to the mammillary bodies and are joined by more fibers from the septal area and dorsal limbic centers (indusium griseum and probably other areas) which have followed a course around the genu of the corpus callosum rather than penetrating it (see Elliot Smith, 1896a,b,c,d, 1897, 1898, 1910b).

D. The Insula

During the development of the medial hemisphere, the differentiation of the neocortex is also taking place. With the overgrowth of the frontal and temporal lobe (Fig. 6) the cortex immediately lateral to the caudal extent of the olfactory tubercle and the middle third of the rhinal fissure is gradually covered by the frontal and temporal operculi. Thus, this lateral portion of the limbic lobe becomes buried deep within the Sylvian fissure—the insula (Elliot Smith, 1902).

The anatomy of the human limbic lobe still maintains its orientation to the foramen of Monro, but becomes distorted from its earlier semisymmetrical orientation by the tremendous overgrowth of the neopallial portion of the cerebral hemispheres. This relative overgrowth of the neopallium is now well documented by the comparative studies of Stephan and Andy (1964).

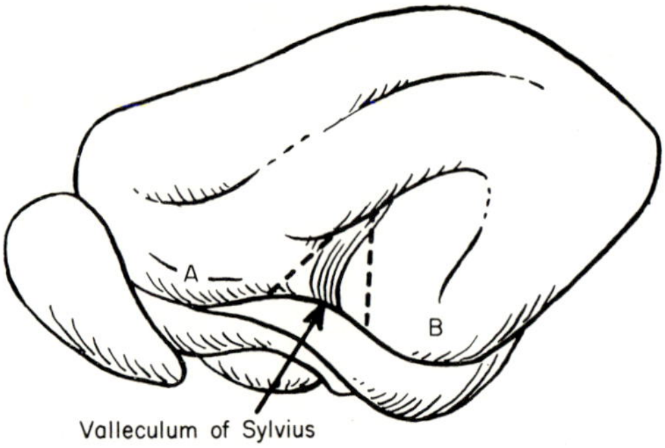

FIG. 6. The development of the insula lateral to the rhinal fissure at the point of the valleculum of Sylvius. A, The frontal lobe and B, the temporal lobe overgrows to form the operculi burying the insula in the Sylvian fissure.

IV. Ontogenetic Development

A. The Telencephalon

The early development of the human brain was clearly depicted by Hochstetter (1919) and little has been added to these gross concepts throughout the years. The major portion of the brain develops rostral to the notochord from that portion of the neural tube related to the prochordal plate (Kingsbury, 1922). In man the prosencephalon has made its appearance at 3.5-mm crown rump length and by 9 mm has differentiated into the diencephalon, two telencephalic vesicles and their connecting link, the telencephalon medium (Hamilton *et al.*, 1947). It is through this initial process of differentiation of the prosencephalon that the basic anatomic configuration of the cerebral hemispheres is created.

It has been suggested that damage to the prochordal plate area will lead to massive defects in the differentiation of the prosencephalon (Mettler, 1947). Although not experimentally documented, the gross evaluation of several human arhinencephalic monsters suggests the way in which the early basic architecture of the telencephalon is created by a possible mid-line cell migration, inducing the telencephalon medium and olfactory bulbs (White and Alvord, 1964). These observations are in agreement with the observations of Hines (1922) that the initial cortical differentiation of the telencephalon is found within the limbic lobe, for in the arhinencephalic monsters the defect is primarily found to be a lack of development of the telencephalon medium (Yakovlev, 1959).

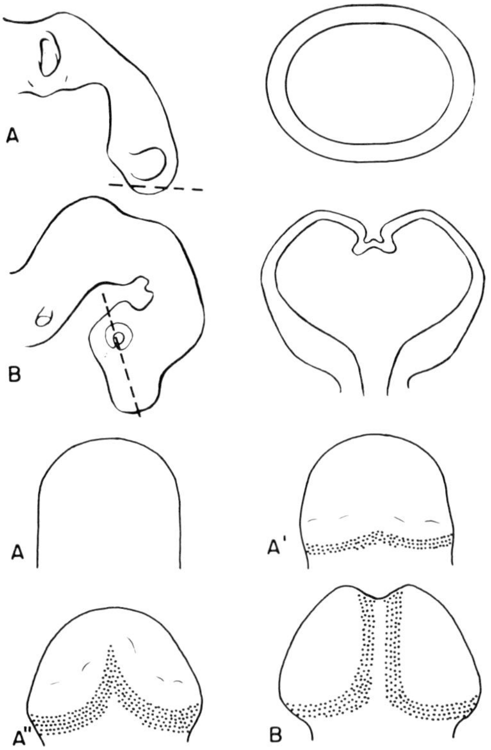

FIG. 7. Diagrammatic representation of the embryologic development of the telencephalon. The upper portion of the figure shows the rostral end at A of a 3.5-mm. CR human embryo and B of a 9.0-mm CR human embryo with a diagrammatic cross section at the level of the hatched line shown to the right, dorsal up. The lower portion of the figure shows a diagrammatic dorsal view of the above embryos at A and B. The stippled area on A′, A″, and B shows the region of cell proliferation forming the velum transversum in A′ and progressively illustrates the hypothesized rostral migration of cells at A″ to separate the telencephalon into two symmetrical halves at B.

Figure 7 shows diagrammatically this early differentiation of the prosencephalon. The telencephalon initially separates from the diencephalon by the development of the velum transversum (Burr, 1922). Hochstetter (1919) and others have pictured this initial evagination as singular, the separation into two lateral vesicles occurring by the later development of a mid-line fissure. How this comes about may be answered by the new concepts of embryonic cell migration as studied with tritiated thymidine (Angevine, 1963,

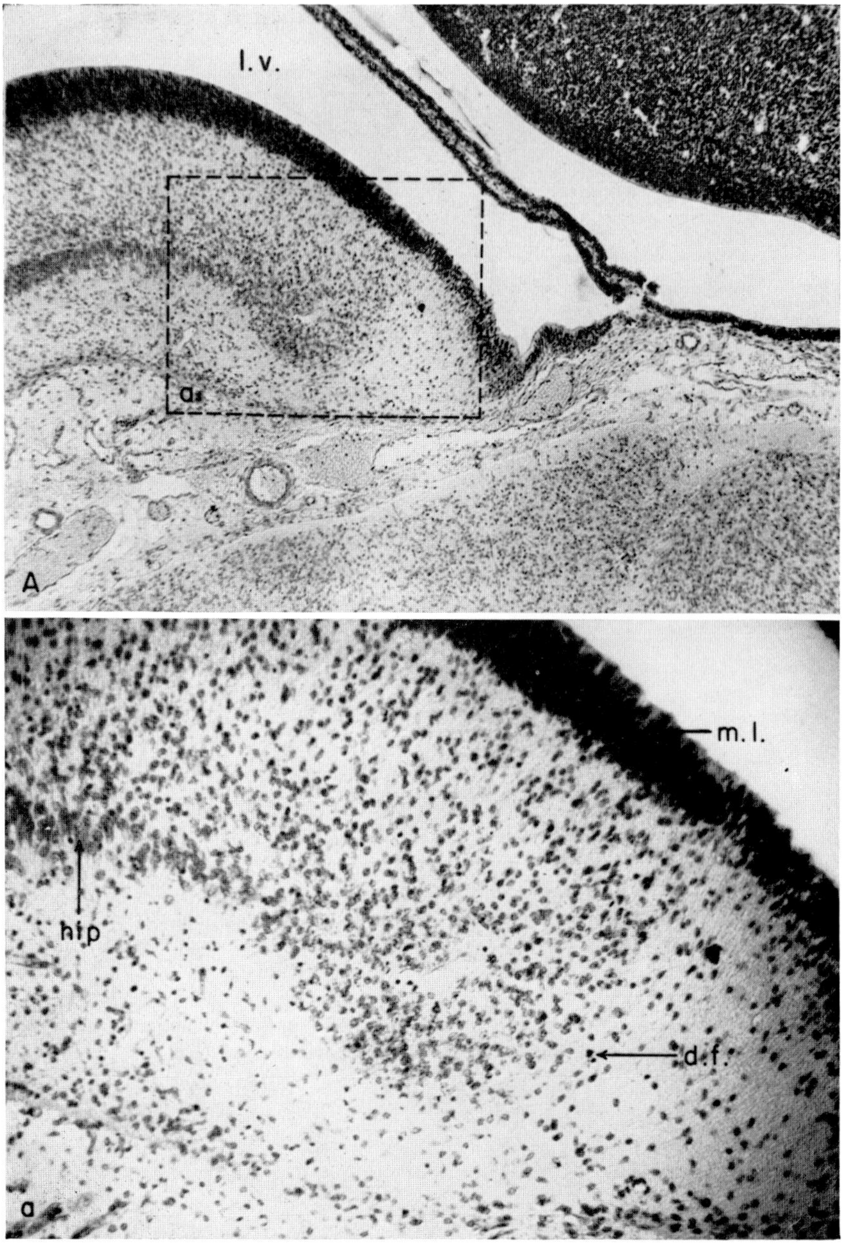

FIG. 8. A, Photomicrograph to illustrate a stage in the early differentiation of the dentate fascia by a migration of small granule cells from the mantle layer of the extreme medial portion of the telencephalon, forming medial to the hippocampal pyramidal cells which have already migrated. a, High-power view of cut out area in A. Abbreviations: d.f., dentate fascia; hip, hippocampus; m.l., mantle layer; l.v., lateral ventricle (65-mm CR human embryo).

1964). These observations have shown that cells move in a systematic fashion from the mantle layer of the hippocampus, set up growth zones, and differentiate into the hippocampal pyramid cells and dentate fascia. The significance of such growth zones has been studied by numerous authors and carefully correlated with the formation of fissures signaling the development of new structures (Kallén, 1951). Figure 8 demonstrates the cell proliferation of the mantle layer in a 65-mm human embryo migrating externally to form the dentate fascia as previously observed by Hines (1922) and documented with tritiated thymidine in the mouse (Angevine, 1964). In Figure 7A′ and A″ the possibility of a similar rostral cell migration from the velum transversum leading to the separation of the telencephalon into two halves is suggested—a hypothesis which may well be illustrated by nature's experiments which lead to the absence or distortion of this normal telencephalic splitting in arhinencephalic monsters (White and Alvord, 1964; Alvord *et al.*, 1963; Yakovlev, 1959; Dekaban, 1959).

The fact that the olfactory bulbs and tracts do not form in these arhinencephalic monsters indicates that this division of the telencephalon may be necessary to induce the telencephalon medium and form a necessary precursor for the induction of the olfactory bulbs. The work of Kundrat (1882) and Yakovlev (1959) has shown that when this separation does not occur the foramen of Monro remains in the region of the velum transversum on the caudal surface of the cerebral hemisphere, and the elements of the limbic lobe develop around it. No mid-line sagittal fissure develops, and a normal telencephalon medium and olfactory lobe are nonexistent. The fact that the archipallium develops from that telencephalic structure created by the velum transversum further indicates that this cerebral tissue may be of earlier origin than the olfactory lobe (Alvord *et al.*, 1963; White and Alvord, 1964). Some support is gained for this hypothesis by the documentation that hippocampus cerebral cortical differentiation is the first known in man (Hines, 1922). Likewise, this hypothesis does not seem to be contradicted from the developmental point of view and in some ways may gain support from it (see Ariëns Kappers *et al.*, 1936).

B. The Limbic Cortex

With the induction of the general framework of the telencephalon, differentiation of the limbic lobe can proceed. Development

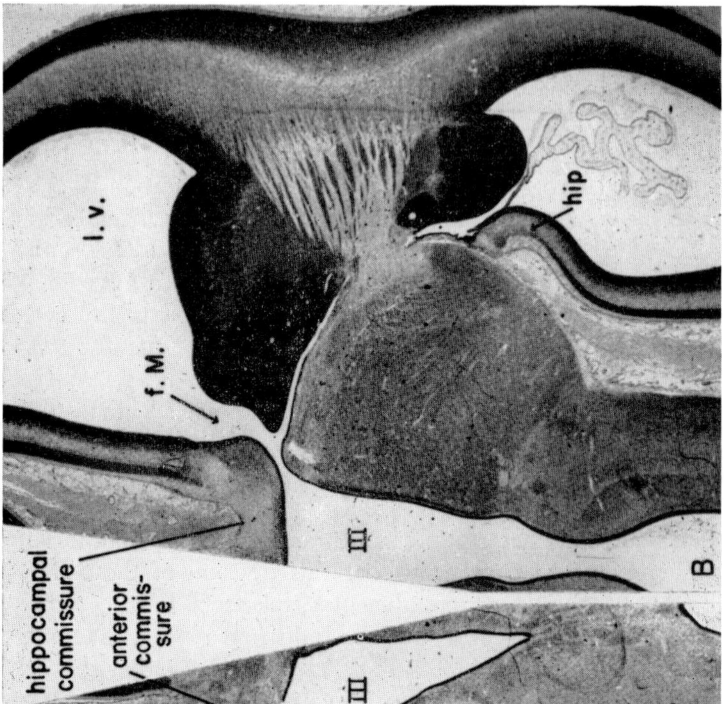

FIG. 9. Low-power photomicrographs of horizontal sections of the developing prosencephalon of a 65-mm CR human embryo to illustrate the independent development of the anterior and hippocampal commissures at A and B, respectively, within the lamina terminalis of the telencephalon medium. Abbreviations: III, third ventricle; f.M., foramen of Monro; hip, hippocampus; l.v., lateral ventricle; S, septal area.

of the hippocampal fissure signals in man and other primates the first attempt at cortical maturation. Hines (1922) submitted this to study in a series of human embryos. She described the early development of the roof plate of the telencephalon medium into choroidal tissue and of the terminal plate into lamina terminalis and its associated septal area. The documentation of the hippocampal fissure as the earliest fissure, and His' (1904) primary fissure as related to the later development of the olfactory bulb, helped orient the gross embryologist to the significance of the early development of the archipallium and its relation to the development of the cerebral cortex (Tilney, 1938).

Concomitant with the development of the cerebral hemispheres, the differentiation of the telencephalon medium takes place (Hamilton *et al.*, 1947). The septal nuclei are formed in conjunction with the anterior commissure, the hippocampal commissure, and finally the corpus callosum (Fig. 9). This is an orderly process and essentially follows the pattern discussed under the phylogenetic development of the commissures (Hewitt, 1962). Lack of development of the corpus callosum leads to gross distortion of the medial hemisphere (Magee and Olson, 1961) and the development of a large medial rostrocaudally oriented bundle of apparently callosal fibers originally described by Probst (1901) running in the depth of the medial archipallium.

There is a rather restricted growth of the hemisphere between the frontal and temporal lobes lateral to the primitive rhinal fissure. This lateral limbic lobe tissue or insula is gradually covered by the opercula (Elliot Smith, 1902; Hochstetter, 1919; Hamilton *et al.*, 1947) creating the great lateral fissure (Connolly, 1940). Concomitantly, the other areas of the limbic lobe are delineated by further cell proliferation and the formation of additional sulci. Subsequent changes are related to cortical maturation and the formation of the various corticoarchitectonic areas of the limbic lobe.

V. Descriptive Limbic Lobe Anatomy

From the historical, phylogenetic, and otogenetic points of view the limbic lobe has one basic thing in common—its roots are in antiquity. Not only has it excited the musings and fancy of the early members in the field of morphology but mother nature has seen fit to develop this area as one of the first, and therefore, primary, structures of the cerebrum. Furthermore, in man with a complex and far advanced cerebral cortex, portions of the limbic lobe are apparently the first to begin to differentiate.

The developed human cerebrum with the commissures removed can readily be thought of as quite similar to a pair of blown-up waterwings—a hollow paired structure, the two halves joined together by an isthmus. The brain stem is held up by or in contact with this winged structure; the diencephalon resting on or in contact with the isthmus (telencephalon medium) and its central cavity freely communicating at the center of the isthmus through the foramen of Monro.

A. The Limbic Cortex

The limbus or immediate medial border of each half of the bulbus telencephalon is that portion bounding the foramen of Monro. It includes one-half of the isthmus (telencephalon medium), the indusium griseum, hippocampus, dentate fascia, and medial amygdaloid (Elliot Smith, 1896d). The direct relationship to the foramen of Monro is illustrated in the following diagram (Fig. 10). The arrangement, like a trunkated sphere, illustrates the laminar nature of the limbic lobe. The inner ring composed primarily of allocortex (Stephan, 1961) is immediately bounded by the transitional elements of the isocortex (juxtallocortex and mesocortex) (von Bonin and Bailey, 1961).

This division is both phylogenetically and ontogenetically sound. As can be noted from the colored drawings of von Bonin and Bailey (1961), the inner ring of cortex is more and more overgrown by the immense growth of the isocortex. This does not mean that the growth of this inner ring tissue is not significant, but rather that its rate of growth is less (Andy and Stephan, 1963). The relationship of the various components of the internal and external rings of tissue are readily appreciated in lower forms (Ariëns Kappers *et al.*, 1936; von Bonin and Bailey, 1961; Stephan, 1961), but not directly evident in the human. The obvious circular relationship of these areas of the medial hemisphere were well known to the German school (Zuckerkandl, 1887, 1888) and recently reiterated in relation to the anterior thalamic to limbic projections by Yakovlev and others (Yakovlev *et al.*, 1960; Locke *et al.*, 1961; Angevine *et al.*, 1962, 1964).

The comparison of the cortical diagram of the limbic lobe in

Fig. 10 to man can be readily applied if one simply eliminates the commissures distorting the telencephalon medium and unfolds the Sylvian fissure. This simple maneuver immediately establishes the intimate relationship of the limbic lobe to the foramen of Monro and again brings the insula, olfactory tubercle, and prepiriform cortex out of the depths of the fissure and onto the ventromedial surface of the hemisphere (Elliot Smith, 1896d, 1902). Similarly, a

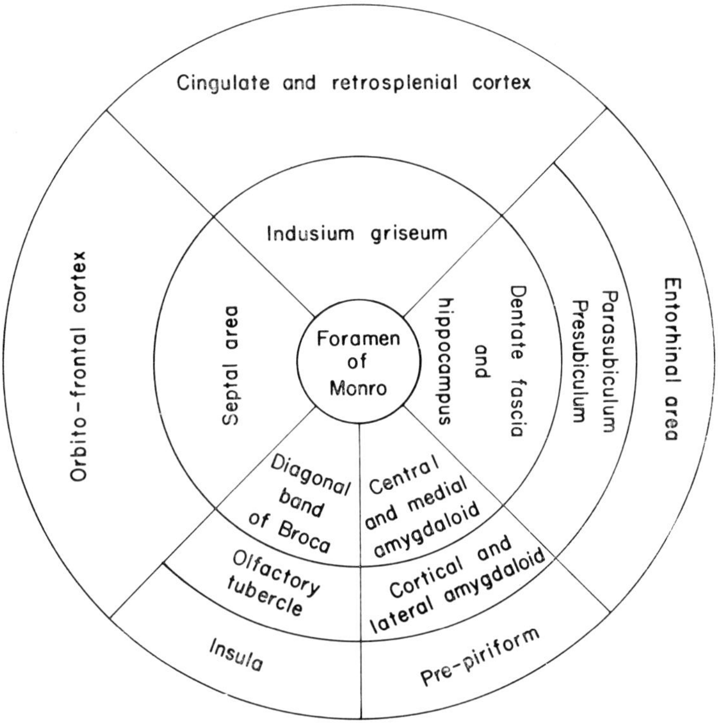

FIG. 10. Circular diagram of the cortical components of the limbic lobe as they border the foramen of Monro.

casual evaluation of the orientation of the fiber tracts deep to this border tissue of the foramen of Monro establishes the same circular orientation (Fig. 11). Likewise, there is a circular projection ring of fibers for the allocortical ring and the juxtallocortical–mesocortical ring—the fornix-diagonal band fibers and the cingulum-unicate fasciculus, respectively. The course of the unicate fasciculus traverses the medial segment of the insula, incorporating this cortex into the outer band of the limbic cortex.

The cortex of the limbic lobe becomes more complex morphologically from the rim of the foramen of Monro peripherally, a point stressed by the majority of the pupils of corticoarchitectonics (Stephan, 1961; von Bonin and Bailey, 1961). Thus, this cortex

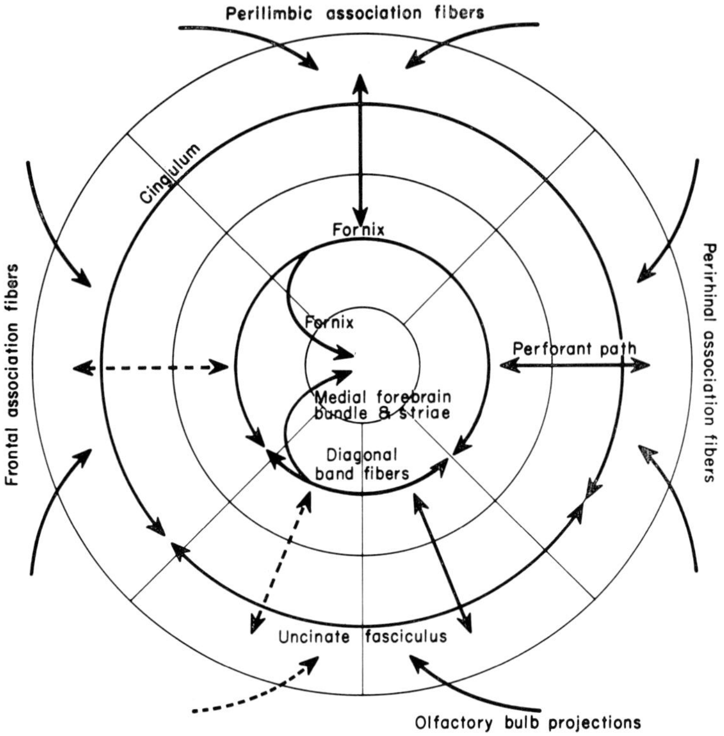

FIG. 11. Circular diagram of the fiber tracts and projection systems within the limbic lobe. See Fig. 10 for names of cortical areas represented.

can be readily separated into definitive corticoarchitectonic areas. This is true for any portion of the limbic rim but vividly demonstrated by the hippocampus and the cortex related to it (Blackstad, 1956; White, 1960; Vaz Ferreira, 1951; Smith and White, 1964). Figure 12 illustrates the limbic cortex of the rat related to the hippocampus and referred to as the hippocampal formation (White, 1960; Smith and White, 1964). This cortex can readily be parceled from medial to lateral by cytoarchitectonic (Krieg, 1946), myeloarchitectonic (Zunino, 1909), or fiberarchitectonic (White, 1960) methods into the dentate fascia, hippocampus, subiculum, presubiculum, parasubiculum, and entorhinal areas. Similarly in

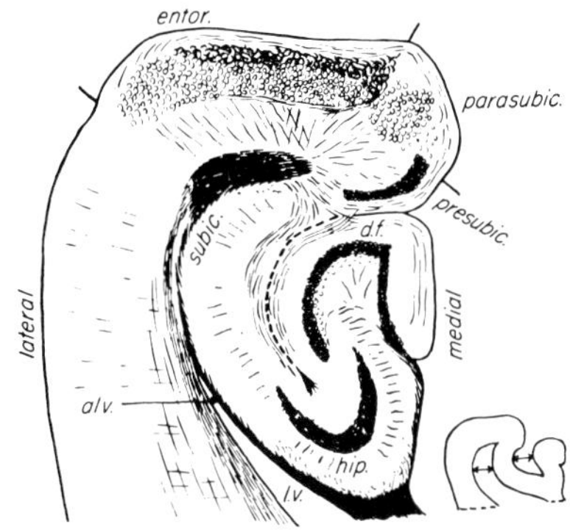

FIG. 12. Diagram of a horizontal section of the rat hippocampal formation to illustrate the medial to lateral orientation of the two rings of the limbic lobe in relation to the hippocampus, refer to Fig. 10. The cut out in the right lower corner has the lateral ventricle and hippocampal fissures opened at the arrows to illustrate further the medial to lateral orientation of the cortical mantle. Compare with the developing hippocampus in Fig. 8 and 9. Abbreviations: alv., alveus; entor., entorhinal area; d.f., dentate fascia; hip., hippocampus; l.v., lateral ventricle; parasubic., parasubiculum; presubic., presubiculum; subic., subiculum.

other areas of the limbus: e.g., the supracallosal gyri can be parceled into the indusium grisium and cingulate cortex; the periolfactory cortex into the diagonal band, olfactory tubercle, and insula; and the periamygdaloid area into the medial amygdaloid, cortical amygdaloid, and prepiriform cortex. This centrifugal differentiation yields progressively more complex cortex which is oriented from medial to lateral and diagrammatically represented in Fig. 10.

B. The Limbic Fasciculi

The interconnecting pathways between these circular components of progressively more complex rings of the limbic lobe have only been partially studied. The unicate fasciculus can be shown grossly to interconnect the medial frontal and temporal lobes traversing the depths of the Sylvian fissure. In the monkey, Nauta (1962, 1964) has demonstrated prefrontal and orbital projections to the cortex of the rostromedial temporal lobe which he feels traverse the medial portion of the uncinate fasciculus. Similar observations have been recorded by Krieg (1954). Definitive studies in the rat (White, 1960), rabbit (Adey, 1951), cat (Smith and White, 1964), and monkey (Adey and Meyer, 1952; Glees *et al.*, 1950) have illustrated caudally directed cingulum fibers associating the cingulate gyrus and medial prefrontal lobe and projecting into the hippocampal formation to end primarily in the presubiculum and parasubiculum. The phylogenetic importance of this frontohippocampal projection tract has recently been stressed. The parasubiculum which receives fibers primarily from the medial surface of the frontal lobe through the cingulum seems to increase in relative size upon ascending the phylogenetic scale from rat to cat, an observation consistent with the relative increase in the size of the frontal lobe between the rat and cat (Smith and White, 1964). The functional correlation of this phylogenetic observation will have to await further confirmation, but it does tend to indicate a possible physiologic correlation.

Input from the remainder of the neocortex to the limbic lobe has been only partially studied morphologically. Neurophysiologic studies using the technique of physiologic neuronography with strychnine or spreading after discharge (Pribram *et al.*, 1950; Pribram and Kruger, 1954; MacLean, 1954) have shown major projections to perilimbic structures which may in turn project into the major limbic rim. Morphologically such pathways have been shown rostrally in relation to the anterior cingulate area (White *et al.*, 1960; Nauta, 1964; DeVito and Smith, 1959; Krieg, 1954; Glees *et al.*, 1950; Showers, 1959) and posteriorly to the perirhinal area just dorsolateral to the entorhinal area (White, 1960). Whether these will remain the sole source of direct neocortical input to the limbic cortex must await further investigation.

Direct projections into the limbic lobe from the olfactory bulbs through the olfactory tracts have been known for a considerable period (Elliot Smith, 1895a; Ariëns Kappers *et al.*, 1936). These projections reach the olfactory tubercle, amygdaloid complex, and prepiriform cortex. Recent studies (Lohman, 1963; Lohman and Lammers, 1963; White, 1962) illustrate that this olfactory bulb projection appears to be confined to paleocortical structures, and, as previously thought from normal studies, the olfactory bulbs do not send direct projections to the septal area (telencephalon medium).

Information is extremely sparse concerning the projections to the insula. The work of Amassian (1951) on evoked potential representation of the viscera to the homolog of the insula in the cat suggests a direct input to the area, but conclusive morphologic information in this regard seems lacking.

The perforant pathway of the corpus callosum has been well documented by early workers (Stieda, 1869; Forel, 1872; Ganser, 1882) and recently studied by Jacobsen (1963). These fibers run from the cingulate gyrus and indusium griseum to the fornix, forming the dorsal portion of the fornix (Elliot Smith, 1896d,e) (fornix superior of von Koelliker, 1894). Likewise, the perforant path of the hippocampus running from the entorhinal area was well known to the older anatomists (von Koelliker, 1894; Ramon y Cajal, 1955) and recently shown by Blackstad (1958) to be composed of projection fibers from the entorhinal area to the molecular layer (layer I) of the hippocampus and dentate fascia. Connections between the prepiriform area and the amygdaloid region are readily demonstrated and have been studied recently in relation to olfactory bulb projections by Lohman (1963) and White (1962). Information is scanty concerning the possible interconnection between the insula and the diagonal band area, as well as possible connections between the orbitofrontal cortex and the septal area. However, the work of Nauta and Valenstein (1958) and Nauta (1962) suggests their presence. For this reason the latter two limbic ring interconnection paths of the limbic lobe are depicted by dotted lines in Fig. 11, further studies being necessary to firmly establish their presence.

C. The Limbic Projection Tracts

The major projection tracts responsible for carrying information into and away from the limbic lobe are three in number: (1) the fornix, (2) the medial forebrain bundle in conjunction with the stria medullaris and terminalis, and (3) the anterior thalamocingulate projections.

The diffuse direct cortical projections of the limbic cortex onto the brain stem (e.g., anterior cingulate projections of Ward, 1948, and entorhinal projections of Adey *et al.*, 1957) and the secondary association fasciculi such as the mammillary peduncle, mammillothalamic tract, and habenulopeduncular tract will not be included here. They are considered by the author to be secondary components of the limbic lobe which are either diffuse in nature or at least one synapse removed from the telencephalic limbic lobe. For this reason they are not considered as immediate primary projection tracts of the limbic lobe. Their significance to the network as a whole should not be neglected, but for purposes of this essay they will be mentioned only in passing (see Adey, 1959; Votaw, 1959; Nauta, 1962, 1964).

Existing information seems to indicate that the major outflow system for the limbic cortex remains the fornix (Nauta, 1956; Valenstein and Nauta, 1959; Votaw, 1959; Guillery, 1956; Powell and Cowan, 1955; Daitz and Powell, 1954; Cragg and Hamlyn, 1957, 1959). This tract has long been known to conduct information from not only the hippocampus but other areas of the limbic portions of the brain through the callosal perforant fibers. Conversely, it also serves to conduct information between the septal area and the hippocampal formation (McLardy, 1955a,b; Andersen *et al.*, 1961a, b; Votaw, 1960; Votaw and Lauer, 1963). In conjunction with the anterior thalamic nuclei (Guillery, 1956; Nauta, 1956) through Gudden's hippocampothalamic bundle it interconnects the hippocampal areas with the cingulate gyrus (White *et al.*, 1960). This major projection bundle of the limbic lobe can no longer be looked upon primarily as an efferent fiber tract for the hippocampus, but rather should be considered as an association fasciculus of the inner ring of the limbic lobe which interconnects various parts of this inner ring in conjunction with the diagonal band of Broca. Concomitantly, the fornix also serves to conduct efferent information out of both rings of the limbic lobe by way of the dorsal and ventral portions of the fornix (Elliot Smith, 1896d,e) to the anterior thalamus, septal area, hypothalamus, and brain stem.

Anatomical studies show that as the fornix approaches the septal area it separates into two distinct bundles in relation to the anterior commissure—the pre- and postcommissural bundles of Huxley (1864). The precommissural portion ends primarily within the lateral septal nuclei (Cragg and Hamlyn, 1959, 1960; Daitz and Powell, 1954; Votaw, 1960; Votaw and Lauer, 1963) whereas the postcommissural bundle partially ends within the septal nuclei related to the anterior commissure and fornix, but is also joined by fibers within the septal area (telencephalon medium) which accompany it to the mammillary bodies of the hypothalamus. Many of these fibers bypass the hypothalamus and join with the medial forebrain bundle to gain access to the brain stem (Guillery, 1956; Nauta, 1956; Valenstein and Nauta, 1959; Daitz and Powell, 1954).

Within the septal area or telencephalon medium begins one of the oldest of the forebrain fiber tracts—the medial forebrain bundle. Through this system numerous short and long fibers project through the hypothalamus into the central core of the brain stem (Nauta, 1956, 1962; Powell, 1963). Likewise, within the telencephalon medium (septal area) is formed the major projection tracts to the epithalamus and striatum—the stria medullaris and stria terminalis. The stria medullaris projects directly into the habenular nuclei, some of its fibers bypassing this nucleus to flow directly into the brain stem (Brodal, 1947; Adey *et al.*, 1957). The stria terminalis interconnects the telencephalon medium with the amygdaloid portion of the striatum. It accompanies the tail of the caudate nucleus caudolaterally to the central nucleus of the amygdala (Nauta, 1962; Valverde, 1963). Although the stria terminalis maintains an association with the caudate nucleus throughout its course it tends to be nothing more than a counterpart of the fornix association system within the inner ring of the limbic lobe, connecting the septal area with the archistriatum.

The thalamocortical connections to the limbic lobe are confined primarily to the anterior thalamus (Rose and Woolsey, 1948; Krieg, 1947), that portion of the thalamus which is in close, gross association with the telencephalon medium. The median nuclei project directly through the septal area to join the cingulum bundle (Nauta and Whitlock, 1954) probably ending diffusely within the fornicate gyrus as a whole (White, 1960). The more lateral anterior nuclei project into the anterior limb of the internal capsule (Krieg, 1947, 1954) to join the cingulum from laterally. Although the anterior nuclei are separated into three distinct nuclear groups in lower forms (Rose and Woolsey, 1948), they become less distinct entities in higher primates (Walker, 1938). Even though it appears that the area of the anterior thalamus is increasing relatively in size with the rest of the brain (Stephan and Andy, 1964), this amalgamation of anterior nuclei is in keeping with the overlapped projection of the various fused components of the nucleus in primates (Yakovlev *et al.*, 1960; Locke *et al.*, 1961; Angevine *et al.*, 1962, 1964) as compared to lower forms where a definite anterior to posterior cingulate orientation is documented (Rose and Woolsey, 1948). Similarly, in lower forms the lateral dorsal nucleus of the thalamus is commonly associated with the parietal lobe (Lashley, 1941). However, in higher forms its close association with the anterior dorsal portion of the thalamus is obvious as it projects primarily to the retrosplenial portion of the cingulate gyrus (Yakovlev *et al.*, 1960; Locke *et al.*, 1961; Angevine *et al.*, 1962, 1964). Again, this seems to represent an apparent phylogenetic differentiation which is leading to a clarification of specific morphologic orientation.

Numerous normal and experimental studies have been conducted on the intimate connections of the fiber projections of the fornix, medial forebrain bundle, striae, and thalamic projections to which the reader is referred for additional details. These are summarized within the works of Ariëns Kappers *et al.* (1936) and Crosby *et al.* (1962). They are not considered within the confines of this discussion which is directed toward establishing a basic concept upon which such specific details can be woven. Similarly, the intimate details of the laminar degeneration patterns, histochemical studies, and submicroscopic observations have been neglected (see Bargman and Schadé, 1963). Likewise, no attempt has been made to consider interrelations of fiber tracts that are not of a first-order nature within the limbic lobe.

VI. Summary and Conclusions

I have taken many liberties with the existing literature and adopted the rules of essay form in order to present as a reviewer a personal opinion of a morphologic concept of the limbic lobe. From a historical point of view the reader is at present caught up in a morass of terminology, which has led to an almost individual approach to the terminology of that portion of the brain now referred to as the rhinencephalon. There is no better illustration of this individualism than in the text of the general discussion on the meaning of the term "rhinencephalon" held as a part of the 3rd International Meeting of Neurobiologists in Keil, Germany, in September 1962 (Bargman and Schadé, 1963).

The concept presented here is based upon a brief historic review of the source of the existing nomenclature adapted to the present concepts of the phylogenetic and ontogenetic development of the human telencephalon. It seems obvious that in the writings of the French school as exemplified by Broca, the German school as ex-

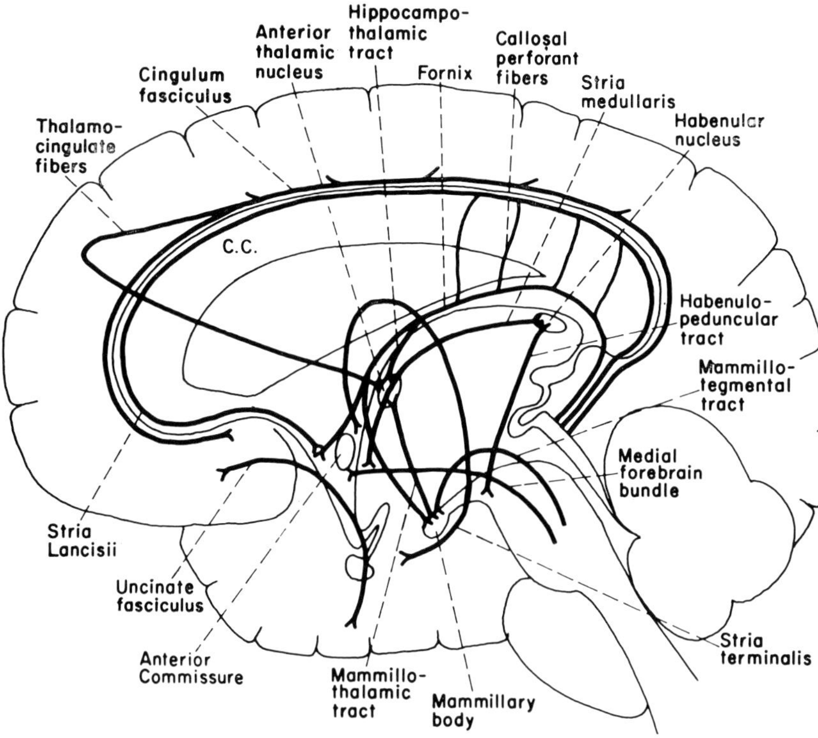

FIG. 13. A summary diagram of the major fiber tracts of the limbic lobe depicted on a distorted medial human hemisphere. Orient with Fig. 1. The extreme medial surface of the temporal lobe is hidden from view by the brain stem covering the termination zones of the stria of Lancisi, fornix, and cingulum. Abbreviation: C.C., corpus callosum.

emplified by Zuckerkandl, the English school as exemplified by Elliot Smith, and the American school as exemplified by Yakovlev that the impression of the limbic lobe as a simple border around the foramen of Monro is not a new one. Why then should we not continue to employ this simple concept of a limbus first utilized in all its simplicity by Willis in 1664? Or, should we continue to confuse the issue by utilizing a term that exemplifies function where over-all function is not known? At present it seems that on this point agreement is in the minority. It is the hope of the author that the concept presented here supports the former question.

Reference to Figs. 1 and 13 diagrammatically summarizes the area of the limbic lobe and its principal connections discussed in this review. No attempt is made to include the secondary projection tracts of the limbic lobe although they are partially diagrammed in Fig. 13 for completeness.

It is concluded that the limbic lobe is formed by the medial border of the telencephalon and incorporates its early precursors, the archipallium and telencephalon medium, in its inner ring. The outer ring is formed by the further differentiation of the cerebral tissue bordering this inner ring—paleopallium ventrally and neopallium dorsolaterally.

Acknowledgments

This work was supported in part by grant number NB-2896 U. S. Public Health Service, National Institute of Neurological Diseases and Blindness. I wish to thank Dr. Med. Theodore Blackstad and Professor Dr. Med. Jan Jansen of the Anatomical Institute, Oslo, Norway and Dr. Arthur A. Ward, Jr., and Mr. Randall Smith of the University of Washington for their inspiration and advice during the gathering of this material. To Mrs. Phyllis Wood for preparing the illustrations and Mrs. Loanna Andersson for typing the manuscript I am indeed grateful.

References

Adey, W. R. (1951). *Brain* **74**, 233.

Adey, W. R. (1959). *Intern. Rev. Neurobiol.* **1**, 1.

Adey, W. R., and Meyer, M. (1952). *J. Anat.* **86**, 58.

Adey, W. R., Sunderland, S., and Dunlop, C. W. (1957). *Electroencephalog. Clin. Neurophysiol.* **9**, 309.

Alvord, E. C., Shaw, C. M., Hayden, R. N., and White, L. E. (1963). *J. Neuropathol. Exptl. Neurol.* **22**, 358.

Amassian, V. E. (1951). *J. Neurophysiol.* **14**, 433.

Andersen, P., Bruland, H., and Kaada, B. R. (1961a). *Acta Physiol. Scand.* **51**, 17.

Andersen, P., Bruland, H., and Kaada, B. R. (1961b). *Acta Physiol. Scand.* **51**, 29.

Andy, O. J., and Stephan, H. (1962). *J. Hirnforsch.* **3**, 230.

Andy, O. J., and Stephan, H. (1963). *Anat. Record* **145**, 201.

Angevine, J. B. (1963). *Anat. Record* **145**, 201.

Angevine, J. B. (1964). *Anat. Record* **148**, 255.

Angevine, J. B., Locke, S., and Yakovlev, P. I. (1962). *Arch. Neurol.* **7**, 518.

Angevine, J. B., Locke, S., and Yakovlev, P. I. (1964). *Arch. Neurol.* **10**, 165.

Arantius, J. C. (1587). Translation found in Lewis (1923).

Ariëns Kappers, C. U., Huber, G. C., and Crosby, E. C. (1936). "The Comparative Anatomy of the Nervous System of Vertebrates, Including Man," reprint, 3 vols., 1960. Macmillan, New York.

Arnold, F. (1851). "Handbuch der Anatomie des Menschen," Emmerling u. Herder, Freiburg im Breisgau, Germany.

Bargman, W., and Schadé, J. P. (1963). *Progr. Brain Res.* **3**, 253.

Beevor, C. E. (1891). *Phil. Trans. Roy. Soc. London* **B182,** 135.
Blackstad, T. (1956). *J. Comp. Neurol.* **105,** 417.
Blackstad, T. (1958). *Acta Anat.* **35,** 202.
Broca, P. (1878). *Rev. Anthropol.* **7,** 385.
Brodal, A. (1947). *Schweiz. Med. Wochschr.* **38,** 971.
Burr, H. S. (1922). *J. Comp. Neurol.* **34,** 277.
Connolly, C. J. (1940). *Am. J. Phys. Anthropol.* **26,** 113.
Cragg, B. G., and Hamlyn, L. H. (1957). *J. Physiol. (London)* **135,** 460.
Cragg, B. G., and Hamlyn, L. H. (1959). *J. Exptl. Neurol.* **1,** 187.
Cragg, B. G., and Hamlyn, L. H. (1960). *J. Exptl. Neurol.* **2,** 581.
Crosby, E. C., Humphrey, T., and Lauer, E. W. (1962). "Correlative Anatomy of the Nervous System." Macmillan, New York.
Daitz, H. M., and Powell, T. P. S. (1954). *J. Neurol. Neurosurg. Psychiat.* **17,** 75.
Dekaban, A. (1959). *J. Neuropathol. Exptl. Neurol.* **18,** 620.
DeVito, J. L., and Smith, O. A. (1959). *J. Comp. Neurol.* **111,** 261.
Ecker, A. (1873). "The Cerebral Convolutions of Man." Appelton, New York.
Edinger, L. (1891). "Structure of the Central Nervous System" (W. H. Vittum, trans.; C. E. Riggs, ed.). Davis, Philadelphia.
Elliot Smith, G. (1895a). *Anat. Anz.* **10,** 470.
Elliot Smith, G. (1895b). *Anat. Anz.* **11,** 91.
Elliot Smith, G. (1896a). *Anat. Anz.* **12,** 119.
Elliot Smith, G. (1896b). *Anat. Anz.* **11,** 49.
Elliot Smith, G. (1896c). *J. Anat. Physiol.* **30,** 465.
Elliot Smith, G. (1896d). *J. Anat. Physiol.* **30,** 157, 185.
Elliot Smith, G. (1896e). *J. Anat. Physiol.* **31,** 80.
Elliot Smith, G. (1897). *Anat. Anz.* **13,** 23.
Elliot Smith, G. (1898). *J. Anat. Physiol.* **32,** 23.
Elliot Smith, G. (1901). *J. Anat. Physiol.* **35,** 431.
Elliot Smith, G. (1902). *J. Anat. Physiol.* **36,** 309.
Elliot Smith, G. (1903a). *Anat. Anz.* **23,** 384.
Elliot Smith, G. (1903b). *J. Anat. Physiol.* **37,** 324.
Elliot Smith, G. (1910a). *Anat. Anz.* **35,** 429.
Elliot Smith, G. (1910b). Lancet **178** (I), 1, 147, 221.
Forel, A. (1872). *Sitzber. Akad. Wiss. Wein, Math.-Naturw. Kl., Abt. III,* **66.**
Foville, A. L. (1844). "Traité complet de l'anatomie, de la physiologie et de la pathologie du système nerveux cérébro-spinal." Masson, Paris.
Freeman, W. J., and Watts, J. W. (1950). "Psychosurgery in the Treatment of Mental Disorders and Intractable Pain." Thomas, Springfield, Illinois.
Fulton, J. F. (1951). "Frontal Lobotomy and Affective Behavior." Norton, New York.
Ganser, S. (1882). *Morphol. Jahrb.* **7,** 501.
Gardner, R. (1881). *J. Anat. Physiol.* **25,** 536.
Glees, P., Cole, J. O., and Whitty, C. W. M. (1950). *J. Neurol. Neurosurg. Psychiat.* **13,** 178.
Guillery, R. W. (1956). *J. Anat.* **90,** 350.
Hamilton, W. J., Boyd, J. D., and Mossman, H. W. (1947). "Human Embryology," Williams & Wilkins, Baltimore, Maryland.

Herrick, C. J. (1920). *J. Comp. Neurol.* **32**, 429.
Herrick, C. J. (1926). "Brains of Rats and Men." Univ. Chicago Press, Chicago, Illinois.
Herrick, C. J. (1948). "The Brain of the Tiger Salamander," Univ. of Chicago Press, Chicago, Illinois.
Herrick, C. J. (1956). "The Evolution of Human Nature," Univ. of Texas Press, Austin, Texas.
Hewitt, W. (1962). *J. Anat.* **96**, 355.
Hill, A. (1893). *Phil. Trans. Roy. Soc. London* **B184**, 389.
Hines, M. (1922). *J. Comp. Neurol.* **34**, 73.
His, W. (1895). "Die anatomische Nomenclatur." Verlag von Veit, Leipzig.
His, W. (1904). "Die Entwicklung des menschlichen Gehirns." Hirzel, Leipzig.
Hochstetter, F. (1919). "Beitrag zur Entwicklungsgeschichte des menschlichen Gehirns." Deuticke, Vienna and Leipzig.
Holmgren, N. (1922). *J. Comp. Neurol.* **34**, 391.
Huguenin, G. (1879). "Anatomie des centres nerveux." Baillière, Paris.
Huxley, T. H. (1864). *Medical Times and Gazette,* March 5, p. 256.
Huxley, T. H. (1894). *In* "The Life of Richard Owen" (Rev. Richard Owen), Vol. II. Appleton, New York.
Jacobsen, C. F. (1935). *A.M.A. Arch. Neurol. Psychiat.* **33**, 558.
Jacobsen, S. (1963). *J. Comp. Neurol.* **121**, 5.
Johnston, J. B. (1913). *J. Comp. Neurol.* **23**, 371.
Kallén, B. (1951). *J. Comp. Neurol.* **95**, 307.
Kingsbury, B. F. (1922). *J. Comp. Neurol.* **34**, 461.
Kingsley, C. (1863). "Water Babies," London. Reprint Altemus, Philadelphia, 1899.
Krieg, W. J. S. (1946). *J. Comp. Neurol.* **84**, 221.
Krieg, W. J. S. (1947). *J. Comp. Neurol.* **86**, 267.
Krieg, W. J. S. (1954). "Connections of the Frontal Cortex of the Monkey." Thomas, Springfield, Illinois.
Kundrat, H. (1882). "Arhinencephalie." Leuschner and Lubensky, Graz, Austria.
Lashley, K. S. (1941). *J. Comp. Neurol.* **75**, 67.
Lewis, F. T. (1923). *J. Comp. Neurol.* **35**, 213.
Locke, S., Angevine, J. B., and Yakovlev, P. I. (1961). *Arch. Neurol.* **4**, 355.
Lohman, A. H. M. (1963). *Acta Anat.* **53**, Suppl. 49.
Lohman, A. H. M., and Lammers, H. J. (1963). *Progr. Brain Res.* **3**, 149.
McLardy, T. (1955a). *J. Comp. Neurol.* **103**, 305.
McLardy, T. (1955b). *J. Comp. Neurol.* **103**, 327.
MacLean, P. D. (1954). *J. Neurosurg.* **11**, 29.
Magee, K. R., and Olson, R. N. (1961). *J. Comp. Neurol.* **117**, 371.
Mettler, F. A. (1947). *J. Neuropathol. Exptl. Neurol.* **6**, 98.
Meynert, T. (1884). "Psychiatrie." Braumüller, Vienna.
Moniz, E. (1936). "Tentatives opératiores dans le traitement de certaines psychoses." Masson, Paris.
Nauta, W. J. H. (1956). *J. Comp. Neurol.* **104**, 247.
Nauta, W. J. H. (1962). *Brain* **85**, 505.
Nauta, W. J. H. (1964). *In* "The Frontal Granular Cortex and Behavior" (J. M. Warren and K. Akert, eds.). McGraw-Hill, New York.
Nauta, W. J. H., and Valenstein, E. S. (1958). *Anat. Record* **130**, 346.

Nauta, W. J. H., and Whitlock, D. G. (1954). *In* "Council for International Organizations of Medical Sciences. Brain Mechanisms and Consciousness." Oxford Univ. Press, London and New York.
Obersteiner, H., and Hill, A. (1890). "The Anatomy of the Central Nervous System." Griffin, London.
Owen, R. (1837). *Phil. Trans. Roy. Soc. London* **pI,** 87.
Owen, R. (1868). "Anatomy of Vertebrates," 3 vols. Longmans and Green, London.
Papez, J. W. (1937). *A.M.A. Arch. Neurol. Psychiat.* **38,** 725.
Pool, J. L. (1954). *J. Neurosurg.* **11,** 45.
Powell, E. W. (1963). *J. Exptl. Neurol.* **8,** 406.
Powell, T. P. S., and Cowan, W. M. (1955). *Brain* **78,** 115.
Pribram, K. H., and Kruger, L. (1954). *Ann. N. Y. Acad. Sci.* **58,** 109.
Pribram, K. H., Lennox, M. A., and Dunsmore, R. H. (1950). *J. Neurophysiol.* **13,** 127.
Probst, M. (1901). *Arch. Psychiat. Nervenkrankh.* **34,** 709.
Ramon y Cajal, S. (1955). "Studies on the Cerebral Cortex" (L. M. Kraft, trans.), Year Book Publ., Chicago, Illinois.
Reichert, K. (1895). "Der Bau des menschen Gehirns." Engelmann, Leipzig.
Rose, J. E., and Woolsey, C. N. (1948). *J. Comp. Neurol.* **89,** 279.
Schwalbe, G. (1881). "Lehrbuch der Neurologie." Besold, Erlangen, Germany.
Showers, M. J. C. (1959). *J. Comp. Neurol.* **112,** 231.
Smith, R. W., and White, L. E. (1964). *J. Comp. Neurol.* **123,** 11.
Solly, S. (1848). "The Human Brain." Lea and Blanchard, Philadelphia, Pennsylvania.
Stephan, H. (1961). *In* "Primatologia" (H. Hofer, A. H. Schultz, and D. Stark, eds.), Vol. II. Karger, Basel.
Stephan, H., and Andy, O. J. (1964). *Am. Zoologist* **4,** 59.
Stieda, L. (1869). *Z. Wiss. Zool.* **19,** 1.
Symington, J. (1892). *J. Anat. Physiol.* **27,** 69.
Tilney, F. (1938). *Bull. Neurol. Inst. N. Y.* **7,** 1.
Todd, R. B. (1839). "The Cyclopedia of Anatomy and Physiology." Longmann, London.
Turner, W. (1890). *J. Anat. Physiol.* **25,** 105.
Valenstein, E. S., and Nauta, W. J. H. (1959). *J. Comp. Neurol.* **113,** 337.
Valverde, F. (1963). *Progr. Brain Res.* **3,** 20.
Vaz Ferreira, A. (1951). *J. Comp. Neurol.* **95,** 177.
Vesalius, A. (1543). "De humani corpis fabrica libri septem." Oporini, Basileae.
von Bonin, G., and Bailey, P. (1961). *In* "Primatologia" (H. Hofer, A. H. Schultz, and D. Stank, eds.), Vol. II. Karger, Basel.
von Koelliker, A. (1894). "Handbuch der Gewebelehre des Menschen." Engelmann, Leipzig.
Votaw, C. L. (1959). *J. Comp. Neurol.* **112,** 353.
Votaw, C. L. (1960). *J. Comp. Neurol.* **114,** 283.
Votaw, C. L., and Lauer, E. W. (1963). *J. Comp. Neurol.* **121,** 195.
Walker, A. E. (1938). "The Primate Thalamus." Univ. of Chicago Press, Chicago, Illinois.
Walker, A. E. (1944). *In* "The Precentral Motor Cortex" (P. C. Bucy, ed.). Univ. of Illinois Press, Urbana, Illinois.
Ward, A. A., Jr. (1948). *J. Neurophysiol.* **11,** 13.

White, L. E. (1960). *J. Comp. Neurol.* **113,** 1.
White, L. E. (1962). *Anat. Record* **142,** 333.
White, L. E., and Alvord, E. C. (1964). *Anat. Record* **145,** 356.
White, L. E., Nelson, W., and Foltz, E. L. (1960). *J. Exptl. Neurol.* **2,** 406.
Willis, T. (1664). "Cerebri Anatome." Martzer and Alleftry, London.
Yakovlev, P. I. (1959). *J. Neuropathol. Exptl. Neurol.* **18,** 22.
Yakovlev, P. I., Locke, S., Koskoff, D. Y., and Patton, R. A. (1960). *Arch. Neurol.* **3,** 620.
Zuckerkandl, E. (1887). "Ueber des Riechcentrum." Enke, Stuttgart.
Zuckerkandl, E. (1888). *Anat. Anz.* **3,** 425.
Zunino, G. (1909). *J. Psychol. Neurol.* **14,** 38.

THE ANATOMOPHYSIOLOGICAL BASIS OF SOMATOSENSORY DISCRIMINATION

By David Bowsher, with the collaboration of Denise Albe-Fessard

Department of Anatomy, University of Liverpool, Liverpool, England, and Centre d'Etudes de Physiologie Nerveuse, University of Paris, Paris, France

> "If we refuse to admit that discrimination is in some way based on different anatomical constituents differently located in the brain, we may as well give up altogether."
>
> R. Granit, 1955

A review of somatosensory neural mechanisms cannot hope to cover in its entirety the immense literature on the subject which has grown up in the last two decades; and in view of the recent publication of the Neurophysiology section of the "Handbook of Physiology," it would be invidious to attempt to do so. Especially when the writers themselves are actively involved in research on these systems, and, therefore, *de parti pris,* they cannot be expected to give equal weight to all views on the subject. Rather, such a review must be both selective and synthetic, and aim to present a particular view which seems to the authors to be, at the time of writing, the most reasonable analysis of the known facts.

Before launching on such an analysis, it would be well to mention briefly some of the limitations of current methodology. Whether data have been collected by anatomical or physiological techniques, they have certain interrelated limitations, of which the gravest are:

1. The electron microscope has revealed, both peripherally and centrally, a very much larger number of neural elements (fibers or fibrils) than can be demonstrated by conventional anatomical, or registered by electrophysiological, techniques. It would be reasonable to assume that nervous functions are subserved by these structures, but at present there is no indication as to what they may be.

2. It is obvious that even the most refined neuroanatomical techniques currently in use fail to demonstrate all of those synaptic endings which, even if properly impregnated, are large enough to be seen by the light microscope, whether degenerated or normal (e.g., Gibson *et al.*, 1955; Gray and Guillery, 1961). Particularly, therefore, when assessing the results of experimental degeneration studies in terms of their possible physiological significance, care must be taken in interpretation. Van Crevel (1958) and Russell and DeMeyer (1961) have drawn attention to the importance of the time-course of axon degeneration. In addition we should consider the possibility of chemical differences as between various types of synaptic ending being a cause of differential impregnability.

3. Peripheral C-fiber activity has been recorded by Zotterman (1939), Iggo (1959, 1962), Douglas and Ritchie (1957, 1959), and others; and Collins and Randt (1958) have been able to record some central effects of C-fiber activity. But this latter is known to exist in far greater profusion than has so far been satisfactorily registered, and its successful analysis urgently awaits further methodological advances.

4. Electrophysiological recordings, although constant and valuable, are in essence only symbolic. They are an outward and electrical sign of an inward and neural event. Recent work is beginning to uncover the nature of neural events [see Hodgkin (1964)], but this does not mean that there may not be important occurrences which are not electrically transduced by conventional recording methods. For example slow dc potentials have recently been recorded, whose significance is not yet fully understood (see O'Leary and Goldring, 1964).

In sum, because various anatomicophysiological data can be crossed-checked, it may justifiably be held that the evidence that we possess is substantially correct; but it is becoming obvious that this evidence is incomplete, and that current methodology is not equipped to collect all the relevant information. Any hypothesis, therefore, that can be put forward at present cannot hope to be more than a partial explanation of the mechanisms under review.

I. The Peripheral System

The welter of literature and the clamor of controversy in recent years rule out the possibility of covering, let alone doing justice to, the whole field in an article of this nature. As has been pointed out by more than one harassed chairman of a symposium, the apparently opposing views of various workers are not, in fact, completely irreconcilable. The mere fact that such heated academic arguments have occurred tends to suggest that the conceptual frame of reference within which the data have been interpreted should perhaps be re-examined. Before attempting to do this, some salient anatomical points should be recalled.

1. Anatomically, two plexuses can be seen in the skin. One is composed of thick myelinated fibers, the other of fine nonmedullated (in the classic sense) fibers. Thick fibers are always accompanied by thin fibers, but there exist other thin fibers which ramify freely, not in association with thick fibers; in other words, there are, as in the peripheral nerve bundle, more nonmyelinated than myelinated fibers.

2. All hair follicles are innervated by at least one medullated fiber. Other myelinated fibers frequently terminate in association with a nonnervous ectodermal structure (for example, see Cauna, 1959), of which structurally the most constant is the pacinian corpuscle.

3. The nonmyelinated fibers may perhaps end freely, or in association with follicular or other nonneural capsules.

4. The cutaneous ramifications of any given axon are of the same order of caliber as one another.

The quarrel has been as to what modalities are subserved by what cutaneous fibers. This further involves the question of what sensations can be felt in the skin, although, as will be seen in this article, it may be that the attempt to correlate objective (extraneous) physiological function with subjective psychological perception lies at the root of one of the major difficulties in this field. It is possible to apply objectively measurable mechanical and thermal stimuli (corresponding subjectively to touch, pressure, heat, and cold) to the skin. Years of careful physiological analyses have shown that within the A (medullated) group, there are fibers that respond specifically either (a) to one of these forms of energy, or (b) to one form at low threshold, and to another at a higher threshold (Maruhashi *et al.*, 1952; Hunt and McIntyre, 1960a). The first recordings from peripheral C (nonmyelinated) fibers (Zotterman, 1939) suggested that they were responsive only to noxious stimuli. Douglas and Ritchie (1957) and Iggo (1959) have now shown that, in fact, there are C fibers specifically responsive to different forms of external energy, and that, indeed, as in the A group, the majority of them are mechanoreceptors (Iggo, 1960). It is of importance, as will appear later, to note that physiological specificity of cutaneous afferent fibers has been demonstrated not only in mammals, but also in amphibia (Maruhashi *et al.*, 1952). Lele *et al.* (1958) have shown that nerves in the skin of *Amphioxus*, which have only fine-caliber endings, as in human cornea, can respond separately to mechanical, thermal, and tissue-damaging stimuli.

The recent researches of Weddell and his collaborators (Weddell *et al.*, 1954) have suggested that there is little, if any, correlation between the histology of cutaneous nerve terminal structures and their physiological specificity. Thus, for example, Lele and Weddell (1956) demonstrated that the human cornea, which contains only bare nerve endings, is sensitive to all sensory modalities that can be recognized. Recent work by Iggo (1963a, 1964) has shown that cutaneous nerve terminals are associated with an organized epidermal or dermal structure. Specifity is conferred on the nerve by the nonnervous structure, which must, therefore, be considered as a specific transducer or at least as responsible for the specific sensitivity of the nerve (Iggo, 1963b).

In addition to touch, pressure, heat, and cold, the fifth classical modality of cutaneous sensation is pain. Although probably resulting from damage of the skin, pain as such cannot be correlated with forms of external energy as can the other cutaneous sensory modalities; its existence is purely subjective. A valid differentiation can be made between pricking pain and diffuse pain. In brief, pricking pain is well-localized, travels rapidly to consciousness, and does not outlast the provoking stimulus. Diffuse pain takes some time to reach consciousness, is poorly localized (particularly in the absence of concomitant tactile stimuli), and almost always considerably outlasts the provoking stimulus. Pricking sensation is normally absent in the buccal mucous membrane on the inner surface of the human cheek—a phenomenon which is put to good use by fakirs; a pinpoint pressed against the cheek from inside the mouth evokes a sensation of pressure, but not of pricking. On the other hand, this region is certainly capable of giving rise to the sensation of diffuse pain. This peripheral dissociation is said to be correlated with an absence of thin fibers in this region of the buccal mucous membrane (Arthur and Shelley, 1959); whatever may prove to be the case, it must have an anatomophysiological basis and this deserves investigation.

It appears that the peripheral fibers that conduct impulses generated by painful stimuli lie not only in the C spectrum, but also in the smaller myelinated group. Thus, in the cat, Hunt and McIntyre (1960c) found a small number of fibers in the Aδ group which responded only to noxious stimuli; and Collins *et al.* (1960), stimulating the exposed sural nerve of man (11 cases), were able to evoke pain at the Aδ threshold. These important findings, taken together with those of Iggo, imply that in both myelinated and nonmyelinated peripheral cutaneous afferent nerves, there are fibers which (individually) are sensitive to each component of the whole range of cutaneous sensory modalities which introspective man is able to perceive.

It seems to have been too often taken for granted (except by Bishop, 1959 and 1960) that if a peripheral nerve fiber is found experimentally to be fired by a particular form of energy, then natural firing of this fiber will always evoke a sensation in consciousness, provided that the impulses are not blocked at some central synapse (descending inhibition, see Hagbarth, 1960). There is no reason why this should be so; indeed, the evidence of comparative anatomy and physiology militates against such a concept; many purely reflex reactions to specific peripheral stimulation are known. Specificity can also be lost centrally because of convergence of peripheral afferents on common central neurons. It is revealed by the well-known fact that the number of dorsal root fibers entering a segment of the spinal cord is greater than the number of secondary fibers ascending from the same segment. In phylogenetic evolution, the development of the peripheral sensory apparatus seems to be in advance of the specificity of the central systems; in this connection may be quoted the following important passage from the masterly essay of Herrick (1948) on the brain of the tiger salamander:

"The several functional systems of peripheral nerve fibers enter the brain in fascicles of the nerve roots, which are physiologically as specific as those of mammals; but at the first synapse this specificity may almost completely disappear, in so far as it has visible structural expression. The root fibers of all sensory systems (except, perhaps, the olfactory) terminate by wide arborizations in a few common fields of neuropil, in each of which several of these systems are inextricably mingled. This neuropil is a common synaptic pool for all entering systems."

There are strong grounds, therefore, for making a distinction between cutaneous afferent and sensory fibers. As all peripheral afferent fibers, in both A and C spectra, show a greater or lesser degree of specificity in their response to external stimuli, the distinction must be made in terms of central connections.

II. The First Central Synapse

The ability of an organism to distinguish between the varieties of sensory information arriving centrally along specifically activated peripheral afferent fibers must depend on the number and synaptic arrangements of second-order neurons within its central nervous system. The salamander (whose brain, according to Herrick, can be roughly considered equivalent in some aspects to that of 6-week human embryo) has such a small number of central neurons that, because of convergence, "the physiological specificity of the root fibers is largely, though not entirely, obliterated at the first synapse" (Herrick, 1948). As, in the course of phylogenesis, greater numbers of central neurons develop, central sorting-out of afferent information becomes possible; and it is this which is known as sensory discrimination. It depends, in the first instance, only on an increase in the number and complexity of synaptic arrangement in second-order, and not higher-order, neurons though, in fact, the two develop *pari passu;* it also depends on the unrelated fact that there is an increase in the complexity of central synaptic arrangements.

Because they are easier to study, both anatomically and physiologically, more recently developed specific systems have been to date the most intensively investigated. In terms of somatic afferent systems, these are the dorsal column–medial lemniscus systems. At the upper end of the evolutionary scale, they exhibit marked modality (or submodality), specificity, and synaptic security (see references below). Both the dorsal columns (Torvik, 1956) and the medial lemniscus (Bowsher, 1958, 1961b; Valverde, 1961a) of mammals have collateral connections, but very few as will be seen below. This in itself is a sign of an advanced system in evolutionary development, for, according to Herrick (1948): "Collateral connections are more numerous and more dispersed in lower forms than in higher."

Although, of course, it is a *sine qua non* of neurophysiology that no synapse exists merely to transmit messages unchanged, it appears that the lemniscal systems approximate more closely in their organization, with modifications, to the now-despised theoretical telephone exchange than do less highly evolved systems. Indeed, since the parallel was first drawn, there have been important developments in the design of telephone exchanges, including selective amplification to increase signal-to-noise ratio (synaptic security), and afferent inhibition on shared lines, which go some way to improve the analogy. It is only in the more primitive neuron systems, still persisting in the highest forms, that this analogy is untenable (see Fessard, 1961).

The dorsal root entry zone remains one of the most baffling links in the afferent chain. Its functional importance cannot be overemphasized, for until we understand the transformations that occur at this level we cannot hope to interpret the modulations that take place at the higher levels. It is perhaps only within the last 5 years that the first glimmering of comprehension has become evident.

Herrick (1948) has pointed out that a neuron system which evolves new connections retains its primitive ones; and that the new connection often involves a long (true) collateral axon, whereas the original connection becomes the "short collateral" whose function has been far too frequently overlooked. Thus it is that the long dorsal column fiber is in reality a collateral, which has recently been shown physiologically (Mallart and Petit, 1963), to possess a "short collateral" connection to dorsal horn cells, as stated by Cajal (1909) and Wall (1961), who by antidromic stimulation in the dorsal part of the dorsal column was able to activate cells in the dorsal horn of the spinal gray matter; and was able to show that these cells are also orthodromically activated by small primary afferent fibers which do not reach the dorsal columns.

It has been stated (Ranson, 1912; Ingvar, 1927) and axiomatically accepted by the textbooks, that the dorsal root enters the spinal cord in two divisions. The medial of these is said to contain only large fibers, whereas the lateral contains both large and (all the) small fibers. However, the examples cited in the preceeding paragraph show that, even if this segregation exists, the possibility of interaction is present at the segmental level of entry.

The first central synapse of myelinated fibers is, therefore, at the "common carrier cells" (Wall) of the dorsal gray horn as well as in the dorsal column nuclei. These cells lie in lamina IV of Rexed (1952), and receive primary afferent fibers of all diameters arranged in microbundles. Long collaterals of the larger of these fibers pass up to establish further primary synaptic connections with the cells of the dorsal column nuclei.

Thus the anatomical differences between these two first-order central neurons lie only in the fiber diameter spectrum of their primary afferents. Whether this alone accounts for their vast functional differences cannot be adequately discussed here; but it lends powerful support to Bishop's (1959) concept of modality segregation according to fiber diameter. Whether they are the only two types of first-order secondary neurons acted upon by myelinated primary afferents is as yet unsettled; probably they are not, for further first-order central neurons seem to be called for to explain the results of analysis of cutaneous input at higher levels.

Arising from first-order central neurons, we may recognize two ascending systems with very different properties. Spivy and Metcalf (1959) differentially stimulated the lateral and medial divisions of the posterior root. Stimulation of the lateral division evoked activity in the ventromedial reticular tegmentum of the midbrain and caused a rise in blood pressure, whereas the medial division alone was shown to activate the ventrobasal thalamus only. These two central systems for us are the extralemniscal and lemniscal, respectively. The lemniscal systems of mammals, caudal to the trigeminal nuclei, consist of the dorsal column–medial lemniscus system, the neospinothalamic fibers (Mehler, 1957), and the older counterpart of the latter, the spinocervicothalamic system of Morin (1955). The quantitative importance in the lemniscal system of the two latter seem to vary in inverse proportion to one another, while both the former are phylogetically recent (see Clezy *et al.*, 1961) and have a partially overlapping thalamic distribution (Bowsher, 1961b).

The extralemniscal systems of mammals, it is submitted, represent the "common fields of neuropil" of lower forms. Their longest fibers are the paleospinothalamic (Mehler, 1957), which are distributed to noncortically dependent thalamic nuclei (Mehler *et al.*, 1956, 1960; Bowsher, 1957a, 1961b; Whitlock and Perl, 1961) and, perhaps, correspond to the nucleus (multi) sensitivus of the amphibian thalamus. The shortest such axons are spino-spinal, and even in man they probably constitute the majority of extralemniscal fibers (see Nathan and Smith, 1959). The cells of origin and termination of these fibers belong to the undifferentiated "common field of neuropil" or "common synaptic pool" of Herrick (1948), which according to most observers constitute some 50% of the neurons in the spinal gray matter of mammals (e.g., Aitken and Bridger, 1961). This central gray core of the spinal cord is continued rostrally as the reticular formation of the brain stem (see Bowsher, 1961a). The longer spino-spinal fibers, by semantic dint of crossing the spinomedullary junction, become spinoreticular. Such fibers, first described in man by Collier and Buzzard (1903), constitute the vast majority of noncerebellopetal long ascending axons in the human spinal cord (Verhaart and Sie, 1957); in lower animals their relative numbers are probably even greater. Within the medial bulbar reticular formation, they terminate in relatively discrete regions in both cat (Rossi and Brodal, 1957) and man (Bowsher, 1962); thence further projections carry impulses to diencephalic cell groups related to those in which direct paleospinothalamic fibers terminate (Nauta and Kuypers, 1958; Albe-Fessard *et al.*, 1962; Bowsher *et al.*, 1962).

It is our thesis, then, that two systems, largely independent of one another between a level above the first synapse and the cortex, are represented in the spinal nerves and their central connections. One of these, the lemniscal, is of recent phylogenetic origin, and signals modality-discriminated information to higher centers. The other, the extralemniscal system, relays through the central reticular core of the neuraxis, which is the modern mammalian remnant of the functionally undifferentiated central nervous system of ancestral vertebrates. Although the extralemniscal reticular system of mammals, as of lower forms, is activated by modality-specific peripheral impulses, centrally it forms the afferent side of Coghill's "total action pattern" system. In other words, whereas the lemniscal system is a true sensory system, the extralemniscal reticular system is an afferent system, not necessarily mediating conscious sensation. In the following pages, it is proposed to examine this hypothesis in greater detail, treating these two systems separately, and devoting a third section to the trigeminal system, which shows special features.

III. The Lemniscal[1] System

The primary afferents of this system show a good degree of submodality specificity, although slowly adapting, tactile receptors have been shown to have a base-line or background activity dependent on skin temperature (Hunt and McIntyre, 1960b; Iggo, 1963a). Pacinian corpuscles [pressure or vibration (McIntyre, 1962) receptors] have been shown to be pure and to possess a "private line" to the spinal cord (Cauna and Mannan, 1961).

The evidence suggests that the highly evolved mechanoreceptors of the A fiber group (including afferents from joint capsules, tendons, and muscle membranes—Hunt and McIntyre, 1960a) have their information handled in an exclusive manner centrally by the most highly developed lemniscal system, that of the dorsal columns and medial lemniscus. The neospinothalamic lemniscal system and perhaps the spino-cervico-thalamic pathway additionally signal thermal and pinprick information, whose primary afferents are found in the smaller myelinated fibers of the A group (Hunt and McIntyre, 1960c; Iggo, 1963a). There are some physiological as well as anatomical differences in the organization of the lemniscal pathways (Fig. 1), which will be pointed out in the ensuing pages, starting with the better-known purely mechanoreceptive system.

A. The Dorsal Column–Medial Lemniscus System

The primary afferent fibers end in a somatotopically organized manner in the gracile and cuneate nuclei (Glees and Soler, 1951), in such a way that the pecunculus is represented lying mediolaterally on its back. In recent years intensive investigations have been carried out on the dorsal column nuclei by Amassian, Gordon,

[1] Lemniscal, for us, means a specific pathway.

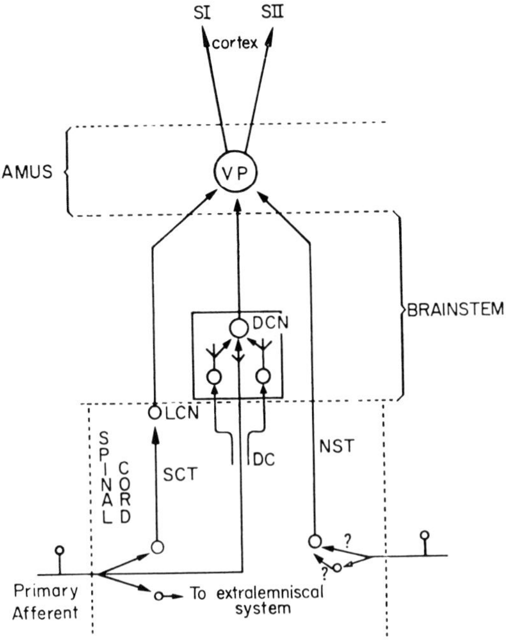

FIG. 1. Diagram of lemniscal systems. Note these systems are crossed, but for purposes of schematic clarity, the decussations are not shown in this figure. Three principal systems are shown relaying through the Ventroposterolateral nucleus of the thalamus (VP) to S I and S II: the spino-cervico-thalamic system (SCT), having an intercurrent synapse in the lateral cervical nucleus (LCN); the neospinothalamic tract (NST), whose importance appears to vary inversely with that of SCT; it is questionable whether the cells of origin of NST are directly or indirectly supplied by primary peripheral afferents; and the dorsal column–medial lemniscus system (DC), which relays both monosynaptically and by way of interneurons in the dorsal column nuclei (DCN).

Kruger, McComas, Perl, and their collaborators. Kruger *et al.* (1961) have demonstrated units in the dorsal column nuclei which respond to joint movements. Perl *et al.* (1962) have demonstrated, in the gracile nucleus of the cat, cells differentially responsive to hair movement, light touch, and vibration or tapping. In addition to the dorsal columns themselves, two other sources of afferent fibers to the dorsal column nuclei are known anatomically. They receive an ascending contribution from the anterolateral columns of the cord (Nauta and Kuypers, 1958; Bowsher, 1962), and a descending one from the sensorimotor cortex (Walberg, 1957; Kuypers *et al.*, 1961). Gordon and his collaborators (Gordon and Paine, 1960; Gordon and Seed, 1961) have shown that there are rostrocaudal differences in the physiological organization of the dorsal column nuclei. Cells in the rostral part of the nucleus have large peripheral receptive fields and do not show any afferent (lateral) inhibition, whereas those in the intermediate part of the nucleus have much smaller cutaneous receptive fields, which exhibit the phenomenon of lateral inhibition. Kruger *et al.* (1961) discussed these observations on a statistical basis; they failed to find afferent inhibition, but considered that, unlike excitation, it may be highly susceptible to the effect of anesthetics. McComas (1963), working with the rat, has adduced evidence that large-field neurons in the caudal part of the gracile nucleus are monosynaptically activated by convergent primary afferent neurons and that these caudal units project secondarily to the more rostrally placed, gracile neurons with small receptive fields. Kuypers (1964) has shown that cells in this caudal part of the nucleus, as well as in the rostralmost section, receive the majority of descending afferents, and either possess more nonlemniscal collaterals or do not contribute to the medial lemniscus. He suggests that they may function, "at least in part, as the interneurones responsible for the pre-synaptic inhibition of relay cells." Gordon (1964) also considers that these cells may act as inhibitory interneurons and has shown that they are uniformly excited by stimulation of the sensorimotor cortex, whereas the intermediately placed, lemniscally projecting, units with small receptive fields and showing afferent inhibition, are inhibited from the sensorimotor cortex (Gordon and Jukes, 1963). That descending afferents to the dorsal column nuclei may be either facilitatory or inhibitory was shown by Towe and Jabbur (1961); descending facilitatory fibers travel exclusively in the pyramidal tract, while inhibitory afferents appear to travel by both pyramidal and extrapyramidal pathways (Jabbur and Towe, 1961).

Thus there is shown to be considerable modification of information at the dorsal column nuclei, as first suggested by Amassian and De Vito (1957). This information is transmitted to the thalamus via the medial lemniscus, which decussates completely (Matzke, 1951; Bowsher, 1958). The chief thalamic end station for the fibers of the medial lemniscus is the ventroposterolateral (VPL) nucleus of the thalamus, in which again there is a complete somatotopic map of the animal. As in the dorsal column nuclei, each skin point projects to an oro-caudal group of cells (Mountcastle and Henneman, 1949, 1952), and the individual neurons are submodality specific (Poggio and Mountcastle, 1963). Just as the fibers of the dorsal columns themselves make no synaptic connections with the brainstem reticular formation (Torvik, 1956), neither does the medial lemniscus give off any collaterals below the mesodiencephalic junction (Bowsher,[2] 1958; Valverde, 1961a). However, some fibers or collaterals of the medial lemniscus terminate in the cell groups (PO of Rose and Woolsey, 1958) lying medial to the medial geniculate nucleus (Bowsher, 1961b). Inferences that this may be the case could be drawn from the physiological observations of Poggio and Mountcastle (1960) and are explicitly suggested by Perl and Whitlock (1961).

VPL and PO show considerable differences in their physiological response properties, as discussed by Poggio and Mountcastle (1960) and Mountcastle (1961). VPL receives only medial lemniscal afferents whereas PO appears to be an area for the interaction of auditory (or vestibular) and somatic signals; it also receives afferents from the superior colliculus in the cat (Altman and Carpenter, 1961).

B. The Spinal Lemniscus: Neospinothalamic and Spino-Cervico-Thalamic Systems

In the amphibian salamander, there are no direct spinothalamic fibers, though such a pathway, interrupted by a relay at the bulbospinal junction, exists (Herrick, 1948). In the marsupial phalanger the spinothalamic pathway is also interrupted at the bulbospinal junction (Clezy *et al.*, 1961); whereas in the marsupial opossum, 2% of anterolateral spinal fibers reach the thalamus (Mehler, 1957). In mammals, the proportion of direct fibers from the cord which reach VPL increases as the phylogenetic scale is ascended (Mehler, 1957). It appears that as the phylogenetic scale is ascended, the interrupted system is progressively replaced by a direct fiber pathway. In the cat, there is a relay in the lateral cervical nucleus (Morin, 1955), from where further fibers project to the contralateral ventrobasal complex of the thalamus. A similar relayed

[2] Re-examination of the material used in this investigation shows that what was then described as the "nucleus of the medial lemniscus," and which receives some lemniscal fibers, is, in fact, the caudalmost part of the PO complex.

pathway exists in the rabbit (Matricali, 1957), while there is no evidence for its existence in man (Verhaart, 1957 cited by Andersson, 1962). The pathway has not been demonstrated in the monkey (Oscarsson *et al.*, 1964), and undoubtedly direct neospinothalamic fibers predominate in this animal (Mehler *et al.*, 1960).

So far as the direct neospinothalamic fibers (spinal lemniscus) in primates are concerned, there is one important anatomical difference as compared with the medial lemniscus. This is that although the majority of fibers are crossed, a certain proportion reach the ipsilateral thalamic VPL (Bowsher, 1957a, 1961b; Mehler *et al.*, 1960). This may occur through failure to decussate in the cord (White and Sweet, 1955), or through redecussation in the medulla (Bowsher, 1957a, 1961b; Mehler *et al.*, 1960) or posterior commissure (Quensel, 1898; Bowsher, 1957a). Within the thalamus itself, fibers of the direct spinal lemniscus are distributed in the same manner, though in lesser quantity, as are those of the medial lemniscus, with which they overlap (Bowsher, 1961b). There is tentative anatomical (Bowsher, 1957b, 1961b) and physiological (Perl and Whitlock, 1961) evidence that, in some cases at least, spinothalamic fibers terminate in relation to different VPL cells than do fibers of the medial lemniscus; this would explain the retention of differential submodality specificity at the thalamic level. Impulses of spinal origin, thought to be neo- rather than paleospinothalamic (Bowsher, 1961b), also terminate in the PO complex (Whitlock and Perl, 1959; Poggio and Mountcastle, 1960). In proportion to the number of fibers reaching VPL, the spinothalamic projection to PO is greater than the medial lemniscal; this is probably also true of absolute numbers of terminations in PO (Bowsher, 1961b).

The cells of origin of spinothalamic fibers lie in the dorsal horn of the spinal gray matter (Edinger, 1889; Foerster and Gagel, 1932). Lundberg and Oscarsson (1962) have described units in the dorsal horn of the cat's spinal cord which they suggest may be cells of origin of the spinothalamic tract. They are activated from contralateral peripheral fields, probably monosynaptically. The cells of origin of the spinocervical tract have been identified by Eccles *et al.* (1960) in lamina IV of Rexed. They are identical with at least one group of Wall's (1960) common carrier cells, which can be collaterally activated by antidromic stimulation of dorsal column fibers. In this respect, it is interesting to note that the average receptive field size of common carrier cells is 2016 mm^2, while that of the gracile hairless skin "touch units" according to Perl *et al.* (1962) is 1818 mm^2; the latter, like the former, do not exhibit afferent inhibition. Spinocervical cells are not influenced from the sensorimotor cortex (Lundberg *et al.*, 1963). Lundberg (1965) describes two types of spinocervical units: (a) those responding only to light touch in a restricted ipsilateral field, and (b) those responding to light touch in a restricted field, and to pressure-pinching from a larger field. Oswaldo-Cruz and Kidd (1964) in a microelectrode analysis of the cat's lateral cervical nucleus, describe 7% of cells with large fields as activated by noxious stimuli.

The medial and direct spinal lemnisci have been shown anatomically (Matzke, 1951; Anderson and Berry, 1959; Mehler *et al.*, 1960; Bowsher, 1961b), and the spino-cervico-thalamic system electroanatomically (Morin, 1955; Andersson, 1962), to terminate in the lateral part of the thalamic ventroposterior nucleus; this, in turn, is known to project to the primary and secondary somatic areas of the cortex (S I and S II) (Macchi *et al.*, 1959). Rose and Woolsey (1958) suggested on the grounds of the inconstant retrograde degeneration in VPL following removal of S II that the thalamic fibers to this area are sustaining collaterals of the projections to S I. The question arises therefore as to the degree of convergence of the various lemnsical systems in and beyond VPL.

It may be true that both dorsal column–medial lemniscal and spino-cervico-thalamic systems project both to S I and to S II; for Andersson (1962) has shown that the body image is represented in both areas where (a) the dorsal columns only are intact, and (b) when these columns only are destroyed. This does not, of course, imply that the same thalamic and cortical units are involved.

In favor of the interpretation that S I mainly reflects dorsal column–medial lemniscus activity, the following points should be considered. The dorsal column–medial lemniscus shows the phenomenon of afferent inhibition, which occurs, as discussed above, at the level of the dorsal column nuclei. In the anterolateral system, Wall (1960) found no afferent inhibition at the level of the common-carrier cells in the dorsal horn of the cord; Perl and Whitlock were unable to demonstrate it in cat and monkey VPL under light barbiturate anesthesia, with the whole cord except for one anterolateral quadrant destroyed. Andersson (1962) found no afferent inhibition in S II units in the cat whose dorsal columns had been destroyed, whereas in the intact animal, 3% of the cells in this area show afferent inhibition (Carreras and Andersson, 1963).

However, it is possible that in the case of convergence of different lemniscal afferents on place-specific cells in VPL, afferent inhibition in the medial lemniscus, taking place in the dorsal column nuclei, is transmitted unchanged across the thalamic synapse; whereas lateral column afferents with no surrounding inhibition, also transfer their information unchanged across the same synapses. This, of course, only applies to those submodality-specific afferents which are common to all lemniscal systems, i.e., to those driven by cutaneous touch-pressure stimulation. This is in accordance with findings in these systems below this level (Table I).

TABLE I
AREA OF CUTANEOUS RECEPTIVE FIELDS OF CAT FOREARM AT VARIOUS LEVELS

Level	Ref.	Area (mean value in mm^2)
Peripheral aff. to common-carrier cells	Wall., 1960	20 (4–180)
Intermediate (hair) gracile cells	Perl *et al.*, 1962	280 (28–900)
	Gordon and Paine, 1960	250
Common-carrier cells	Wall, 1960	2016 (450–5250)
Gracile touch units	Perl *et al.*, 1962	1818

It appears that among the lemniscal systems, the dorsal column–medial lemniscus system has gained a greater degree of accuracy of localization by sacrificing the wider submodality range of the other systems. Perl and Whitlock (1961) found that 3.5% of the units they studied in the monkey thalamus (supplied by only one intact anterolateral column) responded only to noxious stimuli, coming from discrete peripheral receptive fields. Anterolaterally supplied temperature units in VPL have not been numerically investigated.

Macchi *et al.* (1959) have shown that both S I and S II must be removed in order to produce fulminating retrograde degeneration in VPL, though cell changes (and some loss) ensue upon separate removal of S I or S II (Rose and Woolsey, 1958). This suggests that most VPL cells project collaterally to S I and S II. There is some evidence (Mehler *et al.*, 1960; Bowsher, 1961b) that neospinothalamic afferents are chiefly distributed to pars caudalis of VPL (VB of Rose), that is, the part of the nucleus containing small as well as large cells; whereas the medial lemniscus projects equally to both partes oralis and caudalis. Demirjian and Morin (1964) state that the lower-limb projection through the lateral cervical nucleus of the cat overlaps in VPL with that of the gracile nucleus.

Beresford (1962) has shown that the corticothalamic projection to the lateral geniculate body from the visual cortex is the exact reciprocal of the thalamocortical projection. If, as is probable, the same situation holds for the somatosensory relay nucleus, the work of Chandler (1964) is relevant: she finds that while S I projects unilaterally to partes oralis and caudalis of VPL, S II projects only to pars caudalis, but bilaterally, in the cat. Moreover, though both projections show somatotopy, it is less sharply defined in the case of the S II–VPL projection; Carreras and Andersson (1963) point out that the somatotopic projections to S II are less sharply defined than that to S I. Knighton (1950) found, electroanatomically, the posterior part of VPL is that which principally projects to S II.

Joint position sensibility (kinesthesia) is virtually unrepresented except in the dorsal column–medial lemniscus system (see Rose and Mountcastle in "Handbook of Physiology"). However, some anterolateral fibers carry impulses generated in deep tissues, for Perl and Whitlock (1961) found that in monkeys whose whole spinal cord except for one anterolateral quadrant had been destroyed, 10.5% of VPL units were driven by stimuli to deep tissue. This is to be compared with 58% of intact monkey VPL units driven by deep stimuli (Poggio and Mountcastle, 1963); of these, 45% were driven by joint movements. Powell and Mountcastle (1959) found that 59% of the units in S I cortex responded to stimulation of deep tissue, of which 37% were due to joint movement. Thus it can be seen that in the intact animals, the modality relationship between VPL and S I units is very close. Because of the overwhelming numerical preponderance of the medial lemniscus over other lemniscal systems (Glees and Bailey, 1951; Bowsher, 1963) it can reasonably be assumed that, in the intact animal, evoked activity in the thalamus and in S I are mainly a reflection of activity in this system.

A valid comparison of the differential distribution of modality-place-specific neurons between S I and S II can at present only be made for the cat (Table II), as insufficient data exist for the monkey's S II.

Statistically significant analyses do not exist for cat VPL in preparations with only one anterolateral column intact; but Perl and Whitlock (1961) found in such animals only 2 units responding to joint manipulation. Taken together with the previously quoted fact that afferent inhibition is not significantly demonstrable in S II in intact animals and in VPL supplied only by one anterolateral column, a case can be made out for the reflection in S II, in the main, of lemniscal activity other than that conducted via the medial lemniscus.

TABLE II
Distribution of Unit Responses in Cat Cortex

		% Units responding to stimulation of:	
Locus	Ref.	Skin	Deep tissue
S I	Mouncastle, 1957	69	31
S II	Carreras and Andersson, 1963	94	6

Phylogenetically, the oldest lemniscal system is the spino-cervico-thalamic, and the most recent is probably the neospinothalamic. The dorsal column–medial lemniscus system holds an intermediate position, both anatomically and functionally. Thus, spino-cervico-thalamic cord neurons show no afferent inhibition, and are activated by primary peripheral afferents some of whose long collaterals reach caudal gracile cells ("touch units") showing the same properties. Gracile hair units,[3] on the other hand, with smaller receptive fields, show afferent inhibition, and are fired indirectly from the periphery via an interneuron. Conduction in the secondary neurons of the spino-cervico-thalamic system (spino-cervical fibers) is considerably more rapid than in secondary neurons of the dorsal column–medial lemniscus system (medial lemniscus fibers). At higher levels, the spino-cervico-thalamic and neospinothalamic systems have been insufficiently distinguished for valid differentiation to be made. At the cortical level, the nomenclature is unfortunate, for the available evidence indicates that S II is phylogenetically older than S I.

[3] Hairs are peculiar to mammals; but reptiles have dorsal column nuclei.

IV. The Extralemniscal Reticular System

The anatomy and physiology of this system (Fig. 2) is much more complex than that of the lemniscal systems, and despite intensive investigation in the last two decades very much less is

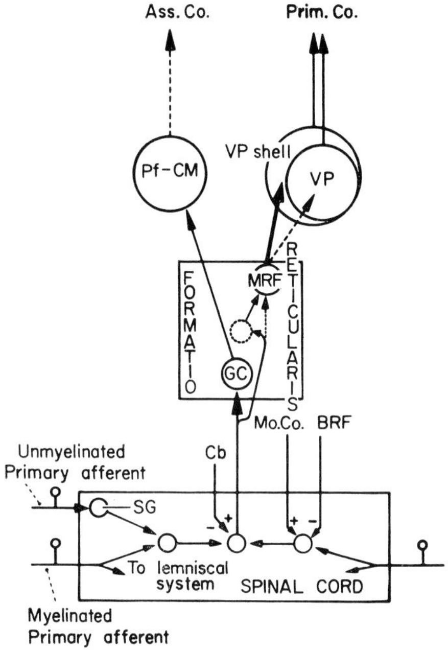

FIG. 2. Diagram of extralemniscal systems. A spinal cord interneuron excited from the motor cortex (Mo. Co.) and inhibited from the bulbar reticular formation (BRF), receives primary afferents directly or indirectly by relay through the substantia gelatinosa (SG). This interneuron sends its axon to a spinoreticular neuron which may be either excited or inhibited from the cerebellum. One spino-reticulo-thalamic pathway relays in the bulbar gigantocellular nucleus (GC) and parafascicular–centromedian complex (Pf–CM) to influence the nonspecific association cortex (Ass. Co.). Other pathways pass either through GC or a more rostral reticular relay (shown in dotted outline), to relay again in the mesencephalic reticular formation (MRF) before passing to cells in VP and its shell showing convergent properties; this activity is finally reflected in cells of the specific primary cortex (Prim. Co.).

precisely known of it than of the lemniscal systems. We do not propose here, for reasons of space, to review in detail the literature already reviewed by Brodal (1957) and Rossi and Zanchetti

(1957). We have already introduced the concept that, in mammals, this system represents a persistence of the nonspecific secondary afferent neuropil of lower forms, and it is our intention in this section to examine the implications of this in greater detail. It is worth recalling that the connections and possible functions of this system had been earlier discussed at the level of the brain-stem reticular formation (Kohnstamm and Quensel, 1908) and intralaminar thalamus (Dejerine, 1910).

The first central neurons of this system would appear to be some of the "common-carrier cells" of Wall (1960) in the dorsal horn of the spinal gray matter. These cells receive anatomical convergence of microbundles of myelinated primary afferent fibers of differing diameter and conduction velocity: their cutaneous receptive field in the cat (forelimb below elbow) lies between 450 and 5250 mm^2 (average 2016 mm^2). Wall has shown that they respond by different discharge patterns to tactile, thermal, and noxious stimuli. In contrast to cells in the dorsal column nuclei (see above), common-carrier cells do not exhibit afferent inhibition. But Wall and Cronly-Dillon (1960) have shown that their threshold for any given submodality of stimulation can be raised by applying a stimulus of another submodality in the same receptive field. More recently, Wall (1962, 1964) has shown that the cells of the substantia gelatinosa, receiving primary unmyelinated peripheral afferents, exert a tonic modulating influence, probably by an interneuron, on the ascending activity from the common-carrier cells. Szentagothai (1964) has recently demonstrated an anatomical basis for this.

Certain homologies exist between Wall's common-carrier cells and some of the units activated by "flexion reflex afferents" of the Lund school (see Oscarsson, 1958). Although their identity has not been proved, it may reasonably be assumed for the purpose of the present argument. Lundberg and Oscarsson (1962) have shown that those cells with axons ascending in the anterolateral columns can be activated from bilateral receptive fields. A pathway descending in the dorsolateral funiculus of the cord can inhibit these cells via an interneuron (Holmqvist *et al.*, 1960); these authors suggest that this descending inhibition [shown by Lundberg *et al.* (1963) to be mediated by the pyramidal tract from the sensorimotor cortex] may serve "to select and restrict the receptive field to parts physiologically needed." Holmqvist *et al.* (1960) also showed that these dorsal horn cells are monosynaptically activated by a ventral descending pathway, shown by Carpenter *et al.* (1963) to be in the ventromedial brain-stem reticular formation.

Thus it can be seen that the first central neuron of the extra-lemniscal pathway is subject to a large number of modulating influences; and it seems certain that not all of these are yet known. The fact that common-carrier cells can be activated by antidromic stimulation of the dorsal columns (Wall, 1961) must mean that they are also the cells which receive the "short collaterals" of large primary cutaneous afferents to the gracile and cuneate nuclei. There exist, however, at least two types of neuron with ascending efferents in the dorsal horn, for Lundberg *et al.* (1963) have shown that the lemniscal spinocervical system, unlike the extra-lemniscal spinobulbar one, is not affected by descending activity from the sensorimotor cortex. It is difficult to imagine, given the great differences in higher distribution and effects, that any spinal lemniscal systems share cells of origin with extralemniscal systems; although it is just possible that the modulating influences could act as a switching device for the channeling of upgoing activity. While awaiting further evidence, it will be assumed for present purposes that spinal extralemniscal neurons are independent of lemniscal neurons except that the existence of lemniscal-extra-lemniscal interaction at spinal segmental level cannot be doubted.

It would thus appear that the first central extralemniscal neuron, which is monosynaptically fired by primary peripheral afferents, has a short (spino-spinal) axon. This is a retention of the anatomical situation that exists in *Amphioxus.* Longer ascending extra-lemniscal neurons are third- (or even subsequent) order, and first appear in lampreys (Ariëns Kappers *et al.,* 1936).

Spivy and Metcalf (1959) showed that the central connections of the purely large-fibered and large- and small-fibered parts of the dorsal root have different central effects. Stimulation of the lateral division of the dorsal root (which probably contains all C and some A fibers) has visceral as well as somatic effects, since it causes "the blood pressure rise known to associate with avoid-ance of noxious stimulation" (Spivy and Metcalf, 1959). Within the common neuropil of the generalized urodele amphibian de-scribed by Herrick (1948), there is an ill-defined and incomplete channeling of information into higher visceral (hypothalamic) and somatic (tectothalamic) centers. Similar interlinked somatic and vegetative neurons have been identified in the developing reticular matter of the human cord (Sukhetzkaya, 1957). So far as the higher (diencephalic) connections are concerned, we shall concentrate on the somatic (thalamic) ones, but it is important not to lose sight of continuous viscerosomatic linkage below this level.

The organization of spinoreticular fibers in the cat has been described by Rossi and Brodal (1957). There is a tendency for spinoreticular terminals to be concentrated in two regions of the medioventral medullary reticular formation. A similar situation appears to exist in man with the addition of a further rostrally placed (mesencephalic), terminal zone (Bowsher, 1962). This illustrates the important principle that the caudalmost connections of an ascending system are phylogenetically the most ancient, whereas more rostral terminals represent either more recently evolved independent neurons, or rostrally projecting collaterals of an older system which retains its caudal connections (cf. the dorsal column fibers). The bulbar reticular regions in which ascending afferents terminate give off further ascending efferent fibers (Brodal and Rossi, 1955). These reticulothalamic connections, originating in the large neurons of the nucleus reticularis gigantocellularis and associated cell groups, terminate in the centromedian–parafascicular complex and the centrolateral nucleus of the thalamic intralaminar nuclear group (Nauta and Kuypers, 1958). In their course rostralward through the brain stem, these fibers are said to occupy the region of the central tegmental fasciculus of Forel (Nauta and Kuypers, 1958; Dennis and Kerr, 1961).

In addition to the spino-reticulo-thalamic pathway, there exist paleospinothalamic fibers passing directly from cord to thalamus (Mehler, 1957). In cat and monkey, they terminate in the same intralaminar nuclei as do reticulothalamic fibers (Anderson and Berry, 1959; Mehler *et al.*, 1960; Bowsher, 1961b); according to Getz (1952), Bowsher (1957a, 1961b), from the physiological results of Kruger and Albe-Fessard (1960) and Whitlock and Perl (1961), and Albe-Fessard and Bowsher (1965), some of these fibers seem also to terminate in the thalamic reticular nucleus. The paleospinothalamic fibers also travel in the central tegmental fasciculus, but it is not certain whether they are independent of spinoreticular neurons or whether they are long ascending collateral branches of these latter. In favor of their complete independence is the fact that local cooling in the bulbar gigantocellular nucleus of the cat greatly diminishes but does not abolish the centromedian–parafascicular response to somatic stimulation (Bowsher *et al.*, 1962). Mallart, Bowsher, and Albe-Fessard (unpublished) have identified units in the reticular relay of the spino-reticulo-centromedian pathway which respond to stimulation of one, two, three, or four limbs. These may explain the positive or negative "preferences" for one or more limbs in the convergent responses found in the centromedian–parafascicular complex of monkeys in the macroelectrode studies of Albe-Fessard and Bowsher (1965).

In addition to medial spinoreticular neurons, there is also a more diffuse spinal projection on the lateral reticular formation of the medulla and pons (Bowsher, 1957, 1962; Anderson and Berry, 1959; Mehler *et al.*, 1960). Nauta and Kuypers (1958) describe fibers ascending from this region which swing medially at the level of the principal sensory trigeminal nucleus to join the central tegmental fasciculus; these neurons have also recently been described in Golgi preparations by Valverde (1961b). According to Nauta and Kuypers (1958), ascending fibers from both medial and lateral bulbar reticular formation relay in the mesencephalic reticular tegmentum and pass from there, via the mammillary peduncle and dorsal longitudinal fasciculus, to the hypothalamus, in addition to the fibers projecting to the thalamus. In so far as a particular visceral afferent pathway can be differentiated from this "common neuropil"; it is probably represented by fibers from the cord to the caudal solitary nucleus (Rossi and Brodal, 1956; Torvik, 1956; Bowsher, 1962); from the caudal solitary nucleus to the dorsal tegmental nucleus (Hawkes, 1960); and from the dorsal tegmental nucleus to the hypothalamus (Guillery, 1959).

In marked contrast to the lemniscal systems, the ascending extralemniscal reticular system, in conformity with its phylogenetic antiquity, shows only partial laterization which is lost at higher levels due to decussation. At almost all levels, after the first synaptic relay, fibers from one side of the reticular core of the neuraxis project to some extent to both sides at higher levels; this is particularly noticeable above the bulbar relay. This implies that the system is developed from a completely nonlateralized neuraxis, such as does not exist alone in modern vertebrates above the level of cyclostomes (Ariëns Kappers *et al.*, 1936). Moruzzi (1954) was the first to show that the mesencephalic reticular formation also receives nonspecific convergent afferents.

The reawakening interest in the brain-stem reticular formation dates from the discovery that it forms the anatomical substrate for activation of the EEG by peripheral afferent stimulation (Moruzzi and Magoun, 1949). We do not intend to deal with this extensive subject here, especially since the relationship between EEG changes and the conscious perception of sensation is an intricate one, and there is certainly insufficient evidence at present to enable us to make any particular correlation between them. For the present purpose, it will suffice to regard EEG changes, either in the direction of slowing of activity or of activation, essentially as a sign of change in ascending reticular activity.

It is interesting to note that stimulation of particular points within the brain-stem reticular formation at different stimulation parameters, can give rise to "slowing" as well as activation of EEG traces (Starzl *et al.*, 1951; Favale *et al.*, 1961; Magnes *et al.*, 1961).

Stimulation, at certain parameters of myelinated peripheral fibers of cutaneous (Pompeiano and Swett, 1962) or vagal (Padel and Dell, 1964) origin, can also produce cortical slow waves.

Pompeiano and Swett (1962) have identified the myelinated peripheral afferent fibers that produce these effects and whose central pathways ascend through the lateral columns of the cord. They found that for cutaneous afferent fibers, low-frequency stimulation of group II fibers alone produced slow activity, whereas high-frequency stimulation of group II fibers produced arousal, which was greatly augmented by stimulation of group III fibers at low or high frequency. Stimulation of group III afferents in muscle nerves also evoked rapid activity.

Before discussing the thalamotelencephalic transfer from the intralaminar nuclei, consideration will be given to other thalamic regions which are activated by extralemniscal signals.

Whitlock and Perl (1959), in the cat, found potentials evoked by stimulation of all four limbs in an ill-defined cell region, including the magnocellular medial geniculate body, situated caudomedial to the lemniscal thalamic relay (VPL). Poggio and Mountcastle (1960) confirmed these findings; designating the receiving area PO after Rose and Woolsey (1958), they attempted to delineate it in anatomical terms. Whitlock and Perl (1959) worked with cats in which only one spinal anterolateral column was spared; Poggio and Mountcastle (1960) worked with intact animals, but felt that transfer to PO was a purely anterolateral phenomenon. However, in their single unit analysis of PO in the intact animal, 9 out of 74 (12%) of units driven by skin stimulation had small restricted contralateral receptive fields; and they state that "some PO cells may respond with latencies as brief as those of the VB cells," as was found with macroelectrodes by Perl and Whitlock (1961). In intact chloralosed cats, Kruger and Albe-Fessard (1960) found some evidence of tactile activation of PO in 11 out of 26 positive macroelectrode explorations. In a study of the modality sensitivity of PO neurons in cat and monkey with only one spinal anterolateral column intact, Perl and Whitlock (1961) state that "light mechanical disturbance of the body integument was the most commonly effective stimulus in exciting discharge of units located within the posterior nuclear group." Their figures make it clear, however, that the peripheral receptive fields for these units are on average larger than those for VPL neurons, and frequently discontinuous. Bowsher (1961b) showed that in the monkey, both the magnocellular and suprageniculate portions of PO receive direct afferents from both the anterolateral quadrant of the cord (spinothalamic fibers) and the dorsal column nuclei (medial lemniscus). Andersson (1962) adduced, as a result of physiological investigations on S II, that PO receives a direct contribution from the medial lemniscus. It may be concluded, therefore, that PO is a mixed region, showing some lemniscal connections and properties, but being primarily an area of nonlemniscal transfer. The only convergent responses in PO with a latency short enough to imply the possibility of lemniscal conduction in the monkey were in the suprageniculate portion (Albe-Fessard and Bowsher, 1965). The dorsal column efferents medial to the main lemniscus bundle in the midbrain, whose properties have recently been described by Gordon and Jukes (1964), may project to PO.

Kruger and Albe-Fessard (1960) observed convergent responses in the ventrolateral thalamic nucleus (VL) of the cat, in that portion immediately superjacent to VPL. Massion *et al.* (1963) have studied the more medial and anterior parts of VL and found convergent preferential responses in this region. In further analysis of convergent responses in the monkey, Albe-Fessard and Bowsher (1965) found them in those regions of VL and LP (lateralis posterior) which overlie VPL. With macroelectrode recordings, these responses could not be evoked by the kind of natural stimuli which normally activates VPL. Latency of response in this "shell" covering VPL is of the same order as in GMmc (medial magnocellular portion of medial geniculate). Mountcastle (1961), in a further elaboration of the work of Poggio and Mountcastle (1960) on PO, indicates that neurons with these properties extend further rostrally above VPL than originally thought. These considerations lead to the speculation that the extralemniscal part of PO and the ventral portions of LP and VL may all be constituent parts of the same functional shell covering the dorsal, dorsomedial, and dorsocaudal aspects of VPL. Further reasons for including these convergent regions in a single functional group will be considered below. The pathways by which extralemniscal impulses are conveyed to this shell are as yet mainly unknown; though it has been noted that stimulation of the mesencephalic reticular formation in a wide area ventral to the level of the central tegmental fasciculus, which carries impulses from lower reticular centers to the parafascicular–centromedian complex, reproduces the extralemniscal effects of VPL stimulation (Covian *et al.*, 1961).

Mallart *et al.* (1961), in a microelectrode analysis of posterior VPL and surrounding regions in the cat, in response to natural stimuli, found that 11 out of 55 somatotopic units in VPL also showed convergence of extralemniscal afferent signals, whereas of 17 units in adjacent areas of VL and LP, 4 showed lemniscal and extralemniscal convergence, and the remaining 13 showed purely extralemniscal responses. Thus VPL and its shell may be considered as a single entity, the whole of which shows extralemniscal properties, but whose inner core (VPL proper) alone possesses, additionally, important lemniscal functions.

This form of organization is also demonstrable in the properties of the thalamocortical projection of VPL and its shell. By an analysis of responses in cat S I cortex to stimulation of (lemniscally conducted) somatotopically represented contralateral limbs and of (extralemniscally conducted) ipsilateral limbs, Jankowska and Albe-Fessard (Albe-Fessard, 1961; Albe-Fessard and Fessard, 1963) were able to show that, in the somatomotor response to contralateral limb stimulation, the main positive deflection is a lemniscal event; but that a part of the surface-positive and -negative components are extralemniscal phenomena. It was subsequently shown that electrical stimulation of VPL proper reproduces the whole (i.e., lemniscal plus extralemniscal components) on the somatomotor cortex, whereas electrical stimulation of the VPL shell reproduced only the extralemniscal components. Stimulation of the centrum medianum (CM) does not reproduce any of the extralemniscal effects in primary somatomotor cortex.

Since stimulation of VPL, either directly or from the periphery, evokes potentials only in the primary somatomotor cortices (including S I and S II), it follows that extralemniscal impulses relayed through VPL and its shell are distributed only to the primary somatomotor cortices; probably principally to S II, where 20% of the units show nonlemniscal properties (Carreras and Andersson, 1963), and to anterior S I (i.e., ? motor) cortex, where 50% of units have extralemniscal properties (Albe-Fessard *et al.*, 1961).

Convergent associative (i.e., heterotopic and heterosensory) phenomena in the nonprimary cortex were first observed in the anterior marginal gyrus of the cat by Amassian (1954). Albe-Fessard and Rougeul (1955, 1958) soon confirmed this and found three further cortical areas—in anterior and posterior zones of the supra-Sylvian gyrus and in the anterior sigmoid gyrus (primary motor area). Eight years later, Thompson *et al.* (1963) were able in almost identical experiments to confirm the findings in all four areas. The primary motor cortex has been carefully analyzed for heterotopic and heterosensory convergence in the cat by Buser and Imbert (1961). Multisensory convergent responses have also been observed on the medial surface of the hemisphere (Bruner and Buser, 1960). Albe-Fessard and Rougeul (1958) also observed that the response characteristics to somatic stimulation of the thalamic center median are very similar to those of the four association areas in the superolateral cortex; and that the cortical effects can be reproduced bilaterally by stimulation of one center median. Relatively short latencies (4 msec) were observed between CM and association cortex in the cat.

In the monkey, Albe-Fessard *et al.* (1959) found two cortical areas of the CM type: the main one is in the superior frontal gyrus, and the other, in the parietal association cortex just behind S I, has a preponderance of upper limb representation. The authors point out that the superior frontal association area is less sharply delimited than in the cat, and that occlusions within it between responses evoked from two limbs are not always total, as in the cat.

Of course, this may merely reflect greater complexity of thalamocortical and subdiencephalic integrating mechanisms. As in the cat, the cortical response pattern can be reproduced by stimulation of CM (at latencies of 8–19 msec).

Two differences may be noted, at the level of the cortex, between what we may call the VPL and CM types of extralemniscal response. First, though the phenomenon of heterotopic convergence is displayed in both, microelectrode analysis in cat (Albe-Fessard, 1961) and monkey (Albe-Fessard and Liebeskind, 1964) shows that although convergence can be observed in neurons encountered in all layers of the association cortex driven by CM, pure extralemniscal properties are only seen in the superficial layers of the primary cortex driven by VPL; deeper layers additionally display somatotopy. Second, the CM-projected association cortex is not only heterotopic, but also heterosensory; in addition to somatic stimuli, it is also activated by visual and auditory stimulation (Buser and Borenstein, 1956, 1959). This heterosensory convergence is a reflection of that already seen at single unit level in thalamic CM (Albe-Fessard and Mallart, 1960). The VPL-projected convergent system, on the other hand, so far as can be judged from preliminary experiments, does not appear to be significantly heterosensory; again, analysis of units in the thalamic VPL shell shows little heterosensory convergence (Massion *et al.*, 1963).

Thus, at the thalamocortical level, the extralemniscal system can apparently be divided into two components: (a) a convergent heterotopic but mainly homosensory system, projected from the ventral mesencephalic reticular formation through VPL and its surrounding shell to the primary somatomotor cortex and (b) an association system, which is both heterotopically and heterosensorially convergent, which projects from a relay in the gigantocellular bulbar reticular formation by way of the central tegmental fasciculus to CM and association (nonprimary) cortex.

The anatomical nature of the centromedian-cortical projection remains in much doubt. Centromedian-cortical latencies in the cat (4 msec) are short enough for monosynaptic conduction to be possible. In the monkey, on the other hand, they were first reported to be considerably longer (10 msec). Albe-Fessard *et al.* (1959) found the latency from periphery to association cortex to have a mean value of 20 msec, whereas the mean of the sum of the latencies from periphery to CM and from CM to cortex was 24 msec. More recently, however, Oswaldo-Cruz (1961) has found CM latencies in *Cebus* of 5–7 msec.

Direct projection of CM to this cortex has been denied by anatomists on the basis of lack of retrograde degeneration following decortication. But since it is now known (Drooglever-Fortuyn and Stefens, 1951; Cowan and Powell, 1955) that the intralaminar thalamic nuclei project to the corpora striata, it is not possible to exclude a collateral projection to the cortex; this would be a sustaining projection as defined by Rose and Woolsey (1958). The latencies found between CM and cortex are a little long for direct connection, but such that the connections could be direct, by small fibers, or indirect with one synaptic relay, by larger fibers. If such a relay exists, its site is unknown, although some structures can be excluded:

1. The corpora striata, although in receipt of intralaminar and cortical afferents (Webster, 1961; Carman, Cowan and Powell, 1963), do not project upon the cortex; they show no retrograde atrophy following decortication.

2. The thalamic reticular nucleus has been cast for the role of relay by some authors. This is because intralaminar and other thalamic efferents certainly pass through it and may establish terminal or collateral connections within it; and because its cells show changes following decortication (Rose, 1952). However, it is unlikely to be a relay because, in the first place, the nucleus reticularis thalami is of ventral thalamic origin; that is to say, it is developed from the basal lamina of the primitive neural tube. In the second place, the changes observed in the cells of the nucleus following decortication are of the type found by Powell and Erulkar (1962) to be due to deafferentation; that is, they may be transneuronal rather than retrograde (Carman *et al.*, 1964).

3. The nucleus ventralis anterior of the thalamus (VA) has been proposed as a possible relay (Hanbery *et al.*, 1955); in the monkey it does project to the region of the superior frontal gyrus. However, a small number of latency measurements made by Kruger and Albe-Fessard (1960) in the cat indicate that it usually responds before CM to peripheral stimulation.

V. The Trigeminal System

Primary afferent neurons of the trigeminal system are of two morphological varieties (Cajal, 1909): many fibers bifurcate proximal to the Gasserian ganglion, sending an ascending branch to the principal sensory nucleus in the pons and a descending branch via the spinal tract to the descending nucleus; a second type of neuron does not bifurcate, but travels caudally in the spinal tract to effect connections in, or in the region of, the descending nucleus.

Recent studies of the distribution of primary trigeminal afferents in the rat have been made by Torvik (1956) and Clarke and Bowsher (1962). They show that in the pons, connections are restricted to the principal sensory nucleus, where they are chiefly axodendritic. In the descending nucleus, on the other hand, primary afferent fibers are distributed beyond the indistinct medial edge of the nucleus into the adjacent lateral and lateroventral reticular formation. Some fibers pass even further medially to make synaptic contact with the gigantocellular reticular nucleus, lying in the central core of the tegmentum. Fibers joining or passing through the descending nucleus from the spinal tract enter as radially arranged microbundles, morphologically reminiscent of those described by Wall (1960) in the dorsal horn of the spinal cord. As in the principal nucleus, axondentric synaptic endings predominate over axosomatic in the descending nucleus; but in the gigantocellular reticular nucleus, the majority of degenerating boutons were seen to be in contact with cell bodies or proximal dendritic processes (Clarke and Bowsher, 1962). In addition to the sensory trigeminal and lateral and medial lateral reticular nuclei, primary afferent trigeminal fibers are also distributed to the nucleus of the solitary tract, to the motor nuclei of the trigeminal and facial nerves, and to ventral horn cells in the upper cervical cord (? spinal accessory nucleus).

Single unit recording in the sensory trigeminal nuclei and adjacent regions of the cat have recently been made by Gordon *et al.* (1961), Kruger *et al.* (1961), Wall and Taub (1962), Kruger and Michel (1962a,b), and Darian-Smith *et al.* (1963a,b). They have demonstrated a somatotopic representation of the face which is continuous throughout the rostrocaudal extent of the nuclei. These units are driven only by mechanoreceptors. Gordon *et al.* (1961), who investigated the caudal descending trigeminal nucleus, found that some 40% of the cells could be activated antidromically from the trigeminal lemniscus, and that afferent inhibition occurred in 6 out of 16 units tested. These authors, together with Wall and Taub (1962), would homologize the descending nucleus with the dorsal horn of the spinal gray matter and the principal nucleus with the dorsal column nuclei; Kruger and Michel (1962a) specifically deny the existence of afferent inhibition in the descending nucleus. This question must at present be regarded as unsettled, but if it be true that there is no afferent inhibition in the somatotopically organized, descending nucleus, homology with the neospinothalamic system is evident. On the basis of embryology (Brown, 1956, 1958, 1960, 1962), morphology (Olszewski, 1950), afferent connections (Torvik, 1956; Clarke and Bowsher, 1962), and efferent connections (Walker, 1938; Torvik, 1957; Nauta and Kuypers, 1958), the most reasonable homologies still seem to be between the principal sensory and dorsal column nuclei, and between the caudal descending nucleus and the cells of origin of the spinal lemniscus. Gordon *et al.* (1961) found cells with very large receptive fields in the lateroventral juxtatrigeminal reticular formation which responded to noxious stimulation; and Lamarche *et al.* (1960) were able to activate cells in the medial gigantocellular reticular formation by noxious stimuli applied to the face. Both these reticular areas receive primary afferent trigeminal fibers (Clarke and Bowsher, 1962). Darian-Smith *et al.* (1963a) also report units with reticular properties along the ventromedial border of the descending nucleus. Thus there appears to be some justification for homologizing the caudal descending trigeminal nucleus and the adjoining reticular formation with the whole of the dorsal horn of the spinal gray matter and the reticular interneurons at its base.

Of particular interest is the fact that both principal and caudal descending trigeminal nuclei are supplied by bifurcating primary afferent fibers, for a similar situation seems to exist for the cells of origin of the two corporal lemniscal systems (medial and spinal) (see Section II). It is tempting to suggest that the cells driven by noxious stimuli from large peripheral fields receive the nonbifurcated descending primary afferents; but at present there is no positive direct evidence to support this conjecture. Sufficient is known, however, of the caudal descending trigeminal nucleus, in its widest morphological sense, to be able to say that it contains cells of both lemniscal and extralemniscal type, as defined in an earlier section of this review; the principal sensory nucleus, on the other hand, probably contains only what we would call lemniscal cells (Torvik, 1957).

In this context, the (secondary) efferent projections of these two portions of the trigeminal sensory complex are of interest. The principal sensory nucleus projects to the medial part of the thalamic ventrobasal complex (arcuate nucleus; VPM) (Walker, 1938; Darian-Smith *et al.*, 1963a). The projections of the caudal descending nucleus and its surroundings are more complex. Some fibers contribute to the trigeminal lemniscus and project to VPM (cf. neospinothalamic lemniscal fibers) (Walker, 1938; Darian-Smith *et al.*, 1963a); some project to the intralaminar thalamic nuclei, in the cat (Nauta and Kuypers, 1958) and in the monkey (Bowsher, unpublished observations) (cf. paleospinothalamic extralemniscal fibers); and there is a very heavy projection medially into the medial reticular formation (Nauta and Kuypers, 1958; Bowsher, unpublished data) (cf. spinoreticular fibers). It should be noted that spinal trigeminal tractotomy (Sjöqvist, 1938), which effectively eliminates pain of facial origin in man, cuts off primary afferents to parts of the trigeminal sensory complex which project extralemniscally.

The fact that the trigeminal sensory nuclei are, as it were, embedded in the lateral brain-stem reticular formation is of interest, because, like the latter, the sensory trigeminal nuclei(particularly the descending) receive an ascending afferent projection from the anterolateral quadrant of the spinal cord (Rossi and Brodal, 1956; Bowsher, 1957a, 1962). Both lateral reticular and descending trigeminal nuclei project to the medial reticular formation, as well as rostrally.

Thus the afferent and efferent connections of the trigeminal complex are such that it may be homologized with the corporal lemniscal systems and the extralemniscal system.

VI. The Cerebral Representation of Pain

It is not our purpose to review even the recent history of physiological thought on this subject, as this has been considered in earlier publications (Bowsher, 1957a, 1963; Bowsher and Albe-Fessard, 1962). We prefer here to take a few salient points of the problem and interpret them in the light of the hypotheses put forward in the present review; this involves slight alteration of some of our earlier views.

Pain appears to consist of two distinct components. The first is a sensation, itself divisible into two: (a) pricking pain (including pinprick, pinching, and itch), and (b) diffuse pain which is of a longer-lasting nature. The second component of pain (c) is an affective phenomenon. Central pain seems to be mainly an affective disorder, and can be dissociated from provoked peripheral pain sensation (Dejerine and Roussy, 1906; Walker, 1943).

a. Pricking pain is well localized. We have previously asserted this to be due, in the normal subject, to concomitant discriminating lemniscal activity. In view of recent findings, we would now propose that it might be also due either to (1) a purely lemniscal spinothalamic projection passing through VPL to orbitary cortex (in the cat) as suggested by Korn and Richard (1964), or (2) to extralemniscal–lemniscal convergence at subtelencephalic level, which is represented in some primary somatomotor cortices.

1. Perl and Whitlock (1961), in the monkey with only one anterolateral cord quadrant intact, found that 3.5% of VPL units which they recorded responded only to noxious peripheral stimuli.

Mountcastle and Powell (1959) found that 12 out of 593 (2%) skin-driven units in the intact monkey's S I cortex responded to noxious stimulation. It is interesting to compare these findings with the results of Penfield and Boldrey (1937), who stimulated the S I cortex in conscious human subjects, and found that 11 out of 426 (2.5%) evoked sensations were described as sharp and localized pain. This would accord also with the persistent reports in the clinical literature (see Garcin, 1937; Marshall, 1951) that discrete lesions within the limits of the sensorimotor cortex can produce analgesia.

As might be inferred from the greater degree of convergence found in the S II cortex, single unit analysis (Carreras and Andersson, 1963, in the cat) reveals a greater proportion of nocisensory cells—18 out of 473 (3.8%) skin-driven units.

2. Within VPL itself, Perl and Whitlock (1961) found 4 units in the cat and monkey which responded to noxious peripheral stimulation. In addition, they found that "units which gave evoked responses to other forms of stimuli applied to certain portions of the body surface were excited by noxious stimuli to much of the body and/or head." These authors, it is true, rejected these units because of the unusualness of the findings.

But this now seems more likely to be true in view of the findings of Mallart *et al.* (1961) that some VPL units show extralemniscal convergence. In the VPL shell (which, like VPL proper, projects to primary sensory or possibly to motor cortex) all units show heterotopic convergence, but many also show extralemniscal–lemniscal convergence; Massion *et al.* (1963) found that 27 out of 72 (37.5%) such units did so in the cat. PO may perhaps also be considered a part (though a specialized one) of the VPL shell, as it also shows these properties. Poggio and Mountcastle (1960) state that 60% of PO neurons in the cat are excited by noxious stimuli (although Perl and Whitlock, 1961, doubt this); some heterosensory (somato-auditory) convergence is also seen in this group (Hotta and Kameda, 1963). This is interesting because many observers consider that noise can cause a "pricking" as well as a "diffuse" pain.

b. Diffuse pain, poorly localized and outlasting the provoking stimulus may be considered to be due to the activation of an extralemniscal system, passing via the brain-stem reticular formation through VPL–VL to a primary cortex such as one or more of the following: S I, S II, motor cortex, and (in the cat) orbitary cortex (Korn *et al.*, 1963). The idea of gross localization within this system is tenable: Massion (1964) has shown that there is some degree of coarse somatotopy within VL in response to afferent stimulation of the tegument. In each of these cortical regions, cells responding to noxious stimuli have been observed. We must assume that under normal conditions these cortical afferent pathways are tonically inhibited at subcortical levels; spontaneous pains appear when this inhibition is removed. It can be compensated only by additional destruction of the alerting system (see below).

c. The affective component of pain, we suggest, is closely allied with diffuse painful sensation. In all cases, the onset of pain sensation is signaled by an alerting system projecting through Pf-CM to nonprimary association cortex, acting in a nonspecific manner. Albe-Fessard and Bowsher (1965) have shown that the monkey Pf-CM complex contains zones of positive and negative preference (in terms of increased or decreased amplitude of response) for particular areas of the body surface; indeed this preference is partially reflected at single unit level in the gigantocellular bulbar reticular formation (Mallart, Bowsher, and Albe-Fessard, unpublished results). Thus the difficulties formerly presented by the existence of gross localization of central pain are removed.

Extensive frontal lobotomies which successfully abolish the affective reaction to pain include the frontal association areas to which Pf-CM projects; we have some suggestive evidence that bilateral removal of this area alone has the same effect as lobotomy insofar as reaction to pain is concerned.

Our suggestion that the purely extralemniscal system passing through Pf-CM adds affective color to primary painful sensation involves the question of effective stimulus for this system. We have stressed throughout that although light somatic stimuli, effective for lemniscal activity, do not evoke activity in this extralemniscal system, effective somatic stimuli for this latter need not necessarily be noxious, but they must be brusque; and they require summation. Mallart (1962) has shown that CM units require temporal or spatial summation of afferent impulses before firing occurs. Such summation is precisely what occurs in peripheral nerves before conscious pain is felt in man (Collins *et al.*, 1960, see above); and common-carrier cells of the spinal cord respond with different spatio-temporal patterns to convergent peripheral afferent impulses, as a time factor is involved. We no longer believe that the passage from consciousness of arousal to that of pain is a quantity-dependent phenomenon within the alerting system (Bowsher, 1957; Bowsher and Albe-Fessard, 1962), but rather that it is a time-dependent process (Massion and Trouche, 1964).

The occurrence of the phenomena discussed above, in peripheral nerves and in central lemniscal and extralemniscal systems may, we believe, be the basis for determining, at conscious level, the quality of painful events.

Acknowledgments

Thanks are due the many neuroanatomists and neurophysiologists who have given of their time to discuss, both personally and by letter, the matters considered in this review; particularly to Professor A. Lundberg, who allowed us to see unpublished manuscripts, and to our colleagues in Paris who have contributed their data to this synthesis. The illustrations were kindly prepared by Mlle. A. Trinson and Mr. D. J. Kidd.

References

Aitken, J. T., and Bridger, J. E. (1961). *J. Anat. (London)* **95**, 38.
Albe-Fessard, D. (1961). *Actualités Neurol.* 3, 23.
Albe-Fessard, D., and Bowsher, D. (1965). *Electroencephalog. Clin. Neurophysiol.* **19**, 1.
Albe-Fessard, D., and Fessard, A. (1963). *Progr. Brain Res.* **1**, 115.
Albe-Fessard, D., and Kruger, L. (1962). *J. Neurophysiol.* **25**, 3.
Albe-Fessard, D., and Mallart, A. (1960). *Compt. Rend. Acad. Sci. (Paris)* **125**, 1040.
Albe-Fessard, D., and Rougeul, A. (1955). *J. Physiol. (Paris)* **47**, 69.

Albe-Fessard, D., and Rougeul, A. (1958). *Electroencephalog. Clin. Neurophysiol.* **10,** 131.

Albe-Fessard, D., Rocha-Miranda, C., and Oswaldo-Cruz, E. (1959). *Electroencephalog. Clin. Neurophysiol.* **11,** 777.

Albe-Fessard, D., Bowsher, D., and Mallart, A. (1962). *J. Physiol.* (*Paris*) **54,** 27.

Albe-Fessard, D., and Liebeskind, J. (1964). *J. Physiol.* (*Paris*) **56,** 271.

Albe-Fessard, D., Dumont-Tyć, D., and Jankowska, E. (1961). *J. Physiol.* (*Paris*) **53,** 243.

Altman, J., and Carpenter, M. B. (1961). *J. Comp. Neurol.* **116,** 157.

Amassian, V. E. (1954). *J. Neurophysiol.* **17,** 39–58.

Amassian, V. E., and De Vito, J. C. (1957). *Colloq. Intern. Centre Natl. Rech. Sci.* (*Paris*) **67,** 357.

Anderson, F. D., and Berry, C. M. (1959). *J. Comp. Neurol.* **111,** 195.

Andersson, S. A. (1962). *Acta Physiol. Scand.* Suppl. 194.

Ariëns Kappers, C. U., Huber, G. C., and Crosby, E. C. (1936). "The Comparative Anatomy of the Nervous System of Vertebrates Including Man." Macmillan, New York.

Arthur, R. P., and Shelley, W. B. (1959). *In* "Pain and Itch" G. E. W. Wolstenholme and M. O'Connor, eds.), p. 84. Churchill, London.

Beresford, W. A. (1962). *J. Hirnforsch.* **5,** 210.

Bishop, G. H. (1959). *J. Nervous Mental Disease* **128,** 89.

Bishop, G. H. (1960). *In* "Cutaneous Innervation" (W. Montagna, ed.), pp. 99. Oxford Univ. Press, London and New York.

Bowsher, D. (1957a). *Brain* **80,** 606.

Bowsher, D. (1957b). *J. Anat.* (*London*) **91,** 611.

Bowsher, D. (1958). *J. Comp. Neurol.* **110,** 135.

Bowsher, D. (1961a). *Brit. J. Anaesthesia* **33,** 174.

Bowsher, D. (1961b). *J. Comp. Neurol.* **117,** 213.

Bowsher, D. (1962). *Psychiat. Neurol.* **143,** 75.

Bowsher, D. (1963). *Toulouse Med.* **64,** 965.

Bowsher, D., and Albe-Fessard, D. (1962). *In* "The Assessment of Pain in Man and Animals" (Keele and Smith, eds.), p. 107. Livingstone for U.F.A.W., London.

Bowsher, D., Albe-Fessard, D., and Mallart, A. (1962). *J. Anat.* (*London*) **97,** 151.

Brodal, A. (1957). "The Reticular Formation of the Brain Stem." Edinburgh.

Brodal, A., and Rossi, G. F. (1955). *Arch. Neurol. Psychiat.* **74,** 68.

Brown, J. R. (1956). *J. Comp. Neurol.* **106,** 393.

Brown, J. R. (1958). *J. Comp. Neurol.* **110,** 105.

Brown, J. R. (1960). *Anat. Rec.* **136,** 171.

Brown, J. R. (1962). *J. Comp. Neurol.* **119,** 55.

Bruner, J., and Buser, P. (1960). *Compt. Rend. Soc. Biol.* **154,** 530.

Buser, P., and Borenstein, P. (1956). *J. Physiol.* (*Paris*) **48,** 419.

Buser, P., and Borenstein, P. (1959). *Electroencephalog. Clin. Neurophysiol.* **11,** 285.

Buser, P., and Imbert, M. (1961). *In* "Symposium on Sensory Communications" (Rosenblith, ed.), p. 607. Wiley, New York.

Cajal, S. R. Y. (1909). "Histologie du système nerveux de l'homme et des vertébrés." Masson, Paris.
Carman, J. B., Cowan, W. M., and Powell, T. P. S. (1963). *Brain* **86,** 525.
Carman, J. B., Cowan, W. M., and Powell, T. P. S. (1964). *J. Anat.* (*London*) **98,** 587.
Carpenter, D., Lundberg, A., and Norsell, U. (1963). *Acta Physiol. Scand.* **59,** 126.
Carreras, M., and Andersson, S. A. (1963). *J. Neurophysiol.* **26,** 100.
Cauna, N. (1959). *J. Comp. Neurol.* **113,** 169.
Cauna, N., and Mannan, G. (1961). *J. Comp. Neurol.* **117,** 309.
Chandler, R. (1964). Thesis, Liverpool.
Clarke, W. B., and Bowsher, D. (1962). *Exptl. Neurol.* **6,** 372.
Clezy, J. A. K., Dennis, B. J., and Kerr, D. I. B. (1961). *Australian J. Exptl. Biol. Med. Sci.* **39,** 19.
Collier, J., and Buzzard, E. F. (1903). *Brain* **26,** 559.
Collins, W. F., and Randt, C. T. (1958). *J. Neurophysiol.* **21,** 345.
Collins, W. F., Nulsen, F. E., and Randt, C. T. (1960). *Arch. Neurol.* **3,** 381.
Covian, M. R., Timo-Iaria, C., and Marseillan, R. F. (1961). *In* "Brain Mechanisms and Learning" (J. F. Delafresnaye, ed.), p. 433. Blackwell, Oxford.
Cowan, W. M., and Powell, T. P. S. (1955). *J. Neurol. Neurosurg. Psychiat.* **18,** 266.
Darian-Smith, I., Phillips, G., and Ryan, R. D. (1963a). *J. Physiol.* (*London*) **168,** 129.
Darian-Smith, I., Proctor, R., and Ryan, R. D. (1963b). *J. Physiol.* (*London*) **168,** 147.
Dejerine, J. (1910). "Sémiologie des affections du système nerveux." Masson, Paris.
Dejerine, J., and Roussy, G. (1906). *Rev. Neurol.* **14,** 521.
Demirjian, C., and Morin, F. (1964). *Anat. Rec.* **148,** 275.
Dennis, B. J., and Kerr, D. I. B. (1961). *Australian J. Biol. Med. Sci.* **39,** 43.
Douglas, W. W., and Ritchie, J. M. (1957). *J. Physiol.* (*London*) **139,** 383.
Douglas, W. W., and Ritchie, J. M. (1959). *In* "Pain and Itch" (C. E. W. Wolstenholme and M. O'Connor, eds.), p. 26. Churchill, London.
Drooglever-Fortuyn, J., and Stefens, R. (1951). *Electroencephalog. Clin. Neurophysiol.* **3,** 393.
Eccles, J. C., Eccles, R. M., and Lundberg, A. (1960). *J. Physiol.* (*London*) **154,** 89.
Edinger, L. (1889). *Anat. Anz.* **4,** 121.
Favale, E., Loeb, C., Rossi, G. F., and Sacco, G. (1961). *Arch. Ital. Biol.* **99,** 1.
Fessard, A. (1961). *In* "Sensory Communication" (W. A. Rosenblith, ed.), p. 585. Wiley, New York.
Foerster, O., and Gagel, O. (1932). *Z. Ges. Neurol. Psychiat.* **138,** 1.
Garcin, R. (1937). *Rev. Neurol.* **69** (*16 ème Reunion Neurol. Intern. Found.*).
Getz, B. (1952). *Acta Anat.* **16,** 271.
Gibson, W. C., Smythies, J. R., Rurkis, V. A., and Morrison, G. E. (1955). *Anat. Rec.* **123,** 239.

Glees, P., and Bailey, R. A. (1957). *Monatsschr. Psychiat. Neurol.* **122,** 129.
Glees, P., and Soler, J. (1951). *Z. Zellforsch.* **36,** 381.
Gordon, G. (1964). *Intern. Brain Res. Organ. Bull.* **3,** 71.
Gordon, G., and Jukes, M. G. M. (1963). *Nature* **196,** 1183.
Gordon, G., and Jukes, M. G. M. (1964). *J. Physiol. (London)* **173,** 263.
Gordon, G., and Paine, C. H. (1960). *J. Physiol. (London)* **153,** 331–349.
Gordon, G., and Seed, W. A. (1961). *J. Physiol. (London)* **155,** 589–601.
Gordon, G., Landgren, S., and Seed, W. A. (1961). *J. Physiol. (London)* **158,** 544.
Granit, R. (1955). "Receptors and Sensory Perception." Yale Univ. Press, New Haven, Connecticut.
Gray, E. G., and Guillery, R. W. (1961). *J. Physiol. (London)* **157,** 581.
Guillery, R. W. (1959). *J. Anat. (Paris)* **93,** 403.
Hagbarth, K. E. (1960). *Ergeb. Biol.* **22,** 47.
Hanbery, J., Ajmone-Marsan, C., and Dilworth, M. (1955). *Electroencephalog. Clin. Neurophysiol.* **6,** 109.
Hawkes, C. H. (1960). Thesis, Liverpool.
Herrick, C. J. (1948). "The Brain of the Tiger Salamander." Chicago Univ. Press, Chicago.
Hodgkin, A. L. (1964). "The Conduction of the Nervous Impulse." Liverpool Univ. Press, Liverpool.
Holmqvist, V., Lundberg, A., and Oscarsson, O. (1960). *Arch. Ital. Biol.* **98,** 60.
Hotta, T., and Kameda, K. (1963). *Exptl. Neurol.* **8,** 1.
Hunt, C. E., and McIntyre, A. K. (1960a). *J. Physiol. (London)* **153,** 74.
Hunt, C. E., and McIntyre, A. K. (1960b). *J. Physiol. (London)* **153,** 88.
Hunt, C. E., and McIntyre, A. K. (1960c). *J. Physiol. (London)* **153,** 99.
Iggo, A. (1959). *Quart. J. Exptl. Physiol.* **44,** 362.
Iggo, A. (1960). *J. Physiol. (London)* **152,** 337.
Iggo, A. (1962). *In* "The Assessment of Pain in Man and Animals" (C. A. Keele and R. Smith, eds.), p. 74. Livingstone for U.F.A.W., London.
Iggo, A. (1963a). *Acta Neuroveget.* **24,** 225.
Iggo, A. (1963b). *Proc. 1st. Intern. Symp. Olfaction and Taste,* pp. 149. Macmillan (Pergamon), New York.
Iggo, A. (1964). *IBRO Bull.* **3,** 64.
Ingvar, S. (1927). *Acta Med. Scand.* **65,** 645.
Jabbur, S. J., and Towe, A. L. (1961). *J. Neurophysiol.* **24,** 499.
Knighton, R. S. (1950). *J. Comp. Neurol.* **92,** 183.
Kohnstamm, O., and Quensel, F. (1908). *Deut. Z. Nervenheilk.* **36,** 182.
Korn, H., Wendt, R., and Albe-Fessard, D. (1963). *Compt. Rend. Acad. Sci.* **256,** 3352.
Korn, H., and Richard, P. (1964). *J. Physiol. (Paris)* **59,** 584.
Kruger, L., and Albe-Fessard, D. (1960). *Exptl. Neurol.* **2,** 442.
Kruger, L., and Michel, F. (1962a). *Exptl. Neurol.* **3,** 139.
Kruger, L., and Michel, F. (1962b). *Exptl. Neurol.* **3,** 157.
Kruger, L., Siminoff, R., and Witkovsky, P. (1961). *J. Neurophysiol.* **24,** 333.
Kuypers, H. G. J. M. (1964). *IBRO Bull.* **3,** 79.

Kuypers, H. G. J. M., Hoffman, A. L., and Beasley, R. M. (1961). *Proc. Soc. Exptl. Biol. Med.* **108,** 634.
Lamarche, G., Langlois, J. M., and Héon, M. (1960). *Can. J. Biochem. Physiol.* **38,** 1163.
Lele, P. P., and Weddell, G. (1956). *Brain* **79,** 119.
Lele, P. P., Palmer, E., and Weddell, G. (1958). *Quart. J. Microscop. Sci.* **99,** 421.
Lundberg, A. (1965). *Progr. Brain Res.* **12,** 135.
Lundberg, A., and Oscarsson, O. (1962). *Acta Physiol. Scand.* **54,** 270.
Lundberg, A., Norsell, U., and Voorhoeve, P. (1963). *Acta Physiol. Scand.* **59,** 462.
Macchi, G., Angeleri, F., and Guazzi, G. (1959). *J. Comp. Neurol.* **111,** 387.
McComas, A. (1963). *J. Physiol. (London)* **166,** 435.
McIntyre, A. K. (1962). *J. Physiol. (London)* **163,** 46.
Magnes, J., Moruzzi, G., and Pompeiano, O. (1961). *Arch. Ital. Biol.* **99,** 33.
Mallart, A. (1962). Thesis, Madrid.
Mallart, A., and Petit, D. (1963). *J. Physiol. (Paris)* **55,** 291.
Mallart, A., Martinoya, C., and Albe-Fessard, D. (1961). *J. Physiol. (Paris)* **53,** 421.
Marshall, J. (1951). *J. Neurol. Neurosurg. Psychiat.* **14,** 187.
Maruhashi, J., Mizuguchi, K., and Tasaki, I. (1952). *J. Physiol. (London)* **117,** 129.
Massion, J., Lelord, G., and Angaut, P. (1963). *J. Physiol. (Paris)* **55,** 166.
Massion, J., and Trouche, E. (1964). *J. Physiol. (Paris)* **56,** 609.
Matricali, B. (1957). *Atti. Soc. Ital. Anat.* **18,** 1.
Matzke, H. A. (1951). *J. Comp. Neurol.* **94,** 439.
Mehler, W. R. (1957). *Anat. Rec.* **127,** 332.
Mehler, W. R., Feferman, M. E., and Nauta, W. J. H. (1956). *Anat. Rec.* **124,** 332.
Mehler, W. R., Feferman, M. E., and Nauta, W. J. H. (1960). *Brain* **83,** 718.
Morin, F. (1955). *Am. J. Physiol.* **183,** 245.
Moruzzi, G. (1954). *In* "Brain Mechanisms and Consciousness" (E. D. Adrian, F. Bremer, and H. H. Jasper, eds.), p. 23. Oxford.
Moruzzi, G., and Magoun, H. W. (1949). *Electroencephalog. Clin. Neurophysiol.* **1,** 45.
Mountcastle, V. B. (1957). *J. Neurophysiol.* **20,** 408.
Mountcastle, V. B. (1961). *In* "Symposium on Sensory Communication" (W. Rosenblith, ed.). Macmillan (Pergamon), New York.
Mountcastle, V. B., and Henneman, E. (1949). *J. Neurophysiol.* **12,** 85.
Mountcastle, V. B., and Henneman, E. (1952). *J. Comp. Neurol.* **97,** 409.
Mountcastle, V. B., and Powell, T. P. S. (1959). *Bull. Johns Hopkins Hosp.* **105,** 173.
Nathan, P. W., and Smith, M. C. (1959). *Brain* **82,** 610.
Nauta, W. J. H., and Kuypers, H. G. J. M. (1958). *In* "Reticular Formation of Brain" (H. H. Jasper, ed.), pp. 3–30. Little, Brown, Boston, Massachusetts.
O'Leary, J. L., and Goldring, S. (1964). *Physiol. Rev.* **44,** 91.

Olszewski, J. (1950). *J. Comp. Neurol.* **92**, 407.

Oscarsson, O. (1958). *Arch. Ital. Biol.* **96**, 199.

Oscarsson, O., Rosén, I., and Uddenberg, N. (1964). *Arch. Ital. Biol.* **102**, 137.

Oswaldo-Cruz, E. (1961). Thesis, Rio de Janeiro, Brazil.

Oswaldo-Cruz, E., and Kidd, C. (1964). *J. Neurophysiol.* **27**, 1.

Padel, Y., and Dell, P. (1964). *J. Physiol. (Paris)* **56**, 415.

Penfield, W., and Boldrey, E. B. (1937). *Brain* **60**, 389.

Perl, E. R., and Whitlock, D. G. (1961). *Exptl. Neurol.* **3**, 256.

Perl, E. R., Whitlock, D. G., and Gentry, J. R. (1962). *J. Neurophysiol.* **25**, 337.

Poggio, G. F., and Mountcastle, V. B. (1960). *Bull. Johns Hopkins Hosp.* **106**, 266.

Poggio, G. F., and Mountcastle, V. B. (1963). *J. Neurophysiol.* **26**, 775.

Pompeiano, O., and Swett, J. E. (1962). *Arch. Ital. Biol.* **100**, 343.

Powell, T. P. S., and Erulkar, S. D. (1962). *J. Anat. (London)* **96**, 249.

Powell, T. P. S., and Mountcastle, V. B. (1959). *Bull. Johns Hopkins Hosp.* **105**, 108.

Quensel, F. (1898). *Neurol. Zentr.* **17**, 482.

Ranson, S. W. (1912). *J. Comp. Neurol.* **22**, 159.

Rexed, B. (1952). *J. Comp. Neurol.* **96**, 415.

Rose, J. E. (1952). *Res. Publ. Assoc. Res. Nervous Mental Disease* **30**, 454.

Rose, J. E., and Woolsey, C. N. (1958). *In* "Biological and Biochemical Bases of Behaviour" (H. F. Barlow and C. N. Woolsey, eds.), p. 127. Univ. Wisconsin Press, Madison, Wisconsin.

Rossi, G. F., and Brodal, A. (1956). *Confinia Neurol.* **16**, 321.

Rossi, G. F., and Brodal, A. (1957). *A.M.A. Arch. Neurol. Psychiat.* **78**, 439.

Rossi, G. F., and Zanchetti, A. (1957). *Arch. Ital. Biol.* **95**, 199.

Russell, J. R., and DeMeyer, W. (1961). *Neurology* **11**, 96.

Sjöqvist, O. (1938). *Acta Psychiat. Neurol. Scand.* Suppl. 17, 1.

Spivy, D. F., and Metcalf, J. S. (1959). *J. Neurophysiol.* **22**, 237–273.

Starzl, T. E., Taylor, C. W., and Magoun, H. W. (1951). *J. Neurophysiol.* **14**, 461.

Sukhetzkaya, M. P. (1957). *Arch. Anat. Gistol. Embryol. (U. S. S. R.)* **34**, 30.

Szentagothai, J. (1964). *J. Comp. Neurol.* **122**, 219.

Thompson, R. F., Johnson, R. H., and Hoopes, J. (1963). *J. Neurophysiol.* **26**, 343.

Torvik, A. (1956). *J. Comp. Neurol.* **106**, 51.

Torvik, A. (1957). *Am. J. Anat.* **100**, 1.

Towe, A. L., and Jabbur, S. J. (1961). *J. Neurophysiol.* **26**, 488.

Valverde, F. (1961a). *J. Comp. Neurol.* **116**, 71.

Valverde, F. (1961b). *J. Comp. Neurol.* **117**, 189.

Van Crevel, H. (1958). Thesis, Leiden.

Verhaart, W. J. C., and Sie, P. G. (1957). *Folia Psychiat. Neurol. Neurochirurg. Neerl.* **60**, 159.

Walberg, F. (1957). *Brain* **80**, 273.

Walker, A. E. (1938). "The Primate Thalamus." Chicago Univ. Press, Chicago.

Walker, A. E. (1943). *Res. Publ. Assoc. Res. Nervous Mental Disease* **23**, 63.

Wall, P. D. (1960). *J. Neurophysiol.* **23**, 197.
Wall, P. D. (1961). *In* "Symposium on Sensory Communication" (Rosenblith, ed.), p. 475. Wiley, New York.
Wall, P. D. (1962). *J. Physiol.* **164**, 508.
Wall, P. D. (1964). *IBRO Bull.* 3, 70.
Wall, P. D., and Cronly-Dillon, J. (1960). *Arch. Neurol.* **2**, 365.
Wall, P. D., and Taub, A. (1962). *J. Neurophysiol.* **25**, 110.
Webster, K. E. (1961). *J. Anat.* (*London*) **95**, 532.
Weddell, G., Pallie, W., and Palmer, E. (1954). *Quart. J. Microscop. Sci.* **95**, 483.
White, J. C., and Sweet, W. H. (1955). "Pain; Its Mechanisms and Neurosurgical Control." Thomas, Springfield, Illinois.
Whitlock, D. G., and Perl, E. R. (1959). *J. Neurophysiol.* **22**, 133.
Whitlock, D. G., and Perl, E. R. (1961). *Exptl. Neurol.* 3, 240.
Zotterman, Y. (1939). *J. Physiol.* (*London*) **95**, 1.

DRUG ACTION ON THE ELECTRICAL ACTIVITY OF THE HIPPOCAMPUS

By Ch. Stumpf

Department of Pharmacology, Emory University, Atlanta, Georgia, and
Institute of Pharmacology, University of Vienna, Austria

I. Introduction

The purpose of this article is to give a short review on the action of drugs on the electrical activity of the hippocampus, excluding the actions of drugs on evoked potentials and evoked seizure discharges. Such a review should probably start with the anatomy, histology, and physiology of the hippocampus, and then proceed to its spontaneous electrical activity and the drug-induced modifications of this activity. However, numerous excellent reviews on the anatomy, histology, and physiology of the hippocampus have been published in the past and it is felt that a new discussion of these topics in this review would at its best be a mere repetition. Instead, the interested reader is referred to the papers by Cajal (1909, 1955) and Lorente de Nó (1934) which may be considered the classical descriptions of anatomy and histology of the rhinencephalon, as well as to the more recently published reviews by Brodal (1947), Droogleever-Fortuyn (1956), Green (1960), MacLean (1954, 1955), Thomalske *et al.* (1957), and others. In fact, the very first paper published in this series was a review dealing with recent studies of the rhinencephalon (Adey, 1959). This review will deal primarily with drug-induced changes of the hippocampus activity, but it will start with a short section on the spontaneous electrical activity of the hippocampus since a knowledge of the normal activity is essential for understanding its drug-induced changes.

The hippocampus has been studied by various investigators for quite different reasons, but there is general agreement on the fact that one of the main advantages of the hippocampus as a tool in neurophysiological and neuropharmacological investigations is the simple and relatively uncomplicated structure of this part of the cortex. Few other brain areas have such a simple structure, one of the exceptions being the prepyriform cortex which is composed of a single sheet of cells (cf. Freeman, 1963). It may be added that probably the simple and well-organized structure of the hippocampus is responsible for its simple pattern of electrical activity, the so-called theta rhythm which appears in the hippocampus under certain experimental conditions. Renshaw *et al.* (1940) are frequently quoted for their statement that the hippocampus is a most suitable area for evoked potential studies. Obviously, it can be argued that for similar reasons the hippocampus might be an ideal model for neuropharmacological investigations.

II. Electrical Activity of the Hippocampus

Under conditions of rest the hippocampus shows a rather inconspicuous EEG pattern consisting of a mixture of slow and fast activities. Under the influence of sensory stimuli both components undergo a drastic change. The resting activity is replaced by a rather regular, sine-wave-like activity for which the term "theta rhythm" will be used here in accordance with Green and Arduini (1954). At the same time there is also a change in the appearance of the fast activity.

A. Slow Activity (Theta Rhythm)

Jung and Kornmüller (1938) first observed the appearance of regular slow waves (4–7 per second) in the rabbit's hippocampus following sensory stimuli. At that time the electrophysiological significance of the ascending reticular system was not yet known. Then, in 1949, Moruzzi and Magoun made the discovery that sensory stimuli cause an excitation of the ascending reticular system thereby producing generalized changes of the EEG which have been termed arousal reaction. Electrical stimulation of this system has the same effect on the cortical activity. In 1954, Green and Arduini published the results of an extensive investigation of the hippocampal electrical activity under various experimental conditions and concluded that the theta rhythm can be regarded as the expression of the arousal reaction in the hippocampus. It can be elicited, in accordance with Jung and Kornmüller (1938), by sensory stimuli as well as by reticular stimulation. The theta rhythm is one of the most regular brain rhythms and, although its shape approaches that of a sine wave to a remarkable degree, significant deviations from a true sinusoid must not be overlooked (Green and Petsche, 1961).

As Green and Arduini (1954) point out, there is some variation in the appearance of the theta rhythm in different species of animals such that, for instance, the theta rhythm is pronounced in the rabbit, almost not detectable in the monkey, and is intermediate in the cat. Undoubtedly, the rabbit with a large and readily accessible hippocampus is an ideal animal for investigations of the hippocampal activity and in this species the occurrence of a regular rhythm during an arousal reaction has been described frequently (Gangloff and Monnier, 1956; Longo, 1956; Longo *et al.*, 1954; Rinaldi and Himwich, 1955d; Sailer and Stumpf, 1957b; and others). However, in other species, as, for instance, in rats (Weiss and Fifková, 1960), guinea pigs (Liberson and Akert, 1953), and cats (Passouant *et al.*, 1955a,b) a regular slow wave activity has also been recorded in the alerted animal.

In clinical electroencephalography the term "theta rhythm" is used to designate a rhythm with a frequency between 4 and 7 per second. In general, the frequency of the hippocampal arousal activity lies, at least in the rabbit, somewhere within these limits. However, under certain experimental conditions or in some species (see below) the frequency of the hippocampal theta rhythm may be lower than 4 per second or higher than 7 per second. Nevertheless, for simplicity, the term "theta rhythm" is used in this article to denote the slow activity which is characteristic of hippocampal arousal reactions, and independent of its frequency.

1. *Properties of the Theta Rhythm*

There is general agreement that in the rabbit the usual frequency of the theta rhythm is 4–7 per second. Some authors (Adey, 1962; Grastyán *et al.*, 1959) found similar frequencies in the cat, whereas others (Bradley and Nicholson, 1962; Tokizane *et al.*, 1959) reported much lower values in this species. When a hippocampal theta rhythm is elicited by arousal stimulus, its frequency gradually decreases while the stimulus is being applied. Thus, the frequency is always highest at the moment of the onset of the stimulus, and this frequency will be called hereafter the "initial frequency" (Sailer and Stumpf, 1957b). The initial frequency depends on the parameters of the stimulation. When the theta rhythm is elicited by reticular stimulation, pulse duration and frequency of this stimulation determine the value of the initial frequency (Mayer and Stumpf, 1958a). In addition, there is a significant linear positive correlation between the logarithm of stimulus voltage and the initial frequency in such a way that a voltage increase of log $V = 0.1$ produces an increase of the initial frequency in steps of 0.81 to 0.99 per second. The regression coefficients of this relationship show only a negligible variation between animals. Strong reticular stimulation may produce a hippocampal theta rhythm with an initial frequency of up to 11 per second. Thus, the frequency of the hippocampal theta rhythm can be regarded as a sensitive index of the degree of reticular excitation. High frequencies indicate a strong excitation of the reticular formation (Sailer and Stumpf, 1957b). An increase of frequency of the theta rhythm due to an increase of intensity of an arousal stimulus has also been mentioned by Tokizane *et al.* (1959) and by Yokota and Fujimori (1964).

It can be shown that the theta rhythm arises in the hippocampus and evidence for this fact will be presented later. This does not mean, however, that the theta rhythm can be recorded from the hippocampus only. Actually, the occurrence of a typical theta rhythm in areas other than the hippocampus, especially in the thalamus and/or parietal cortex, has been described by several authors (Gangloff and Monnier, 1956; Longo, 1956; Longo *et al.*, 1954; Rinaldi and Himwich, 1955d; and others), and for this reason the theta rhythm has sometimes been called "thalamic rhythm." When a monopolar recording technique is employed, the theta rhythm can be recorded from large areas of the rabbit's brain. By means of this technique the potential field of the theta rhythm has been constructed and it has been shown that, although the theta rhythm is present in large areas, its amplitude is largest in the hippocampus. Moreover, a monopolar phase reversal between the theta rhythm recorded from the hippocampus and the one recorded from the overlying neocortex has been found to exist (Petsche and Stumpf, 1960). A zone with no activity at all ("null zone") which may be found only by semimicroelectrode recording, is very narrow and situated at a plane just below the pyramidal cell layer of the hippocampus. The theta waves recorded from above and below the null zone are mirror images, their amplitudes, however, reach different maximal values such that the amplitude in the stratum radiatum is about twice as big as in the stratum oriens (Green *et al.*, 1960). This seems to be a general characteristic of waves that are recorded from the neighborhood of a cell layer forming a curved surface since in such a case the current densities in the concavity can be expected to be higher than in the convexity (Freeman, 1963; Gloor *et al.*, 1963a). The existence of the null zone indicates that the theta rhythm is not propagated in a vertical direction. Moreover, the potential field of the theta rhythm with its null zone proves that this rhythm arises in the hippocampus itself, and it has been concluded that the virtual generator of the theta rhythm lies between the upper surface of the pyramidal cell bodies and the distal regions of their apical dendrites (Green *et al.*, 1960).

The theta rhythm shows the feature of traveling waves. By means of a toposcopical investigation (Petsche and Stumpf, 1960) it has been demonstrated that the theta rhythm shows a spherical propagation with the septum as the center. From there the waves seem to travel through diencephalon and hippocampus as through a homogeneous medium. The velocity of this propagation depends on the theta frequency, increasing with increasing frequency. The average velocity is somewhere near 30 to 40 cm/second. So far no explanation has been offered for this type of slow propagation. At any rate, in the terminology used by Freeman (1963), the theta rhythm may be classified as an ac field which is standing along an axis normal to the hippocampus but moving along its surface. As Freeman (1963) states, a standing ac field is characteristic for several types of simple cortex. In a similar study, but using cross correlation techniques, Adey *et al.* (1960) have shown that the slow waves in the areas CA2 and CA4 of the dorsal hippocampus lead the entorhinal activity by 20 to 35 msec indicating a passage of activity from the hippocampus to the entorhinal area. In the course of approach learning, the direction of this passage was shown by them to be reversed. Thus, in the untrained animal the phase relationships would be consistent with the direction and velocity of spread found by Petsche and Stumpf (1960).

Several studies have been concerned with the action potentials of hippocampal pyramidal neurons. Unit action potentials have been found to occur more or less exclusively in the stratum pyramidale (von Euler and Green, 1960a; Gloor *et al.*, 1963b; Green *et al.*, 1960). Pyramidal neurons show a strong tendency for repetitive firing, especially during a theta rhythm (Green and Machne, 1955; Kandel and Spencer, 1961) and in this case the bursts are frequently but not necessarily correlated to a certain phase of the slow waves (Arduini and Pompeiano, 1955; Green and Machne, 1955; Green and Petsche, 1961; Green *et al.*, 1960). The significance of this correlation will be dealt with in the next section.

2. *Origin of the Theta Rhythm*

Whenever a rhythmic bioelectrical activity is observed, one of the fundamental questions is whether it originates in the area under investigation or in a remote part of the brain. For many years the origin of induced and spontaneous rhythmic activities of the neocortex (especially spontaneous alpha rhythm and spindle bursts) has been discussed (see Bremer, 1958). The question has been asked: "Does the spontaneous activity of the brain originate in the thalamus or in the cortex, or is it a function of their interaction (for instance, via reverberation over closed circuits between them)?" (Bishop, 1949). Obviously, this question could be restated as follows: "Does the theta rhythm originate in the hippocampus or in a subcortical area (for instance, septum), or is it a function of their interaction?" Any hypothesis concerning the origin of neocortical rhythms may be applied in an analogous way to the origin of the hippocampal theta rhythm. It is clear, however, that a hypothesis proven to be applicable to the origin of a neocortical rhythm does not necessarily need to be true for the hippocampal slow waves. Three main concepts concerning the theta rhythm have been developed so far, one by von Euler and Green (1960b), another one by Spencer and Kandel (1962), and a third one by Eccles (1964). Although all these hypotheses are concerned primarily with the nature of the theta rhythm, they have of necessity to make certain assumptions about its origin.

According to von Euler and Green (1960b), the correlation between burst activity of hippocampal neurons and theta rhythm can be explained as follows: The process leading to the generation of bursts starts with a wave of depolarization. During the initial phase of depolarization there is an increased excitability which leads to a series of declining spikes. A further increase of depolarization produces a cathodal depression of the action potentials. Granit and Phillips (1956) had described a similar process in single cerebellar Purkinje cells and called it "inactivation process." In analogy to this event, von Euler and Green (1960b) adopted the same name for the cathodal depression of action potentials in single pyramidal neurons. In such neurons the depolarization is followed by a hyperpolarization. Thus, two kinds of inhibition follow each other. The conclusion drawn by von Euler and Green (1960b) is "that the theta rhythm is due to synchronously occurring 'inactivation processes' in many neurons," and is "generated in the hippocampal formation under the pressure of afferent impulses from the septum and precommissural fornix." Many common features were found to exist between the theta rhythm and inactivation processes. As to the nature of the inactivation processes, Green *et al.* (1961) suggested that these slow potentials are generated by summed postsynaptic potentials.

The tendency of hippocampal pyramidal neurons to fire in bursts and the correlation of these bursts to the theta rhythm was explained by Kandel and Spencer (1961) in a somewhat different way. These authors studied the action potentials of pyramidal neurons by intracellular recording. They found that the action potential is followed by a depolarizing afterpotential (DAP) of a larger magnitude than that described for any other central neuron. In this respect, hippocampal neurons differ in their behavior from motoneurons, the spike potential of which is followed by a brief afterhyperpolarization (Eccles *et al.*, 1957). According to Kandel and Spencer (1961) the excitatory state underlying repetitive firing in the hippocampus pyramidal cell is at least partly maintained by an endogenous process—the DAP that is intrinsic to neuronal membrane. Thus, the cathodal depression occurring when pyramidal neurons fire in bursts is not thought to consist primarily of postsynaptic potentials but rather of an additive depolarization of DAP's, although synaptic potentials can trigger bursts as well. The burst has self-sustaining and self-limiting properties, and it can be shown that the membrane potential repolarizes even in the presence of a long depolarizing pulse. Spencer and Kandel (1962) state that hippocampal neurons possess two properties favorable for the development of a 3 to 7 per second rhythm, namely: first, the time necessary for recovery of spike parameters after a single spike or after a burst is 100–300 msec; second, as found by these authors, hippocampus pyramidal cells possess inhibitory recurrent axon collaterals that produce an inhibition of adjacent neurons for periods up to 200–300 msec. Both these properties would favor the development of a theta rhythm.

Evidence for a recurrent inhibitory pathway with the basket cell as the inhibitory neuron has been presented by Andersen *et al.* (1963), and it has been suggested that this inhibitory mechanism may be responsible for the hippocampal theta rhythm (Eccles, 1964).

All these hypotheses assume the existence of impulses impinging on the hippocampus and thereby producing a theta rhythm. Obviously, Spencer and Kandel (1962) had to assume only "the existence of some uniform and sustained driving force in the form of excitatory synaptic bombardment," whereas for the hypothesis of von Euler and Green (1960b) the arrival of excitatory impulses in a sequence corresponding to the frequency of the theta rhythm would have to be assumed. Recently, a true pacemaker for the theta rhythm has been found to exist in the medial septal nucleus (Petsche *et al.*, 1962). The existence of such a pacemaker supports the hypothesis of von Euler and Green (1960b), but does not contradict the concepts of Spencer and Kandel (1962) or Eccles (1964). Before the properties of this pacemaker can be described, the main inputs of the hippocampus should be discussed.

3. *Significance of the Septum*

Two main fiber systems provide pathways for afferent influxes into the hippocampus: (1) septohippocampal connections, as first described by Ellioth Smith (1910), and later suggested to form a definite pathway (Green and Adey, 1956); (2) entorhinal-hippocampal connections arising as temporoammonic tracts in the entorhinal area and continuing as alvear and perforant path to the hippocampus (Cajal, 1909; Lorente de Nó, 1934). It should be understood that both these systems can also pass impulses in the opposite, i.e., hippocampofugal direction (for a full account on this subject, see Adey, 1959). However, for the production of a theta rhythm, only impulse transmission in the indicated, hippocampopetal direction will be considered. Kandel *et al.* (1961) studied both of these hippocampal inputs and found that the perforant path is the more powerful excitatory input when compared with the forniceal afferents, but they stress that the driving force for the theta rhythm may well come from the septum via the forniceal afferents (Spencer and Kandel, 1962).

Obviously, the theta rhythm is induced in the hippocampus via septohippocampal connections since interruption of septal transmission by lesions (Green and Arduini, 1954) or procaine (Brücke *et al.*, 1959a) abolish the theta rhythm (Fig. 1). Entorhinal ablation had been reported to have a similar effect (Carreras *et al.*, 1955) but, as Adey (1959) points out, this was possibly due to the acute conditions of these experiments. A reinvestigation of the effects of an entorhinal ablation showed no disappearance of the hippocampal slow waves following a click (Adey *et al.*, 1956). Under certain experimental conditions (i.e., in trained animals in the course of approach learning) primary activation of the hippocampus was reported to be initiated from the entorhinal area (Adey *et al.*, 1960). Under normal conditions, however, the septum and hippocampus should be regarded as one entity as far as the theta rhythm is concerned, and it may be concluded that the septum forms an important relay station between the reticular formation and the hippocampus.

The septum is a rather complex structure consisting of many nuclei with probably different functions (see Andy and Stephan, 1961). It is true that a septal lesion abolishes the theta rhythm but it is not necessary to destroy the whole septum or even large parts of it to accomplish this. Instead, only a small area has to be destroyed for this purpose, and this area is situated in the most median part in the center of the septum. A median lesion in this area abolishes the theta rhythm in both hippocampi, whereas with a paramedian lesion the theta rhythm is abolished in the homolateral hippocampus only (Mayer and Stumpf, 1958b). High-frequency electrical stimulation of this area also abolishes the theta rhythm (Brücke *et al.*, 1959b). Thus, all available data indicate that in a small median septal area there must be neurons that send their axons toward the hippocampus and that must pass impulses responsible for the theta rhythm. Therefore, Petsche *et al.* (1962) investigated this area with microelectrodes. In a small area in the median

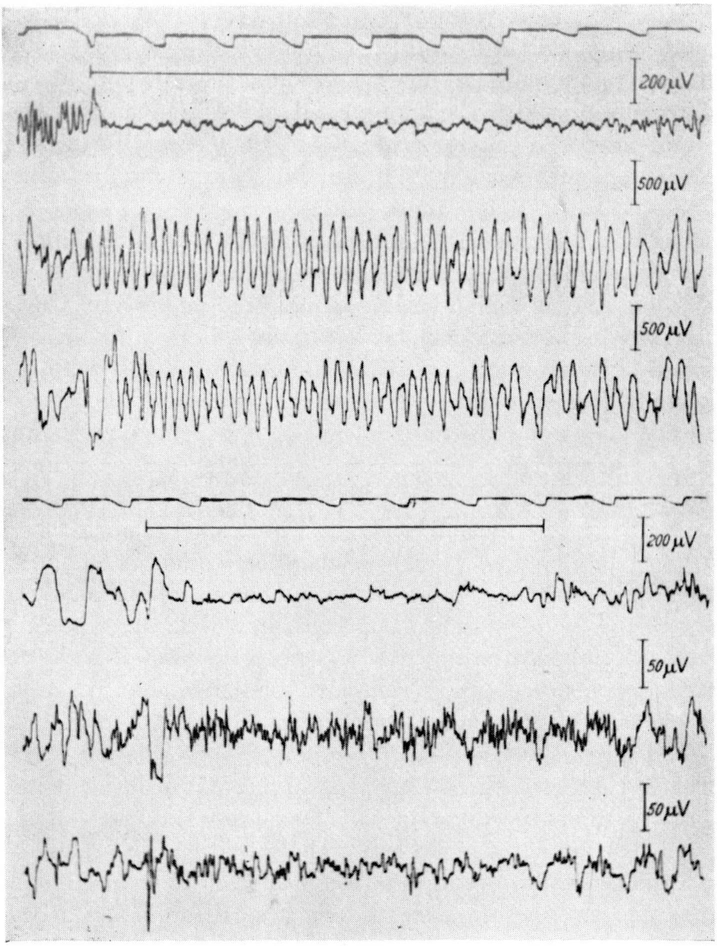

FIG. 1. Neocortical and hippocampal arousal reaction of a rabbit elicited by proprioceptive stimulations (horizontal bars), before (upper part) and after a septal lesion (lower part). EEG recorded from frontal cortex (upper traces), and left and right hippocampus (middle and lower traces). Time markings: 1 second. Note difference in calibration for hippocampus recordings before and after septal lesion. Taken from Mayer and Stumpf (1958b).

part of the septum a group of units was found which show quite a characteristic discharge pattern. When there is a theta rhythm in the hippocampus, these units discharge in bursts and these bursts always occur during a certain phase of the theta waves (Fig. 2). Usually, the phase correlation of the repetitive discharges of these

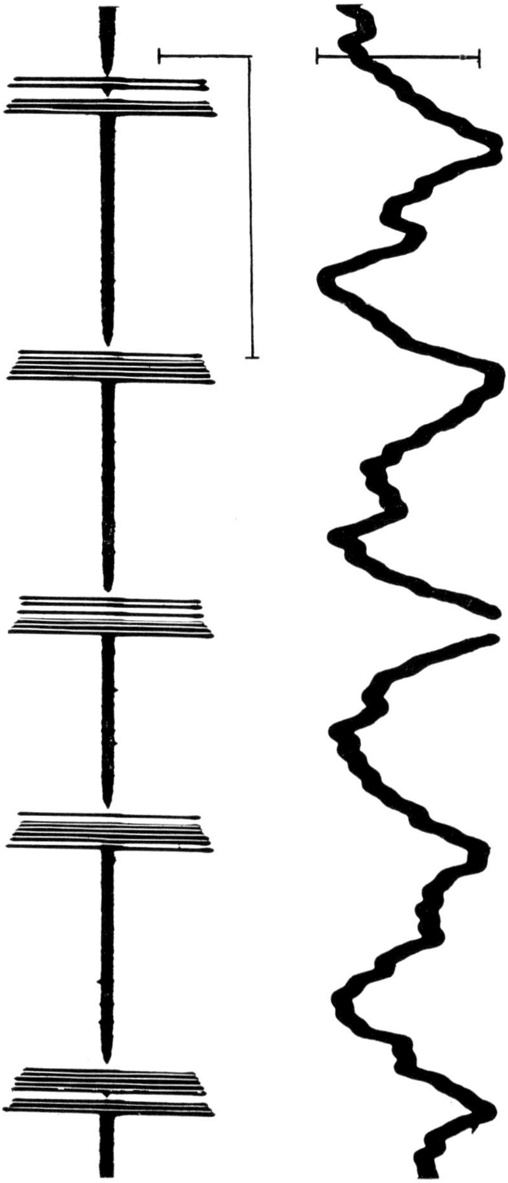

FIG. 2. Action potentials of a single neuron of the medial septal nucleus recorded with an extracellular microelectrode (upper trace), and hippocampal activity recorded with gross electrodes (lower trace) during a theta rhythm elicited by sensory stimulation. Positivity of action potentials down. Voltage calibrations: 1 mv (upper trace) and 0.5 mv (lower trace); time calibration: 250 msec.

cells with respect to the theta rhythm remains constant for long periods of time; in some cases, the discharge pattern of a single neuron was observed for up to 2 hours, and no change of phase correlation occurred. Under certain experimental conditions, the phase correlation may change but this is a rare event. On the other hand, each individual septal neuron may continuously discharge during any phase of the theta wave. When there is no theta rhythm in the hippocampus, the septal neurons discharge irregularly and apparently at random. The neurons firing in a manner just described, are located in the median part of the septum forming a nucleus which was previously described anatomically by various authors under different names: nucleus medialis septi (Cajal, 1909), nucleus parolfactorius (Edinger, 1904), nucleus of the diagonal band (Johnston, 1923; Young, 1936), and pars posterior septi medialis (Loo, 1931).

It is well known that connections between the septum and the hippocampus conduct in both directions. Anatomical evidence for septohippocampal fibers has been presented by many authors, including Ariëns Kappers *et al.* (1936), Bard and Rioch (1937), Cragg (1961), Daitz and Powell (1954), Gerebtzoff (1939, 1941–1942), Mettler (1943), and Morin (1950), although so far there is no agreement on the precise course of these fibers. During the last 10 years several electrophysiological investigations have been carried out which also suggest the existence of septohippocampal projections (Adey *et al.*, 1957; Andersen *et al.*, 1961; Brücke *et al.*, 1959b; von Euler *et al.*, 1958; Green and Adey, 1956; Green and Arduini, 1954). It is true that some of these authors recorded evoked potentials in the hippocampus as a response to stimulation of the dorsal fornix rather than the septum. However, as Andersen *et al.* (1961) point out, it is likely that in these cases the medial septal nuclei were actually stimulated. Green and Adey (1956) suggested a pathway passing through the fimbria to the cells of the dentate gyrus; the axons of the granule cells would relay impulses to the hippocampus pyramidal cells. Further evidence for impulse conduction along this pathway has been presented by von Euler *et al.* (1958). On the other hand, Gloor *et al.* (1963a) rejected this pathway on the grounds that they could not find excitation of granule cells after fimbrial stimulation. Andersen *et al.* (1961) as well as Brücke *et al.* (1963) were able to record clear-cut responses to septal stimulation in the area CA1 of the hippocampus.

However, as Andersen *et al.* (1961) remark, the axons of the dentate granule cells, the mossy fibers, do not reach the areas CA1 and CA2. Therefore, the possibility remains that in addition to the pathway suggested by Green and Adey (1956) there are still other septohippocampal projections. Cragg and Hamlyn (1957, 1959) described ascending fibers in the dorsal fornix, presumably from the septum, which terminate in the subiculum and presubiculum, and Andersen *et al.* (1961) present evidence for a true septohippocampal pathway terminating in the stratum pyramidale and the adjacent part of apical dendrites of area CA1. This site of termination agrees with the findings of von Euler *et al.* (1958).

Summarizing it may be said that whereas all available data indicate the existence of a reticulohippocampal pathway which has the medial septal nucleus as an important relay station, the exact course of the septohippocampal fibers has not yet been determined. Furthermore, since destruction of the mid-line thalamic nuclei also abolishes the theta rhythm (Eidelberg *et al.*, 1959), an ascending reticulohippocampal pathway relaying through these nuclei and projecting from there to the hippocampus (Rose and Woolsey, 1948) has also been assumed. On the other hand, Corazza and Parmeggiani (1963) found no modification of the theta rhythm after coagulation of the thalamic nuclei. According to these authors, the appearance of theta rhythm depends on the integrity of medial hypothalamic structures, indicating "that the afferent system eliciting the hippocampal theta rhythm upon ischiatic stimulation becomes clearly localized only from the hypothalamus and upwards."

B. Fast Activity

Within the last few years data have accumulated which indicate that during rest as well as during an arousal reaction low-voltage activity with frequencies of more than 10 per second occur in the hippocampus EEG of the rabbit (Eidelberg *et al.*, 1959; Gangloff and Monnier, 1956) and cat (Bradley and Nicholson, 1962; Passouant *et al.*, 1956a, 1957; Tokizane *et al.*, 1959). During an arousal reaction this activity appears to be accelerated and superimposed on the theta waves. However, different frequencies have been reported to occur during an arousal reaction: 12–16 per second (Passouant *et al.*, 1956a), 20–25 per second (Tokizane *et al.*, 1959), and 30–40 per second (Bradley and Nicholson, 1962), respectively.

In all the cases mentioned above, the simultaneous occurrence of slow and fast activities has been described. Under certain experimental conditions, however, a low-voltage fast activity appears in the hippocampus EEG as the sole manifestation of an arousal reaction. In these cases the hippocampal arousal reaction is similar to the neocortical arousal reaction to which the term "desynchronization" has been applied. It has been found to occur in response to an arousal stimulus under the following conditions:

(a) According to Grastyán *et al.* (1959), the hippocampal activity of the cat during a novel, unconditioned stimulus is characterized by a desynchronization. The theta rhythm is regarded as the reaction of the hippocampus during an "orienting reaction" in the course of conditioning. Under comparable conditions, Adey *et al.* (1960) found only rarely that short periods of desynchronization preceded the theta rhythm.

(b) In very young cats (Cadilhac and Passouant-Fontaine, 1962) and rabbits (Gogolák *et al.*, 1963), the hippocampal arousal reaction is characterized by a fast, low-voltage activity. The theta rhythm as expression of the hippocampal arousal reaction does not appear until the animals grow older. At a certain age the hippocampus responds to some stimuli with a desynchronization, to other with a theta rhythm (Gogolák *et al.*, 1963).

(c) It has been mentioned previously that septal lesions abolish the theta rhythm (Green and Arduini, 1954). This does not mean, however, that reticular stimulation is ineffective in such animals. Instead, it induces a low-voltage, fast activity in the hippocampus in animals with septal lesions (Mayer and Stumpf, 1958b).

(d) In rats in light barbiturate anesthesia, external stimuli were found to produce a "desynchronization not only in the cortex but also in the hippocampus" (see Section III,A,2,*b*) and rarely the same phenomenon was found to occur in the unanesthetized, curarized rat (Weiss and Fifková, 1960).

(e) In rabbits, reticular stimulations with intensities that exceed a certain value also produce a low-voltage fast activity in the hippocampus (Stumpf, 1965).

In addition to the above effects produced by an arousal stimulus, stimulation of other brain areas has been reported to elicit a desynchronization of hippocampal activity (Brücke *et al.*, 1959b; Torii, 1961; Yokota and Fujimori, 1964).

Thus, there seem to exist at least two patterns of hippocampal responses, theta rhythm with fast activity superimposed on it and desynchronization, as suggested by Torii (1961). Recently, however, Yokota and Fujimori (1964) described four types of hippocampal electrical activity in response to subcortical stimulation: (1) synchronization (i.e., theta rhythm); (2) desynchronization A (i.e., increase in amplitude of fast waves with disappearance of slow waves); (3) desynchronization B (i.e., desynchronization without increase in amplitude of fast waves); and (4) "intermediate response" (i.e., synchronization in response to weak stimulation and desynchronization in response to stronger stimulation). Pattern (1) was found to occur during stimulation of the medial preoptic area, the medial hypothalamic region, and the dorsolateral part of the midbrain tegmentum, pattern (2) during the stimulation of the amygdala and the lateral preoptic area, pattern (3) during stimulation of the bulbar ventromedial reticular formation, and pattern (4) during stimulation of the posterolateral hypothalamic region and the preoptic area. In a recent investigation, the reviewer (Stumpf, 1965) could partly confirm and extend the results reported by these authors. It turned out that any type of hippocampal slow wave pattern (irregular, regularized, or depressed) may or may not be associated with regular fast activity. For instance, reticular stimulations with increasing voltage evoke theta rhythm without regular fast activity, theta rhythm with such a fast activity superimposed on it, and fast activity associated with depression of slow waves (desynchronization); septal stimulation produces depression of slow waves, as originally described by Brücke *et al.* (1959b), with or without fast activity, depending on stimulus voltage. Evidence has been presented that the several different types of hippocampal activity can be explained by assuming the existence of three mechanisms which are able to modify the electrical activity of the hippocampus—one mechanism would produce the theta rhythm, another one would depress the slow waves, and a third one would elicit a regular fast activity. In rabbits with septal lesions, reticular stimulation elicits a regular fast activity as in normal animals, but without theta rhythm. Therefore, it can be concluded that two different reticulohippocampal pathways are responsible for the mediation of theta rhythm and regular fast activity. It has been demonstrated by various authors (von Euler and Green, 1960b; Gloor *et al.*, 1963b; Kandel *et al.*, 1961) that hippocampal pyramidal neurons respond to stimulation of forniceal afferents as well as to stimulation of the perforant path. Moreover, von Euler (1960) stated "that the afferent system from the septum and the perforant path make synaptic contact mainly with different hippocampal neurons." Perhaps, the afferent influx from the entorhinal area is responsible for the mediation of the fast component of hippocampal activity. At the moment, this is a mere speculation and further experimentation is necessary to prove the correctness of this assumption.

III. Pharmacological Studies

Any classification of drugs may be open to criticism. The grouping of drugs adopted here should not be regarded as a rigid classification implying grouping according to common modes of action, but rather as a convenient arrangement which allows the placing of drugs with similar actions on the electrical activity of the hippocampus together. Drugs may produce or inhibit the theta rhythm, they may induce seizures or seizure-like discharges, or they may influence the electrical activity of the hippocampus in other ways. Even with this rather simple classification, overlapping cannot be avoided. For instance, several drugs produce or inhibit the theta rhythm while inducing seizures or seizure-like discharges in the hippocampus, some produce theta effects at one dose and seizures at another.

It is not intended to give here a detailed description of the action of all, or even nearly all drugs known to influence the electrical activity of the hippocampus. There are, however, some specific problems involved relating to drug action on hippocampal activity which will be discussed in the following sections.

A. Drugs That Produce or Inhibit the Theta Rhythm

It has been mentioned before that the theta rhythm has to be regarded as one form of the hippocampal arousal reaction. A great number of drugs are known to influence the EEG arousal reaction in some way, although far more investigations have been carried out on the neocortical arousal reaction than on the hippocampal theta rhythm. Generally, it may be assumed that a drug that induces or inhibits the neocortical desynchronization, will also induce or inhibit the hippocampal theta rhythm. However, this "rule" has several exceptions which will be mentioned later.

It should be clear that a statement such as "a drug inhibits the neocortical arousal reaction caused by reticular stimulation" does not mean very much. Recently, Domino (1962) pointed out that in such a case it is generally assumed that this effect is due to an inhibitory action on the reticular formation itself but that this is not necessarily true. Such an effect may also be caused by an action of the drug on the neocortex or on reticulocortical pathways, and there are several other possibilities which could explain such an inhibition of an arousal reaction. Obviously, the same arguments can be used when it is observed that a drug induces EEG changes similar to those of an arousal reaction. Finally, similar arguments will have to be dealt with when experiments on drug action on the hippocampal theta rhythm are considered. It should be pointed out here that in the case of drug action on the hippocampal theta rhythm one is dealing with a much less complex situation than in the case of drug action on the neocortical arousal reaction. Reticulo-hippocampal pathways can be interrupted by very small lesions (e.g., in the septum) rendering studies on the site of drug action relatively simple. This is not true, however, for pathways from the reticular formation to the neocortex which can only be interrupted by rather large lesions.

1. *Drugs That Produce a Theta Rhythm*

Many drugs are known to produce generalized EEG changes which are characteristic for an arousal reaction, i.e., desynchronization of neocortical activity and theta rhythm in the hippocampus. However, as mentioned before, this does not mean that a drug-induced neocortical desynchronization is always and necessarily associated with a hippocampal theta rhythm. Two examples may illustrate this fact: BAS, the benzyl analog of serotonin (1-benzyl-2,5-dimethylserotonin), a drug with antiserotonin properties, induces in the neocortex of the rabbit a typical alert EEG pattern, but in the hippocampus convulsive-like phenomena rather than a theta rhythm (Rinaldi, 1958). Similarly, LSD, known to produce a flattening of neocortical activity, does not produce a regularization but rather a flattening of the hippocampal activity (Sailer and Stumpf, 1957b). Consequently, the finding that a drug causes a neocortical desynchronization does not necessarily justify the interpretation that this drug produces generalized EEG changes characteristic for an arousal reaction.

Among others, two groups of drugs, cholinergic and adrenergic agents, do produce a desynchronization of neocortical activity and a theta rhythm in the hippocampus, i.e., EEG changes otherwise characteristic for an arousal reaction. It is well known that cholinergic agents may produce an EEG arousal reaction but not a behavioral arousal reaction (cf. Bradley and Elkes, 1957) although behavioral awakening has been observed after intracarotid injection of acetylcholine in the cat encéphale isolé preparation (Bonnet and Bremer, 1937). On the other hand, as will be shown later, the theta rhythm elicited by sensory or reticular stimulation is more similar to the theta rhythm induced by cholinergic agents than to that induced by adrenergic agents.

a. Cholinergic Agents. Acetylcholine (ACh) and the anticholinesterases, eserine and diisopropylfluorophosphate (DFP), are the cholinergic agents which have been used most frequently for electroencephalographic studies and there is general agreement that these three drugs have essentially similar actions. On the other hand, it has been reported that neostigmine does not produce any EEG modifications when given in reasonable doses intravenously and this failure to produce EEG changes has been suggested to be owing to the fact that neostigmine as a quaternary ammonium compound fails to pass the blood–brain barrier (Funderburk and Case, 1951). However, when injected into the carotid artery, Bremer and Chatonnet (1949) found neostigmine effective in changing the electrocorticogram in a manner similar to ACh and eserine. It may be mentioned here that other quaternary ammonium compounds given by the same route of administration have also been found to modify the electrocortical activity (Longo, 1955).

Between 1937, when the action of ACh (injected into the carotid artery in the cat encéphale isolé preparation) on the cortical activity was investigated for the first time (Bonnet and Bremer, 1937), and about 1955, little depth recording was employed in such studies. Surface recording showed that cholinergic agents produce a low-voltage fast activity. Wescoe *et al.* (1948) demonstrated this effect for DFP in cats and monkeys, Bremer and Chatonnet (1949) for ACh, eserine, and neostigmine (all given by the intracarotid route) in the cat encéphale isolé preparation, Funderburk and Case (1951) as well as Bradley and Elkes (1953b) for eserine in the cat, Bradley *et al.* (1953) for DFP also in the cat, and Longo (1955) for ACh injected into the carotid artery in the rabbit. The potency of an anticholinesterase drug in producing a neocortical arousal pattern seems to depend on inactivation of brain pseudocholinesterase rather than on inactivation of brain true cholinesterase (Desmedt and La Grutta, 1957). It has been stated that the electrocorticographic changes produced by cholinergic agents are similar to those seen during an arousal reaction (Bradley and Elkes, 1957; Funderburk and Case, 1951; Longo, 1955) and further experimentation has shown that this similarity is not limited to the electrocorticographic changes. Rinaldi and Himwich (1955d) described the EEG changes after injection of ACh (0.5–5 μg) of DFP (0.1–0.3 mg) into the common carotid artery of rabbits as a typical alert pattern characterized by a fast, low-voltage neocortical activity and a regular, slow "thalamic rhythm." Finally, this thalamic rhythm was identified as hippocampal theta rhythm (Sailer and Stumpf, 1957b). That the regular subcortical rhythm induced by cholinergic agents was first recorded from the diencephalon can easily be explained by the peculiarities of the potential field of the theta rhythm (see Section II,A,1). Petsche and Stumpf (1960) and Monnier (1960) have also recorded a regular slow activity after eserine not only from the hippocampus but from other subcortical areas as well. Intracarotid injection of ACh, eserine, and pilocarpine induce a similar activity (Monnier and Romanowski, 1962). Finally, eserine has been found to produce a theta rhythm in the hippocampus of rats (Bureš *et al.*, 1962) and cats. In the latter species the frequency of theta rhythm was reported to be 2–4 per second rather than 4–7 per second as in the rabbit, but the same frequencies have also been found for slow activity during an arousal reaction (Bradley and Nicholson, 1962).

There are many characteristics which the theta rhythms induced by eserine and by sensory or reticular stimulation have in common. Both slow activities show the same potentials field with a "null zone" at a level just below the pyramidal cell layer, and the same spherical spread with approximately the same velocity (Green *et al.*, 1960; Petsche and Stumpf, 1960). Just as the frequency of the theta rhythm during an arousal reaction depends on the intensity of reticular or sensory stimulation (see Section II,A,1), the frequency of the eserine-induced theta rhythm depends on the dose of eserine. For instance, in the rabbit an eserine dose of 0.1 mg/kg will induce a theta rhythm with a frequency between 4.5 and 5 per second, whereas this frequency will be between 5.5 and

6 per second after a dose of 0.6 mg/kg. After strong reticular stimulation frequencies of 8 per second and more may be obtained. This high a frequency is not possible with eserine, probably because the doses necessary to produce such frequencies would be otherwise toxic (Sailer and Stumpf, 1957b).

With any drug-induced EEG change there is always the question whether the observed effect is due to a direct action of this drug on the brain area under observation or on a remote brain structure. There is much evidence that the eserine-induced theta rhythm has the same origin as the theta rhythm elicited by sensory or reticular stimulation. The following observations demonstrate that the medial septal nucleus is responsible for mediating both kinds of hippocampal slow waves. First of all, it has been shown that after administration of eserine the neurons of the medial septal nucleus discharge in bursts synchronous with the hippocampal theta rhythm just in the same way as they do during a sensory or reticular stimulation (Petsche *et al.*, 1962). As might be expected on the basis of this finding, a septal lesion (or an injection of procaine into the septum) abolishes the eserine-induced theta rhythm (Brücke *et al.*, 1959a; Mayer and Stumpf, 1958b). Probably, these effects are not specific for eserine, nor for cholinergic agents in general. So far no other drug which induces a theta rhythm has been studied as to its action on the firing pattern of septal neurons. It is known, however, that the hippocampal slow waves induced by other drugs (apomorphine, methamphetamine, and nicotine) are also abolished by septal lesions (Mayer and Stumpf, 1958b; Stumpf, 1959). Therefore, it is probably justified to assume that no drug can induce a theta rhythm in animals with septal lesions. This statement would imply that a theta rhythm is in no case caused by a direct action of a drug on the hippocampus itself.

Although a septal lesion abolishes the typical eserine-induced theta rhythm, this does not mean that after such a lesion eserine has not action on the electrical activity of the hippocampus. In such animals, eserine produces fast, low-voltage activity, changing the hippocampus EEG in the same way as an arousal stimulus does following a septal lesion (Fig. 1) (Mayer and Stumpf, 1958b). Recent investigations (Stumpf, 1965) have shown that in the intact rabbit eserine not only produces a theta rhythm but, at the same time, superimposed on it, regular, fast, low-voltage activity which has been discussed in Section II,B. A septal lesion, although abolishing the slow waves, does not change the fast activity.

Finally, a septal lesion modifies the eserine-induced firing pattern of hippocampal pyramidal neurons. During an eserine-induced theta rhythm some pyramidal neurons discharge in bursts correlated to a certain phase of the theta waves just as they do during a theta rhythm induced by reticular stimulation. Generally, the discharge frequency is increased under the influence of eserine (Green *et al.*, 1960). This effect can be abolished by interruption of septal transmission. When, in a rabbit pretreated with eserine, procaine is injected into the septum, theta rhythm and increased discharge rate of pyramidal neurons disappear and later reappear simultaneously (Fig. 3) (Deisenhammer and Stumpf, 1960).

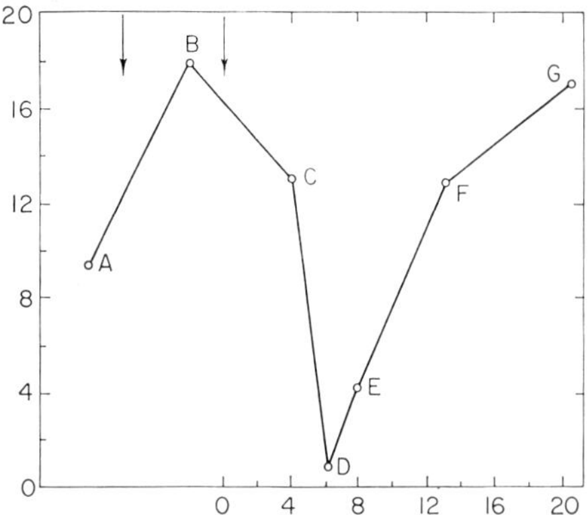

FIG. 3. Discharge rate of hippocampus pyramidal neuron during control period (A), after intravenous injection of 0.25 mg/kg eserine (B), and at various intervals after injection of 0.015 ml procaine (10%) into the septum (C to G). Arrows indicate injections. Abscissa: time in minutes after procaine injection into the septum. Ordinate: number of action potentials per second. Taken from Deisenhammer and Stumpf (1960).

Thus, all available data indicate that the septum plays the same important role for the eserine-induced theta rhythm as it does for that induced by sensory or reticular stimulation. None of the experimental findings mentioned so far requires the assumption that eserine exerts a direct action on the hippocampus itself, this despite the fact that the hippocampus formation has been found to contain quite high concentrations of cholinacetylase (Feldberg and Vogt, 1948) and some pseudo and true cholinesterase

(Burgen and Chipman, 1951), the latter enzyme being located mainly in the regions of the basal dendrites and the proximal parts of the apical dendrites of pyramidal neurons (Gerebtzoff, 1960). Administration of an anticholinesterase should inhibit the cholinesterase and might thereby produce some observable effect if ACh plays any physiological role in the hippocampus. Actually, it has been shown that eserine has a facilitatory action on the response of single hippocampal neurons to septal stimulation, very probably due to a direct action of eserine on the hippocampus itself (Brücke *et al.,* 1963). MacLean (1957) observed slow waves and seizure discharges in the cat's hippocampus after topical application of various cholinergic agents, suggesting that both EEG phenomena are due to a direct action of these drugs on the hippocampus. Unfortunately, these experiments have not been repeated in animals with septal lesions. Drug-induced hippocampal seizure activity can occur in such animals (Stumpf, 1959). If a theta rhythm could be induced in animals with septal lesions by injection of cholinergic agents into the hippocampus, this would be the first case demonstrating a theta rhythm in the presence of a septal lesion and would require a revision of the hypothesis on the origin of the theta rhythm as outlined in Section II,A,2.

From what has been said on the theta rhythm induced by cholinergic agents, it can easily be seen that this rhythm is similar to, if not identical with, the slow activity characteristic for the hippocampus arousal reaction, although a few observations indicate an additional direct action of these agents on the hippocampus itself. However, several precautions must be taken before the identity of these two activities can be taken as granted. First of all, it is not yet established whether these two activities are really identical in every respect. Second, one cannot be sure whether the various effects of cholinergic agents described above are specific for these agents unless other drugs producing a theta rhythm have been studied as well. At least, as mentioned before, the disappearance of a drug-induced theta rhythm after septal lesions is not specific for cholinergic agents. However, it will be seen later that the theta rhythm produced by methamphetamine differs in some respects from that induced by eserine or by sensory or reticular stimulation. Finally, the eserine-induced theta rhythm has been found to be influenced by scopolamine in a somewhat different way than the theta rhythm induced by reticular stimulation (see

Section III,A,2) but so far the explanation for this discrepancy remains obscure.

Reversible functional elimination of the neocortex elicited by spreading depression has no influence on the eserine-induced theta rhythm, as demonstrated by Bohdanecký *et al.* (1963). Similarly, neocortical ablation does not change the theta rhythm during an arousal reaction (Green and Arduini, 1954). However, Bohdanecký *et al.* (1963) maintain that reversible functional elimination of the hippocampus by spreading depression does not influence the theta rhythm recorded from the tegmentum. This unexpected result would imply that an eserine-induced theta rhythm in the brain stem can exist even when the normal function of the hippocampus is eliminated temporarily, therefore requiring the assumption of a second pacemaker for the tegmental theta rhythm. This assumption would require an auxiliary hypothesis, namely, that both pacemakers work completely in phase and synchronously since it has been demonstrated that the theta rhythm in mesodiencephalon and hippocampus forms one coherent activity (Petsche and Stumpf, 1960). Further experimentation is needed before such an assumption can be made with certainty.

b. Adrenergic Agents. The action of epinephrine and norepinephrine on cortical activity has been studied repeatedly but the results of these investigations are conflicting and often contradictory (for a survey of literature see Longo, 1962). On the other hand, there is obviously complete agreement on the actions of *d*-, *l*-, and *dl*-amphetamine and methamphetamine, and it has invariably been found that these sympathomimetics produce EEG and behavioral arousal. This effect has been described in cats (Bradley and Elkes, 1953a, 1957; Funderburk and Woodcock, 1957; Hiebel *et al.*, 1954a; Rothballer, 1957), dogs (Schallek and Walz, 1953), and rabbits (Longo, 1962; Longo and Silvestrini, 1957; White and Boyajy, 1959; White and Daigneault, 1959). Although no detailed studies on the actions of epinephrine and norepinephrine on the hippocampal activity have been reported, the appearance of rhythmic slow waves in the hippocampus after amphetamine and methamphetamine has been demonstrated in the cat (Bradley and Nicholson, 1962) and rabbit (Longo, 1962; Sailer and Stumpf, 1957b). This activity can be abolished by septal lesions (Mayer and Stumpf, 1958b).

Therefore, it appears—and this has been mentioned frequently

—that the EEG changes induced by cholinergic and adrenergic agents are very similar, indeed, being analogous to those occurring during an arousal reaction. However, several differences have been found to exist between the neocortical arousal pattern induced by cholinergic and adrenergic agents, respectively. A discussion of the differential effects of various brain stem transections and of various antagonists on these arousal patterns would be beyond the scope of this review. It may be mentioned, however, that even the distribution of the neocortical desynchronization, induced by eserine and amphetamine, respectively, shows some differences (Longo and Silvestrini, 1957). Therefore, it might be expected that some differences in the hippocampal slow wave patterns induced by cholinergic and adrenergic agents might also exist. In the rabbits, the frequency of the eserine-induced theta rhythm increases with increasing dosage and that of the theta rhythm induced by reticular stimulation with increasing stimulus intensity, whereas the frequency of the methamphetamine-induced theta rhythm remains constant within a range of 5 to 5.5 per second independent of the dose of methamphetamine, even when doses up to 40 mg/kg are used. Moreover, the wave shape of the methamphetamine-induced theta rhythm is considerably more irregular than that of the theta rhythm induced by eserine (Sailer and Stumpf, 1957b), and the addition of reticular stimulation causes a distinct regularization (Longo, 1962). In the cat, Bradley and Nicholson (1962) found much lower frequencies of the theta rhythm induced by amphetamine but, according to these authors, in this species any hippocampal slow wave rhythm tends to have the same frequency between 2 and 4 per second. In the rabbit, again, amphetamine decreases the discharge rate of hippocampal pyramidal neurons, whereas eserine has the opposite effect (Green *et al.*, 1960).

If the above results are compared critically, it must be concluded that only slight differences exist between the theta rhythms induced by some cholinergic and adrenergic agents and that this is generally true for the EEG arousal patterns produced by these two groups of drugs.

2. *Drugs That Inhibit the Theta Rhythm*

A large number of drugs—most anesthetics, hypnotics, tranquilizers, and related drugs, as well as anticholinergic agents—inhibit the neocortical arousal reaction and at the same time depress the theta rhythm of the hippocampus. Important exceptions will be discussed later. As far as the hippocampus arousal reaction is concerned, the effect of subthreshold doses is often far more interesting. It has been mentioned previously (Section II,A,1) that the frequency of the theta rhythm is in some way a quite sensitive index of the excitatory state of the reticular formation. Consequently, it may be expected that drugs which inhibit the arousal reaction, when given in subthreshold doses, will decrease the frequency of the theta rhythm thereby giving a quantitative estimate of the amount of depression. Actually, it has been demonstrated in rabbits that the frequency of the theta rhythm elicited by reticular stimulation is decreased temporarily by hexobarbital, procaine, and chlorpromazine. If, for instance, the frequency is 7 per second during an arousal reaction in the control period, hexobarbital (10 mg/kg) reduces this frequency to about 5 per second during the first few minutes after the intravenous injection (Fig. 4). With all three drugs, the decrease of frequency depends on the dosage and time after administration. Scopolamine shows a different type of action. As long as the scopolamine dose is not high enough to abolish the theta rhythm completely, it will not reduce its frequency during an arousal reaction elicited by reticular stimulation (Brücke *et al.*, 1957). The same type of experiments has been repeated with a theta rhythm induced by eserine instead of reticular stimulation. In this case all four drugs have the same action consisting of a decrease in the frequency of the theta rhythm (Brücke *et al.*, 1958). Urethane has also been shown to influence the eserine-induced theta rhythm in this manner (Stumpf *et al.*, 1962). No explanation can be offered for the difference in action of scopolamine on the theta rhythms induced by eserine and reticular stimulation, respectively. However, it may be stated—obviously with a few exceptions—that drugs which inhibit the arousal reaction tend to decrease the frequency of the hippocampal theta rhythm when given in appropriate subthreshold doses.

Of course, a drug-induced decrease in frequency of theta rhythm per se does not allow any conclusion in terms of site of drug action. It may be due to a depressant action on the reticular formation but it may also be due to such an action on reticulo-hippocampal pathways or on the hippocampus itself. An investigation of the action of drugs that inhibit the arousal reaction, on the burst firing pattern of those septal neurons which trigger the theta

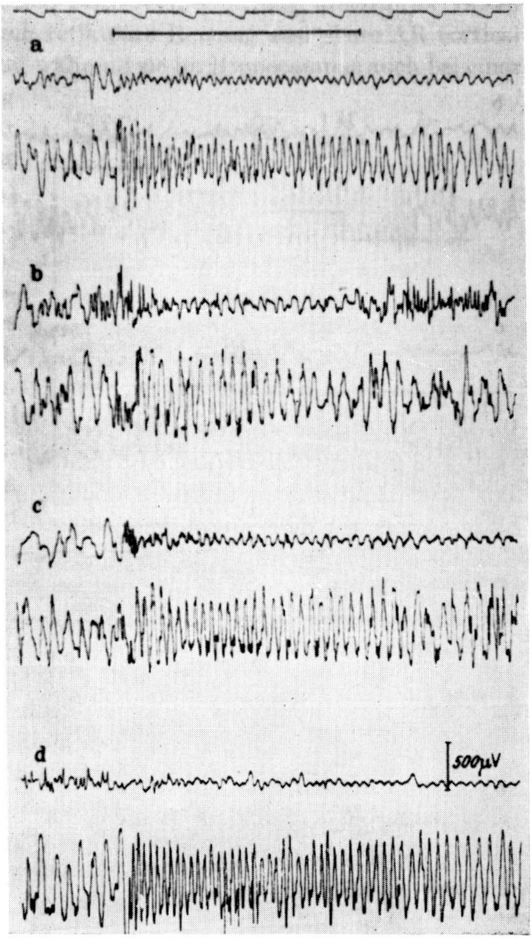

FIG. 4. Neocortical (upper traces) and hippocampal arousal reaction (lower traces) of a rabbit, elicited by reticular stimulations (horizontal bar), before (a) and 5 minutes (b), 12 minutes (c), and 42 minutes (d) after intravenous injection of 10 mg/kg hexobarbital. Time markings: 1 second. Note change in frequency of theta rhythm. Taken from Brücke *et al.* (1957).

rhythm in the hippocampus, at least allows a conclusion as to whether such an action is due to a direct action on the hippocampus or on its afferent pathways. Such investigations have been carried out (Stumpf *et al.*, 1962) and the results will be mentioned later.

a. Anticholinergic Drugs—Atropine and Scopolamine. Atropine and scopolamine produce an electrocortical sleep pattern, they antagonize the EEG changes induced by cholinergic drugs, and they block the electrocortical alert pattern. These effects were first described by Wescoe *et al.* (1948), Bremer and Chatonnet (1949), and Funderburk and Case (1951), and later confirmed repeatedly. Anticholinergic drugs seem to inhibit any activations pattern, be it elicited by reticular stimulation (Rinaldi and Himwich, 1955d), by brain lesions, or by cholinergic and adrenergic agents (White and Daigneault, 1959). The EEG sleep pattern induced by atropine (and scopolamine) is not associated with behavioral sleep; therefore, there is a "dissociation" between EEG and behavior, described in dogs (Wikler, 1952), rabbits (Longo, 1956), and cats (Bradley and Elkes, 1957), whereas in the monkey this dissociation is less marked (Domino and Hudson, 1959). Qualitatively, atropine and scopolamine have similar actions, but in its ability to inhibit the arousal reaction, scopolamine is from 10 to 15 times more potent than atropine (Longo, 1956), and *l*-hyoscyamine is much more potent than its *d*-isomer (Bradley and Elkes, 1957; Domino and Hudson, 1959).

The changes of the hippocampal activity induced by atropine are characterized by an increase in amplitude and replacement of the rhythmic slow waves by an irregular 3–6 per second activity (Bradley and Nicholson, 1962). Such an effect is not specific for anticholinergic drugs but is also seen after administration of various central depressants. In the same way as the neocortical activation pattern is abolished by atropine, this alkaloid also inhibits the rhythmic subcortical activity produced by any arousal stimulus or by cholinergic agents (Bradley and Nicholson, 1962; Longo, 1962; Monnier and Romanowski, 1962; Rinaldi and Himwich, 1955d). However, doses of scopolamine that abolish completely the neocortical arousal reaction elicited by reticular stimulation, have only a slight effect on the theta rhythm without changing its frequency (Brücke *et al.*, 1957). This indicates that the hippocampal arousal reaction is less sensitive to scopolamine than the neocortical arousal reaction.

In contrast to barbiturates, scopolamine does not change the fast component of the hippocampal arousal reaction. This finding suggests that the system responsible for mediation of hippocampal fast activity (see Section II,B) is insensitive for the action of scopolamine (Stumpf, 1965).

The scopolamine-induced changes in the firing pattern of septal neurons in rabbits pretreated with eserine is associated with corresponding changes of hippocampal activity. For instance, after scopolamine, the hippocampal theta rhythm and the typical burst firing pattern of septal neurons disappear simultaneously (Stumpf *et al.*, 1962). It will be shown later (Section III,A,2,*b*) that other drugs that depress the theta rhythm do not necessarily have such an action. The eserine-induced increase in discharge rate of hippocampus pyramidal neurons is likewise abolished by scopolamine (Green *et al.*, 1960). These findings indicate that the inhibition of the theta rhythm is not necessarily due to an action of scopolamine on the hippocampus itself but rather on a lower level.

b. Anesthetics. Bremer (1935, 1936) demonstrated for the first time the fundamentally different action of barbiturates, on the one hand, and of ethyl ether and chloroform, on the other, on the electrocortical activity of the cat. He stressed the similarity of the EEG changes seen under the influence of barbiturates with those observed during natural sleep or in the cerveau isolé preparation. His results were confirmed and extended by Derbyshire *et al.* (1936), Beecher and McDonough (1939), and later by many others. Derbyshire *et al.* (1936) found that tribromoethanol and pentobarbital induce a slow frequency, high-amplitude cortical activity, whereas ether induces a high frequency, low-amplitude activity. As a result of the investigation of 17 anesthetics, Beecher and McDonough (1939) concluded that the first type of EEG modification is in general produced by nonvolatile anesthetics, the second type by volatile anesthetics, whereas a few anesthetics (ethyl urethan, amylene hydrate, and chloroform) were classified as "mixed" anesthetics. It will be seen later that anesthetics belonging to these different groups also have differential actions on the hippocampal activity. To demonstrate this fact, one representative drug or group of drugs belonging to each of the groups mentioned above, will be discussed here—barbiturates as representatives of the nonvolatile anesthetics, ethyl urethan as representative of the "mixed" group, and ethyl ether as a typical volatile anesthetic.

A common property of all anesthetics is their ability to inhibit multisynaptically organized portions of the central nervous system, especially the subcortical arousal mechanisms, and their action on these systems has been regarded as responsible for their generalized effects (Arduini and Arduini, 1954; French *et al.*, 1953). As a consequence of this action, one might expect not only an inhibition of the neocortical arousal reaction but of the hippocampal theta rhythm as well, and, in fact, such an effect was demonstrated early, at least for a barbiturate (pentobarbital), by Green and Arduini (1954). It should be stressed, however, that it has never been stated that anesthetics in general produce a selective inhibition of the brain stem arousal mechanisms. On the contrary, direct actions on the cortex have been reported frequently. Therefore, it may be expected that at least for some anesthetics a direct action on the hippocampus can be demonstrated, too.

Barbiturates. Several investigations have been carried out on the action of barbiturates on hippocampal activity. Longo (1962) described the effect of pentobarbital on the hippocampal activity of the rabbit using a division into three phases for classification of the depth of anesthesia. During the first phase (after 5–10 mg/kg) there is no basic change in hippocampal activity except for slight irregularities of the theta rhythm. During the second phase (after 15–20 mg/kg) the amplitude of hippocampal activity increases and spike-like high-frequency activity may appear. Finally, during the third phase (after 25–30 mg/kg), the hippocampal activity is greatly reduced. Similar changes of hippocampal activity were observed after the administration of phenobarbital, but higher doses were necessary to produce these three phases (20–40, 50–70, and 100 mg/kg, respectively).

An investigation on the effects of sodium pentobarbital on the cat's hippocampus was carried out by Bradley and Nicholson (1962) who report the following changes: after 1–3 mg/kg, no essential change; after 4–7 mg/kg, increase in amplitude; after 8–12 mg/kg, regular 7–10 per second activity together with higher frequencies (15–25 per second) and high-voltage spike activity; after 14–24 mg/kg, a 6–7 per second activity with frequent high-voltage spikes; and after 22 mg/kg and more, spike activity of decreasing frequency with low-amplitude background activity. Similar changes were observed after sodium amobarbital, although higher doses were necessary to induce each change of activity. High-voltage spike activity in the hippocampus has also been observed after sodium thiopental.

Brooks (1962) drew special attention to the "beta activity" (15–50 per second) and spike activity appearing in the cat's hippocampus under light barbiturate anesthesia (defined as an anesthesia just deep enough to prevent spontaneous movement). The three areas where beta activity was found under these conditions were the prepyriform and anterior pyriform cortex, the hippocampus, and the ventromedial thalamic nucleus. In the hippocampus this activity consists of a large amplitude low-frequency (15–25 per second) and a small amplitude high-frequency (35–40 per second) component with its maximal potential gradient in the pyramidal cell layer, this is to say, at a level similar to the maximal potential gradient for the theta rhythm. When the anesthesia deepens, the beta activity is replaced by a spike pattern consisting of biphasic or monophasic spikes which, again, can be recorded from the three areas mentioned above. The potential gradient set up by the field of the biphasic spikes is similar to that of the beta activity. Low voltage, fast activity in barbiturate anesthesia occurring in hippocampus, amygdala, and pyriform cortex was also observed by Kaada (1951). The action of barbiturates on the fast component of hippocampal activity consists of an increase in amplitude and decrease in frequency (Stumpf, 1965). This resulting activity is probably identical with that described by Brooks (1962) as large amplitude low-frequency component of "beta activity" in cats under barbiturate anesthesia.

In summary, it may be said that these are the characteristic features of the action of barbiturates on the hippocampal activity —irregular high amplitude activity associated with a high-frequency component and spikes that depend on the depth of anesthesia. Bradley and Nicholson (1962) regard the high voltage spike activity as a release phenomenon due to the inhibition of the reticular formation. Brooks (1962) puts forward some evidence that under light barbiturate anesthesia the prepyriform cortex acts as a pacemaker for the hippocampal spikes, whereby presumably the biphasic spikes would arise in the region of the pyramidal cell layer, and the monophasic spikes in the region of the dentate gyrus, in response to impulses arriving from the pacemaker. So far no evidence exists for the assumption that the same pacemaker may be responsible for the "beta" or fast activity seen after barbiturate administration.

Barbiturates also increase the threshold for the hippocampus arousal reaction (Green and Arduini, 1954). Low doses decrease the frequency of the theta rhythm induced by eserine or reticular stimulation whereas higher doses abolish this rhythm altogether (Brücke *et al.,* 1957, 1958). Intense afferent stimulation may evoke a fast activity ("desynchronization") in the hippocampus of animals under barbiturate anesthesia (Green and Arduini, 1954; Weiss and Fifková, 1960). Actually, intense reticular stimulation has an unmasking effect on the fact activity by producing a blockade of the slow waves in the unanesthetized animal as well as in the animal under barbiturate anesthesia although, as mentioned above, in the latter case the fast activity is of much higher voltage and slower than in the unanesthetized animal (Stumpf, 1965).

It is generally assumed that the inhibition of the arousal reaction by barbiturates is due to, or at least includes, a depressant action of these drugs on the reticular formation (French *et al.*, 1953; and others). The action of barbiturates on the firing pattern of septal neurons is in agreement with this assumption, at least as far as the hippocampus arousal reaction is concerned. When hexobarbital is given to a rabbit pretreated with eserine, the firing pattern of these neurons is slowed just as it would be by scopolamine. A lower dose of hexobarbital will only reduce the frequency of the theta rhythm while reducing the frequency of the bursts of the septal neurons, whereby the correlation between the burst discharges and the phase of the theta waves remains unchanged. After a higher dose of hexobarbital the eserine-induced theta rhythm disappears, and exactly at the same time the typical burst firing pattern of the septal neurons also disappears. Therefore, it is not necessary to assume that the inhibition of the typical hippocampus arousal reaction by barbiturates is due to a direct action on the hippocampus (Stumpf *et al.*, 1962).

Ethyl urethan. Although urethan is clearly nonvolatile, it was classified by Beecher and McDonough (1939) as belonging to the "mixed group" since it was found to possess many actions characteristic for the volatile anesthetics. In 1937, Pick made a distinction between two different kinds of hypnotics and narcotics, the "brain stem narcotics" and "cortex narcotics," respectively. As these names imply, Pick (1937) assumed that some hypnotics and narcotics would act primarily on the brain stem and others primarily on cortical structures. He classified barbiturates as typical brain stem narcotics. Urethan, however, was considered as a cortex narcotic, or possibly a narcotic which is intermediate in its action between the two groups. Actually, even earlier, Skowroński (1929) had found important differences in the central actions of barbiturates and urethan, respectively. More recently, it has been demonstrated that urethan in anesthetic doses, in contrast to barbiturates, does not completely prevent the (neocortical) arousal reaction in response to reticular stimulation (Longo, 1962).

Hukuhara (1962) investigated the action of urethan on various cortical and subcortical structures of the cat. He found, after administration of 0.75 to 1.0 gm/kg intraperitoneally, irregular, high-voltage activity in the hippocampus and a spindle-like 15 per second activity instead of a theta rhythm in response to reticular stimulation. However, spontaneous periods of slow (3–4 per second), rhythmic, and high-amplitude theta waves may still occur in deepest urethan anesthesia; thus a phenomenon similar to paradoxical sleep may be produced (Gogolák *et al.*, 1964).

The action of urethan on the hippocampal theta rhythm and the firing pattern of neurons of the medial septal nucleus shows characteristic differences when compared with the action of hexobarbital (Stumpf *et al.*, 1962). Eserine was given to rabbits in order to induce a theta rhythm in the hippocampus with the typical burst firing pattern of septal neurons. The action of urethan on this system is classified here into three stages for purely descriptive purposes only. During the first stage (this is after doses up to 1.1 gm/kg intravenously) the frequency and the amplitude of the theta rhythm decrease gradually and low, high-frequency activity tends to predominate in the hippocampus EEG. At the same time, the septal neurons continue to discharge in bursts with unchanged correlation to the theta rhythm. Therefore, the number of bursts occurring during a given time interval decreases in the same way as the number of theta waves during the same time interval. In addition, the number of discharges per burst decreases gradually. During the second stage (this is after doses between 1.3 and 2.7 gm/kg), low, high-frequency activity without theta rhythm can be recorded from the hippocampus and periods of relative electrical silence appear more and more frequently as the urethan dose is increased. The septal neurons, however, show no additional sudden change in their burst firing pattern which might correlate with the absence of the theta rhythm in the hippocampus. Instead, the changes that occurred during the first stage continue during the second stage, this is to say, the number of bursts per second and the number of discharges per burst continue to decrease until, after 2.7 gm/kg, 1 or 2 bursts occur per second, each "burst" consisting of 1 or 2 discharges only. Finally, during the third stage (this is after 2.9 gm/kg) the hippocampal activity is more or less flat and the septal neurons do not fire any more. This urethan dose is near the lethal dose, and a further increase in dose would cause the death of the animal. Interpretation of these results led to the conclusion that a burst firing pattern of the septal neurons can occur even in the absence of a hippocampal theta rhythm. There are a few more examples of such a condition which will be discussed later. At any rate, the fact that such conditions can occur indicates that the hippocampal theta rhythm is the consequence rather than the cause of the septal burst firing pattern. Otherwise there should not be such a pattern when there is no theta rhythm in the hippocampus. From this it follows that if the septal neurons discharge in bursts and at the same time there is no theta rhythm in the hippocampus, as after appropriate doses of urethan, then there may be a block somewhere along the pathways leading from the septum to the hippocampus. Thus, it might be assumed that urethan has a direct action on the hippocampus itself. Likewise it has been shown that under higher doses of urethan the septal neurons discharge in bursts, but these bursts occur at a much lower rate than during the control period. This indicates an additional action of urethan at a lower level in the brain, but this action must be relatively weak, otherwise there could be no burst discharge pattern of septal neurons at all.

Ethyl ether. Ether is mentioned here as a representative of the large group of volatile anesthetics. For a long time it has been known that ether produces low-voltage fast activity in the neocortex during the initial stage of anesthesia. Ever since this effect was noticed, different and sometimes contradictory interpretations have been given to explain it. For instance, Adrian and Matthews (1934) suggested that the main effect of ether and chloroform is "on afferent and efferent pathways rather than on cortical neurons themselves" and similarly Derbyshire *et al.* (1936) concluded that sensory paths are blocked by ether before the cortical activity disappears. To the contrary, Bremer (1935, 1936) assumed a direct depressant action of ether on the cortex and explained the fast activity as a consequence of an increased afferent inflow. The modifications of neocortical activity during inhalation of ether are similar to those occurring during an arousal reaction, and both types of cortical desynchronization are abolished by the same brain stem transections, leading to the hypothesis "that the fast cortical rhythms characterizing the earlier stages of inhalation anesthesia, may be due to a excitatory influence upon the brain stem reticular formation" (Rossi and Zirondoli, 1955). This hypothesis is, of course, contradictory to the assumption that general anesthetic agents, including ether, depress the function of this formation (French *et al.*, 1953) although differences in doses may explain these different interpretations.

A theta rhythm has been recorded from the hippocampus during the initial stage of ether anesthesia simultaneously with desynchronization in the neocortex (Kim and MacLean, 1956; MacLean *et al.*, 1955–1956) and when ether anesthesia becomes deeper, the frequency of the theta rhythm decreases (Longo, 1962). Therefore, the observed modifications of the hippocampal activity during the initial stage of ether anesthesia would be constant with the assumption that ether in low concentrations stimulates the reticular formation and in higher concentrations, when the frequency of the theta rhythm decreases, has a mixed stimulating and depressant effect on this system. However, as Domino and Ueki (1959) correctly point out, it is extremely difficult to describe the actions of ether in such terms, and their paper may be consulted for a detailed discussion on this subject.

Domino and Ueki (1959) found spike-like discharges and other hypersynchronous events in the amygdala, olfactory bulb, posterior hypothalamus, and related rhinencephalic structures of the dog after inhalation of ether and other volatile anesthetics during certain stages of the anesthesia. No records were obtained in these experiments from the hippocampus. Longo (1962) described spike-like discharges in the hippocampus and hypothalamus of rabbits during cyclopropane anesthesia, but not after inhalation of ether. During deep cyclopropane anesthesia hypothalamic seizures may occur. The meaning of the hypersynchronous events occurring in various subcortical structures during anesthesia with various volatile anesthetics is by no means clear.

c. Tranquilizers—Chlorpromazine and Reserpine. It is not a common property of all tranquilizers to inhibit the hippocampal theta rhythm, not even in the case of the two tranquilizers selected for discussion here. Chlorpromazine and reserpine have been selected to stress the dissimilarity rather than the similarity of their action. Despite the fact that a considerable literature on the EEG effects of these two drugs has accumulated during the last

10 years, the results of various investigators and their interpretations are variable and often contradictory. For instance, for chlorpromazine, the original studies demonstrated an "EEG synchronization" and inhibition of the arousal reaction in cats (Hiebel *et al.*, 1954b), rabbits (Longo *et al.*, 1954; Terzian, 1954), and monkeys (Das *et al.*, 1954), whereas later investigations, too numerous to mention here, showed different, often only insignificant EEG changes, and actually even when reinvestigations led to results similar to those found in the original studies, the mechanism of the chlorpromazine action has been interpreted in several different ways. A similar situation exists in the case of reserpine. The following discussion will be confined to studies in which the effects of these drugs on the hippocampal activity was included. It will be seen that in general the hippocampal activity is influenced by chlorpromazine and reserpine in a way analogous to neocortical activity except for the fact that with these drugs seizure-like activity has frequently been found to occur in the hippocampus but not in the neocortex.

Chlorpromazine. All authors who found a synchronization of neocortical activity and an inhibition of the arousal reaction, also reported modifications of the hippocampal activity including inhibition of the theta rhythm. Rinaldi and Himwich (1955c), for instance, described the disappearance of neocortical desynchronization as well as of the regular "thalamic rhythm" after small doses of chlorpromazine in the rabbit, and Longo (1962) has reported similar results. However, a differential sensitivity of the neocortical and rhinencephalic arousal reaction to chlorpromazine was found to exist. In the cat, after chlorpromazine, the intensity of reticular stimulation which elicits an arousal reaction within the limbic system was reported to be more elevated than that which elicits a neocortical arousal reaction (Killam and Killam, 1956). In contrast, in the rabbit, the neocortical arousal reaction is more easily depressed by chlorpromazine than the theta rhythm. After 0.5 mg/kg chlorpromazine, the neocortical arousal reaction due to reticular stimulation is virtually abolished whereas the same stimulation is still effective in eliciting a theta rhythm with slightly reduced frequency; a higher dose (2.5 mg/kg) has a similar effect with the frequency of the theta rhythm being still more reduced (Brücke *et al.*, 1957). Similarly, it was observed that from 1 to 2 hours after 5 mg/kg chlorpromazine, when an "electrographic attention reaction" is induced, it is more pronounced in the rhinencephalon than in the neocortex (Gangloff and Monnier, 1957). Higher doses of chlorpromazine (15 mg/kg and more) produce in the rabbit electrographic changes similar to an arousal reaction and consequently a regularized "thalamic rhythm" (Rinaldi and Himwich, 1955c).

Besides affecting the hippocampal activity as described above, chlorpromazine has another characteristic effect on the hippocampus which consists of the elicitation of seizure-like discharges. Preston (1956) observed such activity in the cat's hippocampus after toxic doses of chlorpromazine (40 to 45 mg/kg). He notes, however, that the hippocampus is not primarily involved in this seizure-like activity. Instead, when the chlorpromazine dose is increased gradually, and increase of spontaneous activity and spike discharges occur first in the amygdaloid nucleus complex, and later similar activity can be recorded from septum and hippocampus. It is not clear whether the seizure-like activity in septum and hippocampus is projected from the amygdala to these structures or is to be regarded as due to volume conduction. Sometimes, spike activity was seen in the hippocampus which could not be related to the activity in the amygdala. At any rate, higher doses were always necessary to produce spike activity in the hippocampus than in the amygdala. Preston (1956) advanced a hypothesis that the effect of chlorpromazine on the spontaneous activity of the amygdala may in some way explain the tranquilizing properties of this drug. Apparently, in the rabbit no seizure-like activity in the hippocampus under the influence of chlorpromazine has been observed so far, despite the fact that the effect of rather high doses have been studied in this species (see above).

Reserpine. Authors who have demonstrated a desynchronizing effect of reserpine on the neocortical activity and who have included recording of the hippocampal activity in their investigations, have consistently found a regular subcortical rhythm. It should be pointed out that the "desynchronization response" has been found to occur at varying times following reserpine injection by different investigators, but the association between neocortical desynchronization and regular, slow subcortical rhythm is unvarying. In the cat, it has been reported that 4 hours after reserpine injection a regular 3.5–4 per second rhythm appears in the hippocampus becoming more conspicuous and slower (2.5–3.5 per second) during the next several hours, and occurring practically continuously after 20 hours; it is always associated with a desynchronized neocortical activity (Kim and MacLean, 1956; MacLean *et al.,* 1955–1956). Similarly, in the rabbit, in hippocampus, thalamus, and occipital cortex, a regular 4–5 per second rhythm was recorded some time after reserpine injection, again associated with a desynchronization of the neocortical activity (Gangloff and Monnier, 1955, 1957; Rinaldi and Himwich, 1955b). On the basis of these findings, the similarity between the reserpine-induced electrographic changes and the "electroencephalographic pattern of alertness" has been stressed (Rinaldi and Himwich, 1955b). It is noteworthy, however, that all authors quoted above agree that the reserpine-induced theta rhythm has a rather low frequency in both cat and rabbit when compared with the frequency seen during alertness. It is generally assumed that the reserpine-induced alert pattern is due to a stimulatory action on the reticular formation; in fact, it can be abolished by brain stem transections (Sailer and Stumpf, 1957a). Under these conditions, the slow frequency of the theta rhythm induced by reserpine might indicate that this stimulatory action is rather weak (see Section II,A,1). Differences between the reserpine-induced EEG pattern and the ordinary arousal pattern have been stressed by Gangloff and Monnier (1957).

In addition to the effects mentioned so far, reserpine influences the hippocampal activity in still another way. In the cat, spontaneous seizures within the limbic system were reported (Killam and Killam, 1956; MacLean *et al.*, 1955–1956; Sigg and Schneider, 1957). In the rabbit, paroxysmal rhinencephalic spike discharges occurring 1 to 2 hours after reserpine were observed by Gangloff and Monnier (1955, 1957), but not by Longo (1962). The origin of these discharges remains unknown. However, it may be significant that under reserpine rhinencephalic seizures appear later than the activation pattern and that the typical reserpine-induced behavioral changes occur when the seizure discharges predominate (Sigg and Schneider, 1957).

B. Drugs That Induce Seizures or Seizure-like Discharges in the Hippocampus

For a long time it has been known (Gibbs and Gibbs, 1936; Green and Shimamoto, 1953; Jung, 1949; Kaada, 1951; Renshaw *et al.,* 1940; and others) that the hippocampus and other rhinencephalic areas are highly seizure-sensitive structures for which the thresholds for elicitation of afterdischarges are much lower than, for instance, in the neocortex. This is true for electrical as well as mechanical stimulation (Liberson and Akert, 1955). Is it to be expected that for this reason drugs with convulsant properties will affect the hippocampus or other rhinencephalic areas first? Obviously not, since several convulsant drugs are known to produce seizure discharges which may or may not involve the hippocampus, but certainly do not originate there. A good example for such an effect is given by Metrazol, a drug which may be regarded as a classical convulsant drug. In a detailed study, Starzl *et al.* (1953) recorded the electrical activity from many cortical and subcortical areas of the cat's brain during seizures induced by threshold doses of Metrazol and found that the seizure discharges start in the cerebral cortex and radiate from there to many deep structures. The hippocampus becomes involved into seizure activity, but only during this radiation from the cerebral cortex. However, the hippocampus and the superior colliculus differ from other subcortical areas in that the seizures activity in these two areas outlasts the end of the cortical fit. This is taken as indication that these areas possess independent capacities for seizure discharges.

When drug-induced seizure activity appears first in the hippocampus or a related rhinencephalic area, the significance of this event can be interpreted in various ways. Preston (1956) pointed out that the excitation of the amygdala by high doses of chlorpromazine theoretically could be the result of the low seizure threshold of the rhinencephalon, but it remains to be explained why the hippocampus is not affected simultaneously, or even earlier than the amygdala. Here it could be argued that some authors (e.g., Kaada, 1951) have found the pyriform-amygdaloid region to be somewhat more sensitive for elicitation of afterdischarges than the hippocampus. Nevertheless, Preston (1956) assumed that the seizure activity in the amygdala after chlorpromazine is probably due not to the nonspecific high seizure sensitivity of this structure, but rather to a more or less specific action of chlorpromazine on it. On the other hand, Tokizane and Sawyer (1957) have suggested that the localized seizure activity in the amygdala and hippocampus during hypoglycemia (see later) can be at least partially explained by the low seizure threshold of these two regions for electrical and chemical stimulation [by cholinergic agents (MacLean, 1957) or hypertonic saline (Sawyer and Gernandt, 1956)]. Thus, the problem is this: Whenever a drug is shown to induce seizure discharges in the brain which start in the hippocampus and/or amygdala, it will be difficult to differentiate between two possibilities, whether the seizure activity started there because these two structures have a low seizure threshold, or because the drug with such an action has a specific affinity for these structures. There may be no generally valid answer to this question. Some drugs certainly do have specific affinities for certain areas of the brain, others may act in a more or less unspecific manner. In the latter case an origin of seizure activity in the rhinencephalon might be expected although, as a consequence of the concepts of Grundfest (1957), low threshold for electrical stimulation may not necessarily be concomitant with low threshold for chemical stimulation.

When pharmacologically induced seizure discharges are recorded from the hippocampus or from any other brain structure, it would certainly be interesting to know whether the seizure activity actually starts there, this is to say, whether threshold doses induce seizure discharges in this structure, and in this structure only. Unfortunately, the experimental setup which would allow such a conclusion, is somewhat difficult to achieve since it would necessitate recording from as many areas of the brain as possible. Even then it might be argued that the recording was not done from the area where the seizure activity actually started. Therefore, whenever pharmacologically induced seizure discharges have been recorded from the hippocampus, there has been no conclusive proof that this is a primary locus. In some cases, however, it has been found that seizure discharges appear in the hippocampus before certain other brain areas become involved. Some of the drugs which have been reported to have such an action will be dealt with here.

It is interesting to note that many drugs which are usually classified as central depressants, cause spike discharges in the hippocampus without affecting the neocortex or other brain structures simultaneously. These drugs have been discussed earlier (see Section III,A,2).

1. *Insulin*

Hypoglycemia caused by the administration of insulin produces significant changes of the electrocortical activity (Goodwin *et al.*, 1938; Moruzzi, 1938). These and later studies offered no clue as to where the seizure activity originates, until Tokizane and Sawyer (1957) were able to demonstrate in the rabbit's brain, seizure activity which originates, and, when the hypoglycemia is not severe, may be confined to the amygdala and/or the hippocampus, especially the dorsal hippocampus. A blood sugar drop to about 50 mg/100 ml is necessary to produce these seizure discharges. Insulin in doses of up to 2000 units with an average of about 1000 units were given and seizures occurred between 1 and 4 hours after the injection. Seizure activity, first confined to the amygdala and/or the hippocampus, may later project to preoptic, hypothalamic, and other brain stem regions. The spread to these brain areas occurs very slowly and takes minutes to be accomplished. A spread of seizure activity to the neocortex or appearance of motor symptoms does not occur until the seizure is quite severe. The projection pattern of the insulin-induced amygdaloid seizure discharges is similar to the projection of amygdaloid seizures elicited by electrical stimulation in the cat, as described by various authors (Gloor, 1954; Naquet, 1954; and others).

Tokizane and Sawyer (1957) assume that hypoglycemia affects the hippocampus and amygdala in a way similar to "subclinical electroshock," that is, when the strength of the stimulus is low, only those brain structures would exhibit seizure activity for which the stimulus intensity just reaches threshold values. These authors have suggested that the beneficial results of insulin therapy may be related to induced subcortical seizures.

2. *Intracarotid Injections of Hypertonic Solutions*

Besides producing other EEG changes, intracarotid injections of hypertonic solutions (0.47 *M* saline or 2.4 *M* glucose in amounts of 2 or 3 ml, injected within a few seconds) sometimes evoke seizure activity in the rabbit's brain which, when it occurs, starts in, or remains confined to, the amygdala or hippocampus (Sawyer and Gernandt, 1956). Preferably, such seizure activity occurs when intracarotid injections of hypertonic solutions are given repeatedly. The same explanation for this preferential site of seizure activity is given by the authors as for the seizure activity induced by hypoglycemia.

3. *Nicotine*

Longo and co-workers (von Berger and Longo, 1953; Longo and Bovet, 1952; Longo *et al.*, 1954) described the changes in electrical activity of neocortex and thalamus produced by nicotine in the normal and encephale isolé rabbit. Small doses were found to produce an activation pattern which, after higher doses (1–3 mg/kg), is followed by seizure discharges. A 5–6 per second rhythmic activity was reported to occur during the activation pattern. In the cat, apparently much higher doses are necessary to produce seizure-like phenomena. In this species, Exley *et al.* (1958) described only "occasional convulsive spikes" in the EEG after intravenous injection of 50 mg/kg nicotine base.

In the rabbit's hippocampus the following sequence of events takes place after intravenous administration of nicotine (Stumpf, 1959): low doses produce, as reported by the Italian workers, an activation pattern and, consequently, a theta rhythm in the hippocampus. The effect of a higher dose of nicotine is illustrated in Fig. 5. Following such doses (0.5–3 mg/kg), again, a theta rhythm appears with a frequency which increases gradually from an initial value of 5 to 6 per second to 7 to 8 per second. Similar changes of hippocampal activity would be observed when reticular stimulation with gradually increasing frequency would be carried out. Following nicotine, after a period of time which usually lasts for about 30 seconds (corresponding to the first phase as described by Longo *et al.*, 1954), the theta rhythm is displaced by a hippocampal seizure activity consisting of spike discharges (first irregular, later very regular with a frequency of about 10 per second) and typical multiple spike and wave discharges similar to those seen in an electrically induced hippocampal afterdischarge. Thereafter, low-frequency spikes appear, followed by a theta rhythm with gradually increasing amplitude. The activity recorded from the overlying neocortex during a nicotine-induced hippocampus seizure is similar to the hippocampal activity and seems to be due merely to volume conduction from the hippocampus. The hippocampus seizure activity spreads slowly to the septum. Seizure discharges in the septum start later than in the hippocampus and last much longer; spike activity can be recorded from the septum

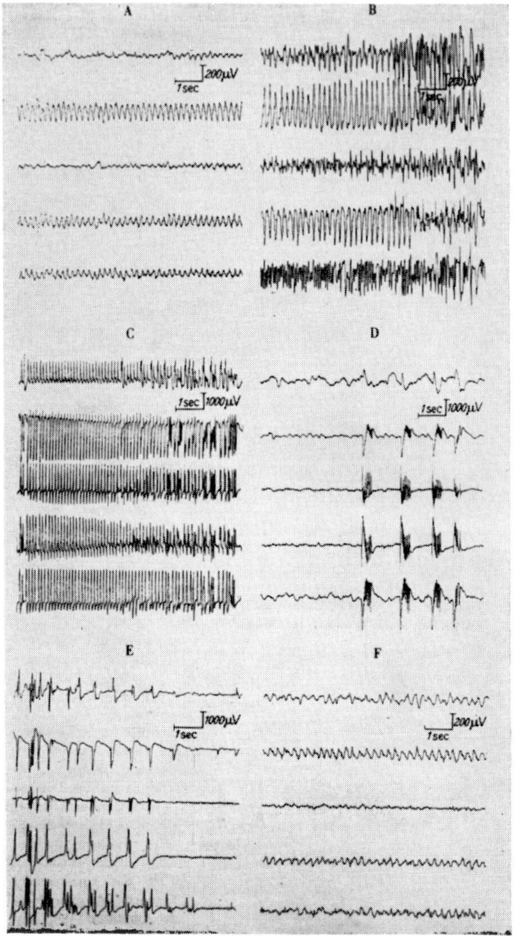

FIG. 5. Hippocampal activity of a rabbit after intravenous injection of 3 mg/kg nicotine bitartrate. A, 6–14 seconds; B, 22–30 seconds; C, 42–56 seconds; D, 64–72 seconds; E, 82–90 seconds; F, 130–138 seconds after injection. Theta rhythm (A) followed by seizure discharges (B to E). Taken from Stumpf (1959).

at a time when in the hippocampus theta rhythm has reappeared again. There is no correlation between the hippocampal seizure discharges and the convulsions of the animal. In animals with septal lesions, the nicotine-induced changes of hippocampal activity become dissociated—the theta rhythm is replaced by a high-frequency, low-amplitude activity, whereas the hippocampal seizure activity appears to be unchanged indicating that the theta rhythm, but not the seizure activity depends on the integrity of the septum. The action of nicotine on the hippocampal activity seems to be relatively specific: lobeline, cytisine, as well as various amino-nicotines, aminobromonicotines, and oxynicotines do not possess such an action although these compounds have nicotine-like actions on peripheral organs. The dose of nicotine necessary to induce hippocampal seizure discharges depends on the room temperature at which the animals are kept for about 24 hours prior to the experiment. Similar results have been reported by Tokizane and Sawyer (1957) for seizure activity due to hypoglycemia. Furthermore, there is a similar correlation between the dose of nicotine and temperature when behavioral convulsions are taken as criterion (Formanek and Lindner, 1960).

An investigation on the action of nicotine on the firing pattern of hippocampal neurons was carried out by Dunlop *et al.* (1960). Nicotine-induced regularization of hippocampal activity is accompanied by an increased firing rate of these neurons whereas they stop firing as soon as the hippocampal seizure activity commences. Therefore, the nicotine-induced theta rhythm is similar in every respect to a theta rhythm induced by eserine. The depression of hippocampal unit activity during nicotine-induced seizure discharges is nonspecific insofar as a similar depression has been observed during electrically induced afterdischarges (von Euler *et al.*, 1958).

Finally, a study on the firing pattern of neurons of the medial septal nucleus after administration of nicotine (Stumpf *et al.*, 1962) has lead to the following results: during the first phase of nicotine action when there is a theta rhythm in the hippocampus, the septal neurons discharge in bursts correlated to the phase of the theta waves, in the same way as during an eserine-induced theta rhythm. For various periods of time after the onset of the hippocampal seizure activity, the septal neurons continue to discharge in bursts as during the initial theta rhythm. Thereafter, the burst firing pattern disappears and the firing pattern is sometimes, but not necessarily, correlated with the hippocampal seizure discharges. From this, and from the effect of a septal lesion, it follows that the nicotine-induced theta rhythm is produced by impulses reaching the hippocampus via the septum whereas this is not true for the hippocampal seizure discharges.

None of the above-mentioned results could support the hypothesis that the nicotine-induced hippocampal seizure discharges are primary in this region. On the other hand, it seems safe to say that from the hippocampus the seizure activity spreads to the septum and radiates to the neocortex although the latter "radiation" may be simply due to volume conduction. Motor convulsions are correlated to the convulsive pattern in the neocortex (Silvestrini, 1958). For a more detailed discussion on this subject the reader is referred to the review by Silvette *et al.* (1962).

4. *Topical Application of Cholinergic Agents*

The experiments discussed under this topic were described by MacLean (1957) who injected cholinergic agents in crystalline form directly into the hippocampus of cats and recorded the hippocampal activity simultaneously and for longer periods after the injection.

Most characteristic are the changes in hippocampal activity obtained after application of carbachol; a few minutes after the injection, a 20 per second rhythmic activity appears either in groups or continuously for longer periods of time, superimposed on the theta rhythm with a tendency to be grouped near the peak of the falling phase of the slow waves. At the peak of drug action (45–60 minutes after injection) high-voltage spikes occur almost continuously. The EEG pattern at the end of drug action is similar to that during the first minutes after the injection until finally the theta rhythm predominates. Acetylcholine and eserine, when injected in combination, but not when given separately, induce changes similar to carbachol although more fleeting. Metacholine evokes a 4 per second theta rhythm with a superimposed fast 35 per second activity. It does not produce hippocampal spikes and for this reason its action is clearly different from that of carbachol or of ACh in combination with eserine. The difference in action between metacholine, on the one hand, and the other cholinergic agents, on the other, is interpreted as owing to the fact that metacholine has a muscarinic action whereas ACh and carbachol have both a muscarinic and nicotinic action.

After topical application of ACh in combination with eserine, and carbachol, electrically induced hippocampal afterdischarges show a prolonged recrudescence. Furthermore, light barbiturate anesthesia also aggravates the carbachol-induced seizure activity. Therefore, it was suggested by MacLean (1957) that electrical stimulation as well as anesthesia might induce a release of ACh.

It will be recalled, as mentioned previously, that barbiturates produce spiking in the hippocampus (see Section III,A,2,*b*). The significance of the fact that cholinergic drugs applied directly into the hippocampus produce a theta rhythm, has been discussed in Section III,A,1,*a*.

5. *Cyclohexamine Derivatives*

Two cyclohexamine derivatives [1-(phenylcyclohexyl)piperidine monohydrochloride, Sernyl; and *n*-ethyl-1-phenylcyclohexylamine monohydrochloride, cyclohexamine), both hallucinogenic drugs (Lear *et al.,* 1959), were found to produce seizure spiking in hippocampus and entorhinal area from 8 to 16 hours after administration, and to abolish the hippocampal theta rhythm during the approach performance few minutes after administration (Adey and Dunlop, 1960).

C. Miscellaneous Drugs

1. *Lysergic Acid Diethylamide (LSD)*

LSD has a highly specific and rather peculiar action on the electrical activity of the brain. The first investigation of the EEG effects of LSD after systemic administration revealed that this drug produces a flattening of the electrocortical activity in the rabbit (Delay *et al.,* 1952). Reinvestigations confirmed this finding in the rabbit (Longo, 1962; Rinaldi and Himwich, 1955a) and cat (Bradley and Elkes, 1953a). Some authors reported that LSD in addition to this effect produces bursts of high-voltage sinusoidal waves with a frequency of about 4 per second in the electrocorticogram of cats (Passouant *et al.,* 1956b) and rabbits (Sailer and Stumpf, 1957b). In a few studies the effects of increasing doses of LSD have been investigated. Rinaldi and Himwich (1955a) maintain that while low doses (10–15 μg/kg) produce a flattening, higher doses of LSD (20–60 μg/kg) cause slow waves and sleep spindles in the electrocorticogram, and Schallek and Kuehn (1959) found a slight decrease of the frequency of the electrocortical activity of cats after 0.1 mg/kg LSD. The significance of these findings remains obscure, but it is known that the LSD-induced EEG changes depend to some extent not only on the dosage but also on the environmental conditions (Bradley and Elkes, 1957). Most investigators, however, found quantitative, but not qualitative, changes of the electrocortical activity under the influence of increasing doses of LSD (Longo, 1962; Passouant *et al.*, 1956b; and others).

The electrocorticogram after LSD is similar to that seen during an arousal reaction. For this reason it has been stated that LSD (in low doses) produces "a long lasting presence of a pattern of alertness, practically indistinguishable from the normal one" (Rinaldi and Himwich, 1955a). Bradley and Elkes (1953a) found many common features in the EEG patterns elicited by LSD and amphetamine, but they emphasized important differences which do exist between these two patterns. Purpura (1957) concluded "that the electrographic picture common to reticular stimulation and the action of LSD does not indicate a direct action of LSD on the brain stem reticular formation, but a diffuse effect on cortical as well as subcortical synapses." It will be seen later that under LSD not even changes of hippocampal activity characteristic for an arousal reaction can be observed.

It will be recalled that the EEG changes during an arousal reaction elicited by sensory or reticular stimulation consist of low voltage, high-frequency activity in the neocortex and high voltage, low-frequency activity (theta rhythm) in the hippocampus (Green and Arduini, 1954). Simultaneous recording from both neocortex and hippocampus after administration of LSD shows that in this case the correspondence between these two activities is lost. In the cat, Passouant *et al.* (1956b) found that whereas LSD has a marked influence on the electrical activity of the neocortex, it scarcely produces any change of the hippocampal activity. In addition, arousal stimuli do not modify this latter activity after LSD. In the rabbit, Sailer and Stumpf (1957b) reported that after LSD the hippocampal activity becomes similar in appearance to the electrocortical activity, this is to say, both activities show a pronounced flattening. Similar results were obtained by Longo (1962) who correctly points out that "the EEG picture evoked by LSD is clearly distinct from the activation pattern seen either after external or reticular stimulations or after administration of the so-called 'desynchronizing drugs,' eserine and amphetamine." According to this latter author, the EEG changes seen under LSD are more similar to the EEG pattern obtained by 5-hydroxytryptophan (see later) or during a spreading depression (Leao, 1944). Doses of LSD necessary to produce EEG changes in direction of the above mentioned pattern start at 20 to 30 μg/kg, and complete flattening of neocortical and hippocampal activity occurs after doses of 100 to 150 μg/kg in the rabbit. LSD not only does not produce a theta rhythm in the rabbit's hippocampus, it also is able to depress the theta rhythm induced by eserine (Sailer and Stumpf, 1957b) or by reticular stimulation (Longo, 1962).

The flattening of the hippocampal activity caused by LSD is associated with a depression of the spontaneous discharges of hippocampal pyramidal neurons. The discharge rate of these neurons is more easily depressed by LSD than is the hippocampus EEG so that, for instance, small doses (10–25 μg/kg) occasionally decrease the spontaneous discharge rate of pyramidal neurons without affecting the hippocampus EEG. Higher doses (100 μg/kg) depress the unity activity completely. When trains of a few theta waves occur occasionally during the action of LSD, this change in hippocampal activity is associated with a rapid increase of the discharge rate of pyramidal neurons. Eserine, given after LSD, may produce a theta rhythm and an increase in the discharge rate of pyramidal neurons, but these effects can again be abolished by another dose of LSD (Fig. 6). The discharge rate of dentate gyrus granule cells is not affected by LSD (Brücke *et al.*, 1961).

The disappearance of the hippocampal theta rhythm and the depression of the firing rate of pyramidal neurons caused by LSD could be due either to an inhibition of the afferent inflow into the hippocampus via the septum, or to an action of LSD on the hippocampus itself. In order to differentiate between these two possibilities, the action of LSD on the firing pattern of septal neurons in rabbits pretreated with eserine has been investigated (Stumpf *et al.*, 1962). Under the influence of eserine the neurons of the medial septal nucleus discharge in bursts and as a consequence a theta rhythm develops in the hippocampus (see Section III,A,1,*a*). LSD in doses of 100 μg/kg abolishes the eserine-induced hippocampal theta rhythm, but does not change the burst firing pattern of septal neurons at all. Thus, under LSD the septal neurons continue to generate impulses which under normal conditions would cause a theta rhythm to arise in the hippocampus. If, nevertheless, no theta rhythm is recorded under the action of LSD, the depression of this activity must be due to an action of LSD on synapses between the septum and hippocampus, or in the hippocampus itself. This hypothesis is supported by the finding that responses to septal stimulation evoked in the hippocampus are depressed by LSD (Brücke *et al.,* 1961). Since, as mentioned earlier, LSD depresses the spontaneous discharges of pyramidal neurons, but not

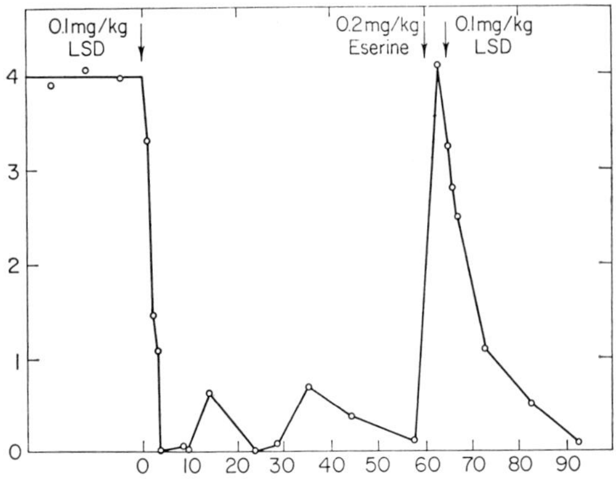

FIG. 6. Discharge rate of a hippocampus pyramidal neuron after intravenous injections of LSD and eserine. Abscissa: time in minutes after first LSD injection. Ordinate: number of action potentials per second. Taken from Brücke *et al.* (1961).

that of granule cells, a depressant action on the synapses formed between septohippocampal fibers and pyramidal neurons might be postulated. LSD is known to block the transmission of many central synapses, but marked differences in the sensitivity of various synapses exist (cf. Evarts, 1957). Curtis and Davis (1962) found that electrophoretically applied LSD depresses the orthodromic excitation of neurons of the lateral geniculate nucleus. In comparing this effect with the depressant action of LSD on hippocampal neurons (Brücke *et al.,* 1961), they discuss the possibility that the transmitter for the excitation of both types of synapses may be the same, or that the action on hippocampal neurons may be due to an antagonism of LSD against the synaptic action of 5-hydroxytryptamine.

In this connection it is worthwhile to mention the results of experiments carried out by Purpura (1957) on the action of LSD on the electrocortical activity of cats. LSD is thought to activate "inhibitory synapses on dendrites that are also available to the transmitter or transmitters that are released by reticular stimulation of the brain stem." It has been shown recently that inhibitory synapses also exist in the hippocampus (Andersen *et al.*, 1963). In summary, the exact mode of action of LSD on hippocampal neurons remains to be explained. It may be concluded, however, that the action of LSD on neocortex and hippocampus is similar in the respect that it is a direct action on the neurons in these structures rather than an action which would modify the afferent inflow.

2. *5-Hydroxytryptamine (5-HT) and 5-Hydroxytryptophan (5-HTP)*

Contradictory results have been reported on the action of 5-HT (serotonin) on the electrical activity of the brain. Longo (1962) found no changes of the electrical activity of the rabbit's brain after intravenous doses of 5-HT of up to 0.1 mg/kg. Higher doses produced an over-all diminution of the brain waves, possibly due to hypotension. He found only minor EEG changes after intracarotid injection of 0.1 to 0.2 mg 5-HT. On the other hand, Mantegazzini (1957) reported a desynchronization of the electrocortical activity in the cat encéphale isolé preparation after injection of 5-HT into the cerebral circulation, comparable to that seen after ACh applied by the same route. A bi- or triphasic action of intravenously administered 5-HT on the EEG (activation—deactivation—activation) has been demonstrated in the cat (Rothballer, 1957) and rabbit (Gangloff and Monnier, 1957). The latter authors emphasized the similarity in the EEG patterns produced by 5-HT and reserpine. During the late phase under the influence of both drugs, a "mixed arousal and relaxation pattern" with a continuous, rather slow (3–5 per second) theta rhythm in the hippocampus, thalamus, and parieto-occipital cortex was found to prevail. It is perhaps surprising that 5-HT when given by intravenous injection, does produce any EEG changes, since passage of 5-HT into the brain is believed to be difficult (Udenfriend *et al.*, 1957) or possible to a limited extent only (Costa and Aprison, 1958). Revzin and Costa (1960), in studying the effect of exogenous 5-HT (1 mg/kg intravenously) on the hippocampal response to amygdala stimulation in a modified cat cerveau isolé preparation, found that this effect does not occur after vagotomy. They point out that "exogenous 5-HT probably does not affect neurons excitability" and has no direct synaptic action in the central nervous system.

5-Hydroxytryptophan, the precursor of 5-HT, readily passes the blood–brain barrier and is decarboxylated in the central nervous system to 5-HT (Udenfriend *et al.*, 1956). The hippocampus has been found to contain rather high concentrations of 5-hydroxytryptamine decarboxylase (Bogdanski *et al.*, 1957). Changes of the hippocampal activity, together with other EEG changes, have consistently been found to occur after 5-HTP administration.

a. Action of 5-HTP on Hippocampal Activity after Intravenous Injection. Costa and Rinaldi (1958) found that in rabbits after intravenous injection of 75 mg/kg of 5-HTP first a slow, high-voltage activity appears in all brain areas including the hippocampus where, at the same time, the theta rhythm disappears. Later, for a period lasting from the second half-hour to the second hour after the injection, the neocortical and hippocampal activity show a marked voltage drop and, therefore, appear more or less flat. During this stage the EEG changes produced by 5-HTP and LSD are very similar (Longo, 1962) although Costa and Rinaldi (1958) deny this similarity. The reason for this disagreement probably lies in the fact that Rinaldi and Himwich (1955a) had not found a flattening of hippocampal activity under LSD, as had other authors, including Longo (1962) (see Section III,C,1).

Other investigators described rhinencephalic spike discharges under the influence of 5-HTP. According to Monnier and Tissot (1958), 10–20 mg/kg cause slow wave activity, whereas higher doses (30 mg/kg) induce a flattening of the neocortical and hippocampal activity, and also (about 1 hour after the injection) spiking in the hippocampus. These findings are similar to those obtained by Domer and Longo (1962) who described the effects of 5-HTP given in form of repeated intravenous injections or by continuous intravenous infusion, on the electrical activity of the rabbit's brain. The first change seen in the hippocampal activity consists of disruption of the theta rhythm whereas higher doses cause spike discharges in the hippocampus at a frequency of 30 to 40 per second. The spiking can also be recorded from the amygdala and fornix, and occasionally it can be activated by external stimuli. In this case the 30–40 per second spike activity is superimposed on the theta rhythm. When single doses are given, a dose of 50 to 100 mg/kg is necessary to produce bursts of hippocampal spikes, whereas with continuous intravenous infusion (5 mg/minute), spiking starts after a total dose of 30 to 50 mg/kg and reaches its maximum after a dose of 75 or 125 mg/kg. During the hippocampal spike discharges the firing rate of hippocampal pyramidal neurons is markedly depressed (de Baran *et al.*, 1963).

It is interesting to note that with 5-HTP, as with other drugs which produce hippocampal spike discharges, these discharges can be recorded from the hippocampus as well as from the amygdala. The depression of the theta rhythm has been assumed to be due to a direct action of 5-HTP on hippocampal neurons (Domer and Longo, 1962). Unfortunately, there are no experimental data available on the action of 5-HTP on the discharge pattern of septal neurons, which would allow a conclusion to be drawn as to whether the disappearance of the theta rhythm under 5-HTP is due to an action similar to that producing the disappearance of this activity under LSD.

b. Action of 5-HTP on Hippocampal Activity after Intracarotid Injection. Costa *et al.* (1960) found that in rabbits intracarotid injection of 22 or 44 mg 5-HTP causes a biphasic EEG pattern in that a neocortical synchronization is followed by desynchronization. During the first stage an irregular activity and, during the second stage, a theta rhythm were found in the hippocampus. It was suggested that 5-HTP acts directly upon some region of the reticular formation. A positive correlation was found to exist between the elevation of 5-HT content in the mesodiencephalon and the EEG changes caused by 5-HTP, and a continuous theta rhythm (and a desynchronization of the neocortical activity) occurred when the 5-HT content in the mid-brain showed a threefold increase. DL-5-Methyltryptophan which is not a precursor of 5-HT neither caused EEG changes nor did it alter the 5-HT content of the brain.

No plausible explanation can be offered for the fact that 5-HTP, when injected intravenously, caused a disappearance of the theta rhythm and rhinencephalic spike discharges whereas, when injected intracarotidly, it induced a late arousal reaction with a theta rhythm in the hippocampus.

3. *Tryptamine*

Tryptamine is mentioned here since its action on the EEG, and especially on the hippocampal activity, is very similar to that of 5-HTP when both drugs are given in comparable intravenous doses to rabbits. Single doses of 15 to 25 mg/kg tryptamine produce in the hippocampus a flattening associated with disappearance of the theta rhythm and occurrence of spiking but, in contrast to 5-HTP, these changes last for about 5 minutes only (Domer and Longo, 1962; Longo, 1962).

The tryptamine-induced depression of the hippocampal theta rhythm is associated with a marked decrease of the spontaneous firing rate of pyramidal neurons. Often, at the peak of tryptamine action, these neurons do not discharge at all. Neurons in the subiculum behave as pyramidal neurons do. The spontaneous firing rate of granule cells of the dentate gyrus, on the other hand, shows frequently a tremendous increase under tryptamine. The firing rate of these neurons may increase to such a frequency that intermittent prolonged partial depolarization of the cell membrane occurs (de Baran *et al.*, 1963). It will be recalled that, under LSD, granule cells also behave differently when compared with pyramidal neurons although no increase in the firing rate of granule cells was observed under LSD. Possibly, the tryptamine-induced discharge pattern of granule cells is in some way related to the high-frequency spike discharges in the hippocampus EEG.

It will be noted that in many respects the actions of LSD, 5-HTP, and tryptamine on the hippocampal activity and unit firing pattern have been found to be similar. In this connection it is of interest that according to Curtis and Davis (1962) all three drugs depress orthodromic excitation of neurons in the lateral geniculate nucleus of the cat when applied electrophoretically close to the neuron under observation.

IV. Conclusions and Summary

The question may well be posed whether any useful conclusions can be drawn from the consideration of the actions of various drugs on only one area of the brain. This may be done, however, if certain limitations are kept in mind. In any event, the consideration of the actions of drugs on the hippocampus has allowed the separation of drugs with probably different modes of actions where this has not been possible by the study of cortical or brain stem rhythms.

The aim of neuropharmacological experimentation of any kind is primarily to clarify the mode and site of action of the drug under investigation. The hippocampus is connected by afferent and efferent pathways with many other brain areas and, therefore, a drug-induced change of hippocampal activity does not necessarily indicate a drug action on the hippocampus itself. For instance, the hippocampus receives impulses from the brain stem reticular formation, as do the neocortex and other brain areas. Consequently, any drug which acts upon the reticular formation, may modify the hippocampal activity, just as it may modify the electrical activity of the neocortex and other brain areas. Problems concerning drug action on the reticular formation have deliberately been touched upon only rarely in this review since changes of hippocampal activity due to the action of drugs on the reticular formation would comprise only a small part of the EEG changes occurring in the brain. However, with some drugs it has been shown that changes of neocortical activity corresponding to an arousal reaction may not justify the assumption that such changes are due to a stimulatory action on the reticular formation. For instance, LSD produces in the neocortex, but not in the hippocampus, electrographic changes corresponding to an arousal reaction.

The most conspicuous hippocampal activity is the 4–7 per second "theta rhythm" which may be elicited by sensory or reticular stimulation, or by various drugs. The properties of this rhythm and its origin have been discussed. Briefly, the theta rhythm shows a monopolar phase reversal at a level just below the pyramidal cell layer indicating that this rhythm is not propagated along an axis normal to the surface of the hippocampus. On the other hand, a slow propagation along this surface does take place. The frequency of the theta rhythm is positively correlated with the intensity of stimulation. The pacemaker for the theta rhythm is located in the medial septal nucleus, the neurons of which discharge in bursts correlated to the phase of the hippocampal theta rhythm. Lesions of this septal nucleus consequently abolish the theta rhythm. Arousal stimuli activate hippocampal fast activity in addition to the theta rhythm, and this fast activity does not depend on the integrity of the septum.

Microelectrode experiments on the firing pattern of hippocampal and septal neurons after drug administration have given valuable information. It has sometimes been inferred that microelectrode experiments do not have much value in pharmacological studies for the simple reason that neurons of the same area or nucleus may react entirely differently to the same drug. Fortunately, this statement seems to be untrue for neurons of the hippocampus and of the medial septal nucleus. With very few exceptions, individual pyramidal cells have been found to react similarly to a given drug; likewise, individual granule cells react similarly though, of course, pyramidal cells and granule cells may react differently in response to a single drug. Septal neurons, moreover, react in a like manner without exception. Probably, this is a consequence of the fact that the hippocampus is one of the most uniform structures within the brain, and together with the medial septal nucleus apparently forms one functional entity.

Drugs may modify the hippocampal activity in various ways: some drugs produce a theta rhythm; some inhibit the theta rhythm; some produce seizure-like discharge patterns; and some cause a flattening of the hippocampal activity. Rather than attempting a complete coverage of all drugs known to influence hippocampal activity, a few drugs representing each type of action have been discussed in order to outline the problems involved.

Many drugs produce a theta rhythm—some cholinergic and adrenergic agents, nicotine in low doses, ethyl ether and reserpine during certain phases of their action, and chlorpromazine in high doses. In all these cases, the hippocampal theta rhythm is associated with low-voltage, high-frequency activity in the neocortex. In these cases, neocortical and hippocampal activity resemble the modifications seen during the usual arousal reaction. The data presented in this review can neither support nor contradict the hypothesis that some or all of the above drugs produce a pure arousal reaction. It is known, however, that in all cases investigated so far a drug-induced theta rhythm is abolished by septal lesions. Therefore, in all of these cases, the theta rhythm cannot be due to an action on the hippocampus itself. For eserine and nicotine, it has been demonstrated that these two drugs influence the septal neurons to adopt a burst firing pattern which apparently triggers the theta rhythm. Therefore, an action on these septal cells, or, more likely, on a lower level, has to be postulated. Slight differences have been found to exist between the theta rhythms induced by eserine and methamphetamine. The theta rhythm elicited by sensory or reticular stimulation is more similar to the rhythm induced by eserine than to that induced by methamphetamine.

Some anticholinergic drugs, anesthetics, and tranquilizers inhibit the theta rhythm. Low doses of such drugs usually decrease the frequency of a theta rhythm induced by reticular stimulation or eserine. Scopolamine is a notable exception in that it does not decrease the frequency of a theta rhythm elicited by reticular stimulation while reducing the frequency of the eserine-induced theta rhythm. With scopolamine and barbiturates the depression of the eserine-induced theta rhythm is associated with corresponding changes in the firing pattern of septal neurons. Thus, the action of these drugs on the hippocampal activity may be assumed to be due to an action on the septal neurons, or, more likely, on a lower level. Urethan has a different type of action under similar experimental conditions: at a dose level that completely abolishes all regularized hippocampal activity, the septal neurons continue to discharge in bursts although at a much lower rate. Consequently, an additional direct action of urethan on the hippocampus may be postulated.

Seizure activity occurs in the hippocampus after insulin, nicotine, cyclohexamine derivatives, and intracarotid injection of hypertonic solutions. Seizure activity or at least spiking has also been reported to occur after barbiturates, ethyl ether, high doses of chlorpromazine, reserpine, 5-HTP, and tryptamine. Such discharges have frequently been found in hippocampus and/or amygdala, sometimes, as after high doses of chlorpromazine, apparently starting in the amygdala. The nicotine-induced hippocampal seizure discharges are associated with a depression of pyramidal neuron activity and are not changed by septal lesions. This is probably true for other drug-induced seizure activities as well. Two explanations for the preferential site of drug-induced seizure discharges have been discussed. One explanation assumes that the low seizure threshold of rhinencephalic structures is responsible; the other one assumes a specific affinity of a drug for these structures. Certain cholinergic agents injected into the hippocampus have been found to produce theta rhythms and seizure discharges. Further experimentation is needed before these theta rhythms can be postulated to be due to a direct action on the hippocampus.

LSD has a unique action on hippocampal activity. Under LSD neocortical and hippocampal activity show a pronounced flattening of the hippocampal activity which is associated with a depression of the spontaneous firing of pyramidal neurons. Since LSD does not affect the eserine-induced burst firing patterns of septal neurons and, nevertheless, depresses the hippocampal theta rhythm, it is postulated that the latter effect is due to a direct action on the hippocampus itself, probably on synapses formed between septo-hippocampal fibers and pyramidal neurons. Tryptamine and 5-HTP induce a similar flattening of the hippocampal activity and, in addition, spike discharges associated with depression of pyramidal neuron activity. Under LSD and tryptamine, single neuron activity of the dentate gyrus is influenced in a different manner than pyramidal neuron activity; the granule cells of the dentate gyrus are scarcely influenced by LSD whereas their firing is markedly accelerated by tryptamine.

Acknowledgment

The author is greatly indebted to Dr. Harry L. Williams for reading the manuscript and for helping with the presentation.

References

Adey, W. R. (1959). *Intern. Rev. Neurobiol.* **1,** 1.

Adey, W. R. (1962). *Colloq. Intern. Centre Natl. Rech. Sci.* (*Paris*) No. 107, p. 203.

Adey, W. R., and Dunlop, C. W. (1960). *J. Pharmacol. Exptl. Therap.* **130,** 418.

Adey, W. R., Merrillees, N. C. R., and Sunderland, S. (1956). *Brain* **79,** 413.

Adey, W. R., Sunderland, S., and Dunlop, C. W. (1957). *Electroencephalog. Clin. Neurophysiol.* **9,** 309.

Adey, W. R., Dunlop, C. W., and Hendrix, C. E. (1960). *Arch. Neurol.* **3,** 74.

Adrian, E. D., and Matthews, B. H. C. (1934). *J. Physiol.* (*London*) **81,** 440.

Andersen, P., Bruland, H., and Kaada, B. R. (1961). *Acta Physiol. Scand.* **51,** 17, 29.

Andersen, P., Eccles, J. C., and Løyning, Y. (1963). *Nature* **198,** 540.

Andy, O. J., and Stephan, H. (1961). *J. Comp. Neurol.* **117,** 251.

Arduini, A., and Arduini, M. G. (1954). *J. Pharmacol. Exptl. Therap.* **110,** 76.

Arduini, A., and Pompeiano, O. (1955). *Arch. Sci. Biol.* (*Bologna*) **39,** 397.

Ariëns Kappers, C. U., Huber, G. C., and Crosby, E. C. (1936). "The Comparative Anatomy of the Nervous System of Vertebrates Including Man," Vols. I and II, 1845 pp. Macmillan, New York.

Bard, P., and Rioch, D. McK. (1937). *Bull. Johns Hopkins Hosp.* **60,** 63.

Beecher, H. K., and McDonough, F. K. (1939). *J. Neurophysiol.* **2,** 289.

Bishop, G. H. (1949). *Electroencephalog. Clin. Neurophysiol.* **1,** 421.

Bogdanski, D. F., Weissbach, H., and Udenfriend, J. (1957). *J. Neurochem.* **1,** 272.

Bohdanecký, Z., Weiss, T., and Fifková, E. (1963). *Arch. Intern. Pharmacodyn.* **143,** 23.

Bonnet, V., and Bremer, F. (1937). *Compt. Rend. Soc. Biol.* **126**, 1271.
Bradley, P. B., and Elkes, J. (1953a). *J. Physiol.* (*London*) **120**, 13P.
Bradley, P. B., and Elkes, J. (1953b). *J. Physiol.* (*London*) **120**, 14P.
Bradley, P. B., and Elkes, J. (1957). *Brain* **80**, 77.
Bradley, P. B., and Nicholson, A. N. (1962). *Electroencephalog. Clin. Neurophysiol.* **14**, 824.
Bradley, P. B., Cerquiglini, S., and Elkes, J. (1953). *J. Physiol.* (*London*) **121**, 51P.
Bremer, F. (1935). *Compt. Rend. Soc. Biol.* **118**, 1241.
Bremer, F. (1936). *Compt. Rend. Soc. Biol.* **121**, 861.
Bremer, F. (1958). *Physiol. Rev.* **38**, 357.
Bremer, F., and Chatonnet, J. (1949). *Arch. Intern. Physiol.* **57**, 106.
Brodal, A. (1947). *Brain* **70**, 179.
Brooks, D. C. (1962). *Am. J. Physiol.* **202**, 1221.
Brücke, F., Sailer, S., and Stumpf, C. (1957). *Arch. Exptl. Pathol. Pharmakol.* **231**, 267.
Brücke, F., Sailer, S., and Stumpf, C. (1958). *Arch. Exptl. Pathol. Pharmakol.* **232**, 433.
Brücke, F., Petsche, H., Pillat, B., and Deisenhammer, E. (1959a). *Arch. Exptl. Pathol. Pharmakol.* **237**, 276.
Brücke, F., Petsche, H., Pillat, B., and Deisenhammer, E. (1959b). *Arch. Ges. Physiol.* **269**, 319.
Brücke, F., Gogolák, G., and Stumpf, C. (1961). *Arch. Exptl. Pathol. Pharmakol.* **240**, 461.
Brücke, F., Gogolák, G., and Stumpf, C. (1963). *Arch. Ges. Physiol.* **276**, 456.
Bureš, J., Bohdanecký, Z., and Weiss, T. (1962). *Psychopharmacologia* **3**, 254.
Burgen, A. S. V., and Chipman, L. M. (1951). *J. Physiol.* (*London*) **114**, 296.
Cadilhac, J., and Passouant-Fontaine, T. (1962). *Colloq. Intern. Centre Natl. Rech. Sci.* No. 107, p. 429.
Cajal, S. R. Y. (1909). "Histologie du système nerveux de l'homme et des vertebres," Vol. II, 993 pp. Maloine, Paris.
Cajal, S. R. Y. (1955). "Studies on the Cerebral Cortex (Limbic Structures)" (Trans. by Lisbeth M. Kraft), Vol. XI, 179 pp. Year Book Publ., Chicago, Illinois.
Carreras, M., Macci, G., Angeleri, F., and Urbani, M. (1955). *Boll. Soc. Ital. Biol. Sper.* **31**, 1.
Corazza, R., and Parmeggiani, P. L. (1963). *Helv. Physiol. Pharmacol. Acta* **21**, C10.
Costa, E., and Aprison, M. (1958). *Am. J. Physiol.* **192**, 95.
Costa, E., and Rinaldi, F. (1958). *Am. J. Physiol.* **194**, 214.
Costa, E., Pscheidt, G. R., van Meter, W. G., and Himwich, H. E. (1960). *J. Pharmacol. Exptl. Therap.* **130**, 81.
Cragg, B. G. (1961). *Exptl. Neurol.* **3**, 388.
Cragg, B. G., and Hamlyn, L. H. (1957). *J. Physiol.* (*London*) **135**, 460.
Cragg, B. G., and Hamlyn, L. H. (1959). *Exptl. Neurol.* **1**, 187.
Curtis, D. R., and Davis, R. (1962). *Brit. J. Pharmacol.* **18**, 217.

Daitz, H. M., and Powell, T. P. S. (1954). *J. Neurol. Neurosurg. Psychiat.* **17,** 75.

Das, N. N., Dasgupta, S. R., and Werner, G. (1954). *Arch. Intern. Pharmacodyn.* **99,** 451.

de Baran, L., Gogolák, G., Longo, V. G., and Stumpf, C. (1963). *J. Pharmacol. Exptl. Therap.* **139,** 337.

Deisenhammer, E., and Stumpf, C. (1960). *Arch. Exptl. Pathol. Pharmakol.* **239,** 481.

Delay, J., Lhermitte, F., Verdeaux, G., and Verdeaux, J. (1952). *Rev. Neurol.* **86,** 81.

Derbyshire, A. J., Rempel, B., Forbes, A., and Lambert, E. F. (1936). *Am. J. Physiol.* **116,** 577.

Desmedt, J. E., and La Grutta, G. (1957). *J. Physiol.* (*London*) **136,** 20.

Domer, F. R., and Longo, V. G. (1962). *Arch. Intern. Pharmacodyn.* **136,** 204.

Domino, E. F. (1962). *Ann. Rev. Pharmacol.* **2,** 215.

Domino, E. F., and Hudson, R. D. (1959). *J. Pharmacol. Exptl. Therap.* **127,** 305.

Domino, E. F., and Ueki, S. (1959). *J. Pharmacol. Exptl. Therap.* **127,** 288.

Droogleever-Fortuyn, J. (1956). *Acta Neurol. Psychiat. Belg.* **56,** 115.

Dunlop, C. W., Stumpf, C., Maxwell, D. S., and Schindler, W. (1960). *Am. J. Physiol.* **198,** 515.

Eccles, J. C. (1964). "The Physiology of Synapses," 316 pp. Springer, Berlin.

Eccles, J. C., Eccles, R. M., and Lundberg, A. (1957). *Nature* **179,** 866.

Edinger, L. (1904). "Bau der nervösen Zentralorgane," 398 pp. Vogel, Leipzig.

Eidelberg, E., White, J. C., and Brazier, M. A. B. (1959). *Exptl. Neurol.* **1,** 483.

Ellioth Smith, G. (1910). Quoted by Adey *et al.* (1960).

Evarts, E. V. (1957). *Ann. N. Y. Acad. Sci.* **66,** 479.

Exley, K. A., Fleming, M. C., and Espelien, A. D. (1958). *Brit. J. Pharmacol.* **13,** 485.

Feldberg, W., and Vogt, M. (1948). *J. Physiol.* (*London*) **107,** 372.

Formanek, K., and Lindner, A. (1960). *Wien. Klin. Wochschr.* **110,** 461.

Freeman, W. J. (1963). *Intern. Rev. Neurobiol.* **5,** 53.

French, J. D., Verzeano, M., and Magoun, H. W. (1953). *A.M.A. Arch. Neurol. Psychiat.* **69,** 519.

Funderburk, W. H., and Case, J. (1951). *Electroencephalog. Clin. Neurophysiol.* **3,** 213.

Funderburk, W. H., and Woodcock, R. T. (1957). *J. Pharmacol. Exptl. Therap.* **119,** 148.

Gangloff, H., and Monnier, M. (1955). *Experientia* **11,** 404.

Gangloff, H., and Monnier, M. (1956). *Electroencephalog. Clin. Neurophysiol.* **8,** 623.

Gangloff, H., and Monnier, M. (1957). *Helv. Physiol. Pharmacol. Acta* **15,** 83.

Gerebtzoff, M. A. (1939). *J. Belge Neurol. Psychiat.* **39,** 205.

Gerebtzoff, M. A. (1941–1942). *J. Belge Neurol. Psychiat.* **41–42,** 199.

Gerebtzoff, M. A. (1960). *In* "Structure and Function of the Cerebral Cortex" (D. B. Tower and J. P. Schade, eds.), p. 334. Elsevier, Amsterdam.
Gibbs, F. A., and Gibbs, E. L. (1936). *A.M.A. Arch. Neurol. Psychiat.* **35**, 109.
Gloor, P. (1954). *Electroencephalog. Clin. Neurophysiol.* **6**, 711.
Gloor, P., Vera, C. L., and Sperti, L. (1936a). *Electroencephalog. Clin. Neurophysiol.* **15**, 353.
Gloor, P., Sperti, L., and Vera, C. L. (1963b). *Electroencephalog. Clin. Neurophysiol.* **15**, 379.
Gogolák, G., Petsche, H., and Stumpf, C. (1963). *Arch. Ges. Physiol.* **277**, 166.
Gogolák, G., Petsche, H., and van Zwieten, P. (1964). *Arch. Exptl. Pathol. Pharmakol.* **249**, 446.
Goodwin, J. E., Lloyd, D. P. C., and Hall, G. E. (1938). *Proc. Soc. Exptl. Biol. Med.* **38**, 897.
Granit, R., and Phillips, C. G. (1956). *J. Physiol.* (*London*) **133**, 520.
Grastyán, E., Lissák, K., Madarász, I., and Donhoffer, H. (1959). *Electroencephalog. Clin. Neurophysiol.* **11**, 409.
Green, J. D. (1960). *In* "Handbook of Physiology" (J. Field, ed.), Sec. I, p. 1373. Am. J. Physiol. Soc., Washington, D. C.
Green, J. D., and Adey, W. R. (1956). *Electroencephalog. Clin. Neurophysiol.* **8**, 245.
Green, J. D., and Arduini, A. (1954). *J. Neurophysiol.* **17**, 533.
Green, J. D., and Machne, X. (1955). *Am. J. Physiol.* **181**, 219.
Green, J. D., and Petsche, H. (1961). *Electroencephalog. Clin. Neurophysiol.* **13**, 847.
Green, J. D., and Shimamoto, T. (1953). *A.M.A. Arch. Neurol. Psychiat.* **70**, 687.
Green, J. D., Maxwell, D. S., Schindler, W. J., and Stumpf, C. (1960). *J. Neurophysiol.* **23**, 403.
Green, J. D., Maxwell, D. S., and Petsche, H. (1961). *Electroencephalog. Clin. Neurophysiol.* **13**, 854.
Grundfest, H. (1957). *Ann. N. Y. Acad. Sci.* **66**, 537.
Hiebel, G., Bonvallet, M., Huvé, P., and Dell, P. (1954a). *Semaine Hop. Paris* **30**, 1880.
Hiebel, G., Bonvallet, M., and Dell, P. (1954b). *Semaine Hop. Paris* **30**, 2346.
Hukuhara, T. (1962). *Arzneimittel-Forsch.* **12**, 1133.
Johnston, J. B. (1923). *J. Comp. Neurol.* **35**, 337.
Jung, R. (1949). *Arch. Psychiat. Nervenkr.* **183**, 206.
Jung, R., and Kornmüller, A. E. (1938). *Arch. Psychiat. Nervenkrankh.* **109**, 1.
Kaada, B. R. (1951). *Acta Physiol. Scand.* **24** Suppl. 83, 1.
Kandel, E. R., and Spencer, W. A. (1961). *J. Neurophysiol.* **24**, 243.
Kandel, E. R., Spencer, W. A., and Brinley, F. J., Jr. (1961). *J. Neurophysiol.* **24**, 225.
Killam, K. E., and Killam, K. F. (1956). *J. Pharmacol. Exptl. Therap.* **116**, 35.

Kim, C., and MacLean, P. D. (1956). *Electroencephalog. Clin. Neurophysiol.* **8,** 524.
Leao, A. A. P. (1944). *J. Neurophysiol.* **7,** 359.
Lear, E., Suntay, R., Pallin, I. M., and Chiron, A. E. (1959). *Anesthesiology* **20,** 330.
Liberson, W. T., and Akert, K. (1953). *Electroencephalog. Clin. Neurophysiol.* **5,** 320.
Liberson, W. T., and Akert, K. (1955). *Electroencephalog. Clin. Neurophysiol.* **7,** 211.
Longo, V. G. (1955). *Experientia* **11,** 76.
Longo, V. G. (1956). *J. Pharmacol. Exptl. Therap.* **116,** 198.
Longo, V. G. (1962). "Rabbit Brain Research," Vol. II, 130 pp. Elsevier, Amsterdam.
Longo, V. G., and Bovet, D. (1952). *Boll. Soc. Ital. Biol. Sper.* **28,** 612.
Longo, V. G., and Silvestrini, B. (1957). *J. Pharmacol. Exptl. Therap.* **120,** 160.
Longo, V. G., von Berger, G. P., and Bovet, D. (1954). *J. Pharmacol. Exptl. Therap.* **111,** 349.
Loo, Y. T. (1931). *J. Comp. Neurol.* **52,** 1.
Lorente de Nó, R. (1934). *J. Psychol. Neurol.* **46,** 113.
MacLean, P. D. (1954). *J. Neurosurg.* **11,** 29.
MacLean, P. D. (1955). *Psychosomat. Med.* **17,** 355.
MacLean, P. D. (1957). *A.M.A. Arch. Neurol. Psychiat.* **78,** 113.
MacLean, P. D., Flanigan, S., Flynn, J. P., and Stevens, J. R. (1955–1956). *Yale J. Biol. Med.* **28,** 380.
Mantegazzini, P. (1957). *Arch. Intern. Pharmacodyn.* **112,** 199.
Mayer, C., and Stumpf, C. (1958a). *Experientia* **14,** 143.
Mayer, C., and Stumpf, C. (1958b). *Arch. Exptl. Pathol. Pharmakol.* **234,** 490.
Mettler, F. A. (1943). *J. Comp. Neurol.* **79,** 185.
Monnier, M. (1960). *Arch. Intern. Pharmacodyn.* **124,** 281.
Monnier, M., and Romanowski, W. (1962). *Electroencephalog. Clin. Neurophysiol.* **14,** 486.
Monnier, M., and Tissot, R. (1958). *Helv. Physiol. Pharmacol. Acta* **16,** 255.
Morin, F. (1950). *J. Comp. Neurol.* **92,** 193.
Moruzzi, G. (1938). *Compt. Rend. Soc. Biol.* **128,** 1181.
Moruzzi, G., and Magoun, H. W. (1949). *Electroencephalog. Clin. Neurophysiol.* **1,** 455.
Naquet, R. (1954). *Electroencephalog. Clin. Neurophysiol.* **6,** 711.
Passouant, P., Passouant-Fontaine, T., and Cadilhac, J. (1955a). *Compt. Rend. Soc. Biol.* **149,** 164.
Passouant, P., Cadilhac, J., and Passouant-Fontaine, T. (1955b). *J. Physiol. (Paris)* **47,** 715.
Passouant, P., Passouant-Fontaine, T., and Cadilhac, J. (1956a). *Compt. Rend. Soc. Biol.* **150,** 779.
Passouant, P., Passouant-Fontaine, T., and Cadilhac, J. (1956b). *Compt. Rend. Soc. Biol.* **150,** 2237.

Passouant, P., Passouant-Fontaine, T., and Cadilhac, J. (1957). *Compt. Rend. Soc. Biol.* **151**, 2166.
Petsche, H., and Stumpf, C. (1960). *Electroencephalog. Clin. Neurophysiol.* **12**, 589.
Petsche, H., Stumpf, C., and Gogolák, G. (1962). *Electroencephalog. Clin. Neurophysiol.* **14**, 202.
Pick, E. P. (1937). *Klin. Wochschr.* **16**, 1481.
Preston, J. B. (1956). *J. Pharmacol. Exptl. Therap.* **118**, 100.
Purpura, D. P. (1957). *Ann. N. Y. Acad. Sci.* **66**, 515.
Renshaw, B., Forbes, A., and Morison, B. R. (1940). *J. Neurophysiol.* **3**, 74.
Revzin, A. M., and Costa, E. (1960). *Am. J. Physiol.* **198**, 959.
Rinaldi, F. (1958). *J. Nervous Mental Disease* **126**, 272.
Rinaldi, F., and Himwich, H. E. (1955a). *J. Nervous Mental Disease* **122**, 424.
Rinaldi, F., and Himwich, H. E. (1955b). *Ann. N. Y. Acad. Sci.* **61**, 27.
Rinaldi, F., and Himwich, H. E. (1955c). *Diseases Nervous System* **16**, 133.
Rinaldi, F., and Himwich, H. E. (1955d). *A.M.A. Arch. Neurol. Psychiat.* **73**, 387, 397.
Rose, J. E., and Woolsey, C. N. (1948). *J. Comp. Neurol.* **89**, 279.
Rossi, G. F., and Zirondoli, A. (1955). *Electroencephalog. Clin. Neurophysiol.* **7**, 383.
Rothballer, A. B. (1957). *Electroencephalog. Clin. Neurophysiol.* **9**, 409.
Sailer, S., and Stumpf, C. (1957a). *Arch. Exptl. Pathol. Pharmakol.* **230**, 378.
Sailer, S., and Stumpf, C. (1957b). *Arch. Exptl. Pathol. Pharmakol.* **231**, 63.
Sawyer, C. H., and Gernandt, B. E. (1956). *Am. J. Physiol.* **185**, 209.
Schallek, W., and Kuehn, A. (1959). *Arch. Intern. Pharmacodyn.* **120**, 319.
Schallek, W., and Walz, D. (1953). *Proc. Soc. Exptl. Biol. Med.* **82**, 715.
Sigg, E. B., and Schneider, J. (1957). *Electroencephalog. Clin. Neurophysiol.* **9**, 419.
Silvestrini, B. (1958). *Arch. Intern. Pharmacodyn.* **116**, 71.
Silvette, H., Hoff, E. C., Larson, P. S., and Haag, H. B. (1962). *Pharmacol. Rev.* **14**, 137.
Skowroński, V. (1929). *Arch. Exptl. Pathol. Pharmakol.* **146**, 1.
Spencer, W. A., and Kandel, E. R. (1962). *Colloq. Intern. Centre Natl. Rech. Sci.* (*Paris*) No. 107, p. 71.
Starzl, T. E., Niemer, W. T., Dell, M., and Forgrave, P. R. (1953). *J. Neuropathol. Exptl. Neurol.* **12**, 262.
Stumpf, C. (1959). *Arch. Exptl. Pathol. Pharmakol.* **235**, 421.
Stumpf, C. (1965). *Electroencephalog. Clin. Neurophysiol.*, **18**, 477.
Stumpf, C., Petsche, H., and Gogolák, G. (1962). *Electroencephalog. Clin. Neurophysiol.* **14**, 212.
Terzian, H. (1954). *Rev. Neurol.* **91**, 445.
Thomalske, G., Klinger, J., and Woringer, E. (1957). *Acta Anat.* **30**, 865.
Tokizane, T., and Sawyer, C. H. (1957). *A.M.A. Arch. Neurol. Psychiat.* **77**, 259.
Tokizane, T., Kawakami, M., and Gellhorn, E. (1959). *Electroencephalog. Clin. Neurophysiol.* **11**, 431.

Torii, S. (1961). *Japan. J. Physiol.* **11,** 147.
Udenfriend, S., Bogdanski, D. F., and Weissbach, H. (1956). *Federation Proc.* **15,** 493.
Udenfriend, S., Weissbach, H., and Bogdanski, D. F. (1957). *Ann. N. Y. Acad. Sci.* **66,** 602.
von Berger, G. P., and Longo, V. G. (1953). *Boll. Soc. Ital. Biol. Sper.* **29,** 431.
von Euler, C. (1960). *In* "Structure and Function of the Cerebral Cortex" (D. B. Tomer and J. P. Schade, eds.), p. 272. Elsevier, Amsterdam.
von Euler, C., and Green, J. D. (1960a). *Acta Physiol. Scand.* **48,** 95.
von Euler, C., and Green, J. D. (1960b). *Acta Physiol. Scand.* **48,** 110.
von Euler, C., Green, J. D., and Ricci, G. (1958). *Acta Physiol. Scand.* **42,** 87.
Weiss, T., and Fifková, E. (1960). *Electroencephalog. Clin. Neurophysiol.* **12,** 841.
Wescoe, W. C., Green, R. E., McNamara, B. P., and Krop, S. (1948). *J. Pharmacol. Exptl. Therap.* **92,** 63.
White, R. P., and Boyajy, L. D. (1959). *Proc. Soc. Exptl. Biol. Med.* **102,** 479.
White, R. P., and Daigneault, E. A. (1959). *J. Pharmacol. Exptl. Therap.* **125,** 339.
Wikler, A. (1952). *Proc. Soc. Exptl. Biol. Med.* **79,** 261.
Yokota, T., and Fujimori, B. (1964). *Electroencephalog. Clin. Neurophysiol.* **16,** 375.
Young, M. W. (1936). *J. Comp. Neurol.* **65,** 295.

EFFECTS OF DRUGS ON LEARNING AND MEMORY[1]

By James L. McGaugh and Lewis F. Petrinovich

Department of Psychobiology, University of California, Irvine, California, and Department of Psychology, State University of New York, Stony Brook, Long Island, New York

I. Introduction

The discovery and preparation of drugs with psychological effects has occupied the interest and energy of humans since the beginning of recorded history. Only in recent years, however, have systematic attempts been made to discover the nature and bases of drug effects on behavior. Experimental research in psychopharmacology began around the turn of the century. Shortly after the first demonstrations that animal behavior could be studied systematically, researchers in several laboratories began to adopt the newly developed techniques for use in drug research. Much of the early research was motivated by applied medical questions. Research with animals provided a means of investigating the behavioral ef-

[1] The preparation of this review was supported by research grant MH-07015 from the National Institute of Mental Health, United States Public Health Service, and by research grant GB-1672 from the National Science Foundation.

fects of prolonged use of common drugs such as alcohol, barbiturates, morphine, nicotine, and caffeine (e.g., Macht and Leach, 1929; Barnhardt, 1936a,b). In addition, it was recognized that the techniques used in studies of animal behavior might be used to search for drugs with beneficial effects on human behavior. Much current research in psychopharmacology is a direct consequence of interest in drug treatment of human behavior disorders (e.g., see reviews by Herz, 1960; Ross and Cole, 1960; Cook and Kelleher, 1963).

Recent years have seen increasing use of drugs as research tools. Drugs, together with other techniques such as lesions and electrical stimulation, are now used in investigations of the brain functions that underlie behavior (Russell, 1960, 1964). Such researches are based on the assumption that knowledge of drug effects on behavior, together with knowledge of drug mechanisms of action, can provide clues to the nature of the basic physiological mechanisms.

Although there have been numerous studies of drug effects on learning during the past several decades, research in this area has been particularly active during the past few years. This review summarizes representative studies of the effects of drugs on learning and memory in infrahumans. It is not comprehensive, but instead emphasizes research concerned with the bases of drug effects on learning and memory and the relevance of the findings to current concepts of memory storage mechanisms.

A. Performance, Learning, and Memory

The most crucial problem in research concerning drug effects on learning and memory is that of distinguishing drug effects on *learning* from other effects of drugs on performance. What distinguishes learning from performance? It is clear that when the word "learning" is used, it refers to a change in behavior which is brought about through practice. It is also clear that not all changes in behavior that appear to occur as a function of practice should be included. Changes in performance as a result of physical growth, effects of fatigue, or changes in motivation are clearly not instances of learning.

The distinction between learning and performance was brought into sharp relief by experiments on latent learning. In an early latent learning experiment, Blodgett (1929) gave three groups of rats one trial each day in a simple maze. One group was rewarded in the goal box on all trials, a second group was not rewarded until the seventh day and then on each subsequent day, and a third group was only rewarded beginning on the third day and then daily. The animals in the first group showed a gradual drop in errors at the outset, whereas the error scores for the other two groups remained high until the day after the first time they found food. At that point the error scores dropped very suddenly and were almost immediately comparable to the scores of the first group. Therefore, it appears that the animals in the second and third groups had been learning much more than their performances had indicated during the nonrewarded trials, but that the learning had remained "latent" (i.e., not indicated by performance) until the reward was introduced. Subsequent experiments (e.g., Tolman and Honzik, 1930) obtained essentially similar results. [See Thistlethwaite (1951) for a review of the extensive latent learning literature.] These findings indicate quite clearly that although learning must be inferred from performance, learning is not always evident in performance records.

Often, the problem of defining those changes in behavior which can be considered as evidences of learning is solved by offering an operational definition in which the term learning is defined by a set of operations. These operations usually are measurements and procedural descriptions which establish conditions for use of the term. Strict operationism maintains that ". . . in general, we mean by any concept nothing more than a set of operations; the concept is synonymous with a corresponding set of operations" (Bridgman, 1928). Objections have been raised to the application of strict operationism because it is deemed fundamentally circular (Popper, 1959). Nevertheless, regardless of the position taken about strict operationism, it is inescapable that any concept that is to be studied empirically must, at the point of experimentation, have an operational *translation*. Usually, when operationally translating the concept "learning," some arbitrary performance criterion must be chosen. It has been shown that the nature of this criterion can affect greatly the results obtained. The conclusions drawn from a study may be entirely specific to the criterion chosen. For example, Herz (1959) has shown that anticholinergic drugs will abolish a conditioned avoidance response early in the acquisition process, but that they have no effect on a well-established response.

Studies of learning typically emphasize improvement in performance with repeated trials. Thus learning is usually identified by responses which are repeated. As the findings of the latent learning studies indicate, however, learning can occur without the repetition of specific "correct" responses. Further, in many studies evidence of learning is based on observations of variations in responding. In response alternation learning (e.g., Petrinovich and Bolles, 1957) and one-trial avoidance learning (e.g., Essman and Jarvik, 1960), degree of "memory" is indicated by the tendency of the animals to avoid making a previous response. The nature of the memory trace or "engram" underlying the capacity of animals to either repeat or vary their responses as a consequence of experience has been the focus of many recent psychopharmacological studies. The main interest has centered on the nature of the processes involved in memory storage. This research has required the development of techniques for distinguishing those drug effects on learning that are due to effects on memory storage from other effects due to attentional, perceptual, and motor influences. Failure to provide for such distinctions can readily result in faulty inferences concerning the bases of drug effects on performance.

Influence of Research Focus

Research concerning drug effects on behavior tends to be focused alternatively on either pharmacological questions or on psychological questions. Most of the research employing operant conditioning techniques is done with a pharmacological focus. The operant response is often chosen as an assay technique because it is very reliable and easily quantified. The effects of various drugs may be evaluated by a study of the changes in the rate and pattern of response in the light of variables in the reinforcement schedule. This kind of research yields sets of performance curves which can be compared to one another readily. These comparisons make possible the classification of drugs in terms of behavioral effects. However, this approach often uses the rate of performance of a strongly established response as the dependent variable. The animals are usually pretrained on a simple reinforcement schedule until very stable rates of responding are obtained before the drug conditions are introduced. Consequently, the results are not very informative about the acquisition process. This is, or course, a result of the focus of the research. The emphasis in such work is on factors affecting the performance of highly learned responses, and usually no inference is drawn regarding the nature of any underlying psychological or psychophysiological principles concerning learning.

A much smaller amount of research has been done using a psychological focus. Here, the goal is to study psychological or psychophysiological processes, such as the necessary and sufficient conditions for the storage of memory traces and for their retrieval. With this focus, the drug becomes but one of many tools. Research with a psychological focus tends to be characterized by closer attention to the problems of operational translation (see above). This permits systematic study of the basic parameters involved in learning, such as the effect of the relative massing or distribution of practice.

With the above principles in mind, let us review some early examples of drug research on learning. The merits, as well as the shortcomings, of this work will serve as an introduction to the current survey which follows.

B. Early Examples of Drug Research on Learning

In this section some of the earlier studies of drug effects on learning are discussed rather briefly. These are a reasonably representative but not comprehensive sample of the earlier research.

1. *Thiamine*

As indicated in the Introduction, much of early drug research was concerned with applied problems. Research with thiamine was based on an interest in the possible enhancing effect of supplementary thiamine on the intellectual functioning of retarded children, as well as on a more general interest in the effects on learning of a substance known to be essential to cerebral metabolism. Several studies have indicated that young rats deficient in thiamine are inferior to normal rats in maze learning as well as in classical conditioning (Maurer, 1935; C. Poe *et al.*, 1937; E. Poe *et al.*, 1939; Biel and Wickens, 1941). Stevens (1937) found that thiamine deficiency occurred before the animals were 30 days old. Dietary replacement of thiamine was found to improve the learning of thiamine-deficient rats (O'Neill, 1949). Other work (Marx, 1948b) indicated that supplementary thiamine did not enhance the learning of normal rats. In fact, in the latter study, the treated rats were inferior to controls on a retention test given 2 weeks after the original training.

Although the results of these studies are not entirely consistent, the findings seem to suggest that (1) thiamine deficiency impairs learning, (2) the amount of impairment is related to the age at which the depletion occurs, (3) the deficiency can be overcome by replacing thiamine in the diet, and (4) supplementary thiamine does not enhance the learning of normal rats.

These studies highlight the difficulties that occur in studies using chronically affected subjects. Thiamine-deficient animals and normals differ in physical strength, level of motivation, hunger, etc. Therefore, it is difficult, if not impossible, to distinguish those performance effects that are due to influences on strength, etc., from those which might be due to changes in memory storage mechanisms. See the discussion above on the differences between performance, learning, and memory.

2. *Glutamic Acid*

Glutamic acid has been the subject of a great deal of experimentation and controversy since the initial study of Zimmerman and Ross (1944). These investigators reported that rats given a glutamic acid supplement (200 mg/day) learned a maze faster than did controls. Albert and Warden (1944) also reported facilitating effects of glutamic acid on rats' performances of a pedal-pushing problem. These findings led to a flurry of animal studies (Hamilton and Maher, 1947; Marx, 1948a, 1949; Stellar and McElroy, 1948; Porter and Griffin, 1950, 1951; Pilgrim *et al.*, 1951; Zabarenko *et al.*, 1951), all of which reported negative results. Contrary to the negative evidence just cited there were a few positive studies on human mental defectives. All these, however, can be questioned on methodological grounds (see Astin and Ross, 1960). There was also one study reporting beneficial effects of glutamic acid on the performances of the offspring of rats given the supplement during pregnancy (Sweet, 1951).

In the midst of the controversy, Hughes and Zubek (1956, 1957) reported some results which seemed to introduce some order into the conflict. They pointed out that the Zimmerman and Ross (1944) control animals appeared to be duller animals than those employed in other studies. This led them to suspect that differences between strains of rats in initial learning ability might be the cause of the conflicting data and that glutamic acid might facilitate the learning ability of dull animals but have no effect on bright ones. To test this hypothesis they administered 200 mg of monosodium glutamate (MSG) to groups of rats from the McGill bright and dull strains. The supplements were given daily from the time the animals were weaned (25 days of age) until they were 65 days of age. In learning and relearning (60 days later) the Hebb-Williams closed-field maze, the animals from the dull strain which had received MSG were significantly better than their controls. There was no difference between the treated brights and the control brights.

After these encouraging findings, however, Hughes *et al.* (1957) published a subsequent study of the effect of varying dosages of glutamic acid on the learning ability of the McGill bright and dull rats. In this study, supplementary feeding of 500 mg of MSG daily did not affect learning. They also found, much to their alarm, that the 200-mg dosage, which was effective in the first studies, did not have a significant effect. The only difference in the experiments was that the first two studies used animals from the F_{10} and F_{11} generations of brights and dulls, whereas the later study was done with animals from the F_{12} generation. They doubted that this was the reason for the difference in results, however, because the control animals were approximately equal in both studies. [Rosenzweig *et al.* (1960) also found no effect on learning using glutamic acid with descendants of the Tryon maze-bright and maze-dull rats.] Hughes *et al.* (1957, p. 255) concluded, "It is obvious from these results that the action of glutamic acid on learning ability is not as simple as it first appeared and that numerous variables affect it, variables whose influence only future research can clarify." This statement provides an adequate summary of the findings about the effects of glutamic acid on learning.

It is not entirely clear why glutamic acid was expected to affect learning. Glutamic acid is one of the nonessential amino acids and is readily synthesized by mammals in amounts large enough to make the organism independent of an outside source (Waelsch, 1955). Further, it is doubtful that ingested glutamic acid enters the brain when administered to *normal* animals (Waelsch, 1952), although it may do so in some pathological states such as deep insulin hypoglycemia (Himwich and Petersen, 1958). McIlwain (1955) has pointed out that in cerebral cortex tissue from laboratory animals, glutamic acid does not support the respiratory response to applied electrical impulses as do glucose or pyruvates. He also pointed out, however, that it does have this action with human cerebral tissues. Thus, species differences might account for some of the conflicting data, since some studies were on humans and some were on rats.

3. *Barbiturates*

Most early research with barbiturates also was motivated by applied questions. Early experiments on the effects of barbiturates on learning indicate, for the most part, that barbiturate administration impedes learning. Boughton (1942) found that the learning of food-motivated rats was retarded by injections of phenobarbital administered prior to each training session. However, Jones and Jones (1943) did not find that phenobarbital (80 mg/kg) had any effect on rats' discrimination, learning, retention (1 month later), or reversal learning. The drugged animals were significantly poorer than controls on retention of the reversal habit 1 month after the reversal learning. Jones and Jones argued that the earlier studies on the effect of barbiturates on learning (Mendenhall, 1940; Omwake, 1933; Williams and O'Brien, 1937) cannot be accepted without qualification, because all employed food or water deprivation as motivation. In an earlier study, Jones (1943) found that phenobarbital (80 mg/kg) has a direct effect on food and water intake and on eating habits. Drugged male rats ate less food and ingested more water.

Similar results have been reported for other barbiturates. For example, O'Kelly and Weiss (1955) found that rats dosed with pentobarbital (20 mg/kg sc) drank more than did controls. Schmidt (1958) also found increased drinking by female rats given pentobarbital (3–15 mg/kg sc). It should be mentioned, however, that Alexander and Siegel (1947) report (in abstract form only) that male rats given an unspecified amount of pentobarbital intraperitoneally drank significantly *less* than did controls.

Relatively long-term impairment of performance has been found with repeated injections of pentobarbital. Mendenhall (1940) has shown that pentobarbital injections retarded learning, even though the injections were discontinued 40 days before the beginning of training. Rats were dosed with pentobarbital (0.020–0.102 gm/kg) every other day starting at the age of 37 days (110 injections). It was found that the treated rats performed significantly less well than controls in both learning and relearning (50 days after attainment of criterion) a maze.

In other work with pentobarbital, a single injection has been found to have long-term impairing effects. Armitage (1952) found that if mother rats were injected with 6 mg of pentobarbital 19½ days after breeding, their progeny were significantly poorer learners at 90 days of age than were the progeny of undrugged mothers. Williams and O'Brien (1937) found that rats given daily intraperitoneal injections of pentobarbital (0.024 gm/kg increased after 4 weeks to 0.102 gm/kg) were inferior to controls in learning a multiple-U-maze, even though the drugged animals were dosed *after* each day's run.

In a study using escape from water as motivation, Marx and Ederstrom (1950) found distinct retardation in learning with female rats treated daily with 40 mg/kg of pentobarbital for 4 weeks after weaning, but no impairment was found with male rats. The animals were allowed a 4-day rest period between the last drug injection and the learning tests in order to permit recovery from immediate effects of the drug. Marx and Ederstrom (1950) reanalyzed the data of Williams and O'Brien (1937) and found that the retarding effect of pentobarbital was limited to the male subjects. This is quite puzzling, because mature females are said to be more susceptible to barbiturates than males (Himwich, 1951), and also because Marx and Ederstrom (1950) found only their female rats to be affected.

Dews (1955a) reported that pentobarbital (1.0–5.2 mg/kg) does not affect simple discriminations (e.g., red light *vs.* blue light) in dosages which are sufficient to reduce the rate of responding by pigeons, but does impair more complex discriminations, even in small dosages which do not affect the rate of responding.

The weight of evidence from these early studies leads to the conclusion that barbiturates do impair learning, despite the difficulties with motivation which may vitiate some of the studies. The experimental contradictions that appear in the literature can be summarized as follows: The contradictory results related to sex differences reported by Williams and O'Brien (1937) and Marx and Ederstrom (1950) await resolution. There is the question regarding the nature of the effect of barbiturates on water intake. The cause of the impaired learning performance of adult rats who had received barbiturates in infancy is unsettled. This impairment of learning persists long after the injections have been discontinued. Marx and Ederstrom (1950) allowed 4 days recovery, Mendenhall (1940) allowed 40 days, and Armitage (1952) allowed over 90 days, yet all reported impaired learning. None of these experimenters investigated the possibility that either prenatal injections or a series of injections during infancy might have produced damage to the central neural tissue. The impairment of later learning might also be the result of impaired perceptual functioning during development. A large number of studies have reported that animals raised in an impoverished sensory environment learn more slowly than those reared in a normal or enriched environment (see Epstein, 1964, for a review of this). Since it is not possible, on the basis of the studies considered here, to rule out the possibility of neural damage or to separate effects on the storage process from other performance effects, no clear conclusions can be drawn from these studies. More recent studies of the effects of barbiturates are discussed below (Sections III,A,1 and III,B,1).

4. *Amphetamine*

Amphetamine is a potent sympathomimetic amine and stimulant of the central nervous system. Animals given large amounts of amphetamine exhibit tremors, restlessness, increased motor activity, agitation, and sleeplessness (e.g., Brown and Searle, 1938; Zieve, 1937). Because of these stimulant properties, interest arose in the effect of amphetamine on learning and performance. Several studies have indicated that amphetamine impairs rats' learning. Minkowsky (1939) found that 0.5 mg/kg of amphetamine sulfate impaired rats' learning of a water maze. When saline injections were substituted there was a decrease in the error score; upon reinstatement of the drug, performance deteriorated. Other early studies also reported impairing effects of amphetamine on performance. Dispensa and Barrett (1941) found that, although performance on a water maze was not affected for 1 to 2 hours after injections of amphetamine (0.25–1.00 mg/kg), the experimental animals were inferior to the controls on retention tests given 3½–5 hours after injections. Ewing *et al.* (1952) found no differences between control groups and experimental groups given either 1.0 or 0.5 mg/kg of *d*-amphetamine, or 8.0 or 4.0 mg/kg of *l*-amphetamine, in either the amount of time or the number of errors required to learn a multiple-T-maze. However, when larger doses were given to animals already trained, the time to run the maze and the number of errors required to attain the criterion increased with increasing dosage. The rank order of effectiveness of the drugs was as follows (greater to least): *d*-amphetamine, methamphetamine, *dl*-amphetamine, *l*-amphetamine.

Amphetamine also impairs discrimination. Alpern *et al.* (1943) showed that administration of 20 or 30 mg/kg of amphetamine sulfate to dogs 20 minutes before conditioning trials produced a decrease in differentiation between excitatory and inhibitory stimuli. This was true both for a secretory reflex and for shock-avoidance conditioning. Dews (1955b) trained pigeons to peck for an intermittent reinforcement when a red stimulus was present and not to respond when a blue one was present. The ratio of responses to the two stimuli was not changed by injections of 0.1–3.0 mg/kg of methamphetamine. When the task complexity was increased by changing the stimulus-reinforcement contingencies, there was a decrease in differentiation with injections of 0.3, 0.52, and 1.0 mg/kg.

In general, the findings of these experiments indicate that amphetamine impairs learning and performance. The amount of impairment seems to be related to the complexity of the task. More recent studies (Section III,C,1) indicate that, under appropriate conditions, learning may be enhanced by injections of amphetamine.

5. *Curare*

Older studies of the effect of curare on learning used various South American arrow poisons which contained many alkaloids and other substances. Thus, there were possible confounding effects due to varying kinds and amounts of noncurare materials.

Later studies used erythroidine alkaloids which have actions similar to those of curare. The most recent studies have used *d*-tubocurarine which produces the same flaccid paralysis as crude curare or erythroidine. The purified alkaloid produces only paralysis and does not produce insensibility or anesthesia, although other substances present in the crude preparations may have the latter effects. Smith *et al.* (1947) have confirmed experimentally that a wide variety of sensory stimuli are experienced by humans paralyzed with *d*-tubocurarine and that these sensations can be accurately described after recovery.

The interest of investigators in curare was stimulated by the possibility of discovering whether or not overt responding is necessary for learning to take place. During the curare-induced immotility, the animal cannot perform any skeletal responses.

In the first study of the effects of curare on conditioning, Harlow and Stagner (1933) subjected cats and dogs to a skeletal conditioning procedure under curare. Afterward, these investigators found no evidence of training when the animals were tested without drug. They found no learning of the skeletal response and no evidence of an effect of extinction trials given while the animals were curarized. They concluded that cortical activity was not depressed, however, since a pupillary response could be conditioned and extinguished in the curarized animals.

Using a more refined technique, Girden and Culler (1937) subsequently reported evidence of learning under curare. Their results also indicated that there was "dissociation" of the learning between the normal and the curarized state. The conditioned response was a twitch of the semitendinosus muscle rather than the gross bodily response used by Harlow and Stagner. They found that responses learned in the normal state could not be elicited when the dogs were curarized and responses learned in the curarized state could not be elicited in the normal state. In both cases, upon reinstatement of the condition under which the response was learned, the conditioned response reappeared. They suggested that the curare inhibited normal cortical dominance and that the conditioning then occurred at subcortical levels. In support of this interpretation, Girden (1940) found no evidence of dissociation in animals with ablations in sensory cortical areas. The cortex appears to be necessary in order to obtain dissociation with curare. Dissociation has also been demonstrated with erythroidine paralysis (Girden, 1947).

Here the matter remained until several other investigators (Lauer, 1951; Black *et al.*, 1962; Solomon and Turner, 1962) reported that with *d*-tubocurarine, learning during the paralyzed state does transfer to the normal state. Black (1958) has also found that dogs given extinction trials while immobilized by *d*-tubocurarine subsequently required fewer trials to extinguish a habit previously learned in the normal state than did dogs which had not received extinction trials under *d*-tubocurarine. Solomon and Turner (1962, pp. 216–217) conclude that, "Animal subjects can acquire discriminative instrumental response tendencies without the overt responses themselves being exercised in the presence of the discriminative stimuli."

In reply to a suggestion by Smith (1964) that the *d*-tubocurarine may not have produced total striate paralysis, Black and Lang (1964) reported evidence that animals can learn (as indicated by subsequent retention tests) while under *d*-tubocurarine even when electromyograms show consistent blocking of skeletal responses.

It seems, therefore, that skeletal responses are not essential for learning to occur. The research on curare seems to have answered the original theoretical question. It would, however, be of great value to test directly the possibility that dissociation is obtained with crude curare or erythroidine but not with *d*-tubocurarine. Dissociation has received no further attention until just lately. Recent research on this phenomenon is discussed below.

II. Methodological Problems

A. Complexities of Drug Influences

Even a cursory examination of the literature concerned with drug effects on learning and memory reveals that the methodological problems are immensely complex. The following discussion does not cover all of the complexities to which experimenters must be alert, but dwells on those which appear to be the most serious and whose effects can be documented.

1. *Dissociation*

The dissociation effect has been mentioned in the context of the early curare studies. This refers to the condition in which habits learned by animals in a drugged state do not transfer to the normal state, but can be evoked again whenever the animal is drugged. Dissociation can also occur from the normal to the drugged state. This is a serious problem whenever interest is centered on the retention of habits learned under the influence of drugs in order to determine whether or not the drug affects memory storage processes. If an animal has learned a habit under the influence of a drug and then shows no retention of the habit when retested in the normal state, it is difficult to be certain that no vestige of the experience exists unless additional control groups are included to evaluate whether or not dissociation has occurred. Dissociation was first demonstrated by Girden and Culler (1937) using crude curare and by Girden (1942) using erythroidine. Recently, Sachs *et al.* (1962) have found that conditioned avoidance learning in rats is facilitated by injections of chlordiazepoxide. The rats trained with the drug showed virtually no retention when tested without the drug, although the learning response reappeared when the drugged state was reinstated. On the other hand, the performance of control rats trained without the drug deteriorated when they were tested 20 minutes after injections of chlordiazepoxide. Similar dissociation was reported by Otis (1964) in a study of the effects of chlorpromazine on the learning and retention of a shock avoidance habit by rats. Overton (1964) also found dissociation with pentobarbital in a study of learning and retention of a shock avoidance habit in a T-maze by rats. In addition to total dissociation between drugged and nondrugged states, he found partial dissociation between drugged states not sufficiently different from each other to produce total dissociation. The more similar two drugged states were, the more complete the transfer of training between them. Overton suggests that the performance decrements are not due simply to sensory cue changes.

The basis of dissociation could be, as Girden and Culler (1937) supposed, that different neural units are mediating the learning in drugged and nondrugged states. Another possibility, as Otis argues, could be that the dissociation is due to an altered stimulus input to the storage mechanisms during the drugged state, even though the external stimulating environment is the same. Therefore, responses learned to the same stimulus cues when drugged would not transfer to the normal state, although, according to his hypothesis, the storage mechanisms are not affected in either case. Overton interprets the dissociation effect to be due to a disruption of complex central mediating processes. The change in a drugged state is assumed to modify the timing and routing of nerve impulses within those mediating processes to a degree that would disrupt them but still leaving brain function sufficiently intact so that new mediating processes could come into action. These new mediating processes would be specific to the drugged state. Therefore, no transfer would occur and the dissociation effect would be observed. It is not possible, at present, to decide between these alternative explanations.

2. *Peripheral and Central Effects*

The theoretical significance of the effects of a given drug on learning and memory depends on whether the primary action of the drug is on the receptor or effector systems or on the central nervous system. Any drug that has only peripheral effects can still cause an indirect alteration in central nervous system function by modifying the input to the central nervous system. Conversely, any drug which has only central effects can produce alterations in peripheral nervous system function because of the general dominance of the central nervous system. For example, if a drug acts to increase receptor sensitivity, then drug-induced differences in the rate of learning would bear on the issue of the effect of varying the intensity or quality of input to the storage system. If the drug is shown to enhance the sensitivity of central nervous system synaptic mechanisms, then drug-induced differences of learning in rats would bear more directly on the nature of the storage system itself.

The usual approach to this problem has been to assess the effects of drugs on various forms of behavior which are known to be related to various aspects of learning (e.g., Petrinovich, 1963). However, Carlton (1963) has suggested an approach which might prove to be more satisfactory. He used closely similar drugs, of which some have both central and peripheral effects while others, which do not cross the "blood–brain barrier" very well, are much less active in the brain but retain potent peripheral actions. The latter then provide a proper control for assessing the central-acting drug.

3. *Dose–Response Effects*

One of the most serious defects of the existing literature concerning the effects of drugs on behavior is the lack of systematic data on dose–response relations. Frequently, drug studies employ one arbitrarily chosen dosage of a drug, assess the effect of this single dosage on behavior and then offer generalizations about the nature of the drug's effect on behavior. The particular dosage level may be chosen because it is some fraction of the minimal lethal dosage or of the LD_{50}, or because it produces no noticeable side effects, or because it is some fraction of the dosage that produces noticeable side effects. The choice of dosage level is sometimes based on determinations made in some other investigator's laboratory even though the strain and/or species of animals is different, and despite the fact that different strains can vary greatly in sensitivity to various drugs, as discussed below. Even in the same strain, the behavioral effect of a drug can be completely different, depending on the dosage chosen. Stratton and Petrinovich (1963) have reported that the effect of physostigmine, an anticholinesterase agent, on the rate of alley-maze learning depends on the dosage level. Small doses of the drug have no effect on learning, larger doses enhance learning, and still larger doses disrupt learning. In view of the above, it is mandatory that a broad range of dosages be employed in any study in which the aim is to gain an over-all understanding of the effects of the drug on a given behavioral system.

4. *Tolerance and Sensitization*

Another troublesome factor with some drugs is that the effects change with repeated administration. Either increasing tolerance or increasing sensitivity may be encountered. Often, either the problem is ignored (e.g., Jones and Jones, 1943; Marx and Ederstrom, 1950) or the investigator has to revise the dosage to try to maintain a given behavioral effect. Williams and O'Brien (1937) increased from 0.087 to 0.102 gm/kg phenobarbital after 4 weeks, Mendenhall (1940) increased from 0.02 to 0.024 gm/kg, from 0.050 to 0.060 gm/kg, and from 0.087 to 0.102 gm/kg after 35 injections (one every other day). The results are very difficult to interpret, because the major independent variable is varying at an undetermined rate.

5. *Strain and Species Differences*

It is now widely recognized that great caution must be exercised when generalizing from either pharmacological or behavioral results obtained from only one species. Differences in the basic neurochemical substrates, differences in neural and anatomical structure, and differences in receptor and effector capabilities are evident between species, and all these make generalizations hazardous. For example, Thiessen *et al.* (1961) presented data which were intended to bear on the way in which strychnine sulfate enhanced maze learning by rats, as reported by McGaugh and Petrinovich (1959). The dosage used in the Thiessen *et al.* study (1 mg/kg) was chosen because it was the same dosage used by McGaugh and Petrinovich. However, the former study was done on mice and the latter on rats. In one strain of mice, at least, the LD_{50} for strychnine is less than one-half of that for one strain of rats (Longo *et al.*, 1959). Yet the results are taken by Thiessen *et al.* to cast doubt on the interpretation of McGaugh and Petrinovich, because the mice received injections of the drug ". . . in amounts previously shown to improve learning" (Thiessen *et al.*, 1961, p. 494). (For a complete discussion of this study, see McGaugh and Petrinovich, 1963a.)

Less widely recognized, however, are the less obvious, but equally important differences which exist between strains of the same species. Great differences in the results of behavioral manipulations are known to exist among representatives of the same species (Fuller and Thompson, 1960; Rosenzweig *et al.*, 1960). This point is often ignored, and, as a result, comparison of different studies and evaluation of the evidence on which different experimental conclusions are based are quite difficult.

B. Problems of Behavioral Taxonomy

1. *Side Effects*

Any investigator who has studied the effects of drugs on any aspect of behavior is aware that side effects of drugs must be considered carefully in interpreting results. We have already mentioned Carlton's (1963) use of pairs of drugs of which one member is primarily central-acting and the other mainly peripheral-acting. If such pairs are not to be found within some families of drugs, one must rely on behavioral assessment of the drug's effects on those aspects of behavior known to be related to learning effectiveness. In some instances, drugs may enhance the performance of responses rather than affect the storage mechanism. For example, this might occur as a result of a change in hunger motivation or in emotionality. Therefore, measurements of hunger, emotionality, sensory thresholds, etc., are sometimes undertaken. This provides some information and hence a certain degree of control, but, unfortunately, different behavioral measures of what is presumed to be the same variable often do not correlate with one another. For example, Miller *et al.* (1950) have shown that measuring hunger by determining the amount of food eaten by rats will sometimes give a different answer than does measuring either how much work they will do for food or the amount of quinine required to stop them from eating. Yet all these factors are assumed to be measures of hunger. Miller and Barry (1960) argue that it is important to use a battery of diversified tests whenever attempting to measure the effect of a drug on such things as level of motivation or emotionality.

2. *Apparatus Factors*

The type of apparatus chosen to study the effect of a drug on behavior can also influence the results. This is a serious consideration, since usually only one type of problem and apparatus is used to measure learning, and generalizations are based on the results thus obtained. Small differences in the design of a maze can produce discrepant results in studies of the effects of drugs on learning. For example, since the addition of retracing doors has been shown to increase the reliability of mazes (Leeper, 1932), it should be easier to detect drug-induced differences in performance in a maze with retracing doors. Similarly, any differences in the manner of presenting the stimulus cues in a discrimination problem can be critical. Lashley (1930) found that rats could learn a pattern discrimination in fewer than 100 trials if the patterns were placed so that the rat had to jump at the stimulus cards to reach the goal. Fields (1928) had previously found that if the patterns were placed so that the rat merely went toward the visual stimulus and then under it, the discrimination required 800 trials.

3. *Procedural Factors*

As mentioned earlier, many strategies have been employed to overcome the difficulties created by differential motivational states induced by drugs. Motivation may be based on approach or avoidance; if a drug is known to influence thirst, and not hunger, then hunger motivation might seem to be appropriate for studying the effect of that drug on learning. This is not satisfactory, however, because factors influencing one drive state can affect the other indirectly (Verplanck and Hayes, 1953). One way of handling this problem would be to train animals with the drug, then to test them without the drug, and compare them with nondrug controls which have received the same training. The difficulty with this is that there might be dissociation from the drugged to the nondrugged state. Often, avoidance motivation such as escape from shock or cold water are used in an attempt to circumvent these problems with approach motivation. These are not necessarily satisfactory procedures either, because drugs that influence the motivational states of animals in any way tend also to influence metabolic rates, which in turn affect muscular strength and endurance, body temperature, stress tolerance, and other basic bodily functions. Still another solution to this problem has been to use classical conditioned responses in an attempt to minimize the effect of most motivational influences (e.g., Biel and Wickens, 1941; Headlee and Kellogg, 1941).

Drug effects on performance have been shown to be influenced by the specific training procedure used. For example, McGaugh *et al.* (1961) have shown that the effects of drugs on learning by different strains of rats depends on the degree of distribution of practice in the training trials. Recently, Terrace (1963a) has developed a technique which permits discrimination learning to proceed without any errors occurring. The technique insures that the animal always responds to the correct stimulus and never responds to the incorrect stimulus. When discrimination is learned in this way without errors, such things as sporadic bursts of responding to the negative stimulus do not have an opportunity to occur as they do with other methods. Terrace (1963a,b) has demonstrated that chlorpromazine or imipramine disrupt visual discrimination by pigeons only if the discrimination is learned *with* errors.

III. Drug Influences on Learning and Memory

A. Drug Impairment of Learning

As we have pointed out, there are many ways in which drugs can influence an animal's performance. If a drug impairs the rate of error elimination in a maze-learning task, this, quite obviously, does not necessarily mean that the compound interferes with the storage of information in the nervous system. The drug could impair performance by decreasing motivation, producing ataxia, decreasing arousal and attention, impairing sensory processes, or by generally debilitating the animal. Similarly, a drug *improving* maze acquisition could do so in a variety of ways unrelated to those involving memory storage. Enhanced motivation and increased alertness and motility are several possible influences. The problem of specifying the nature of a drug's influences on acquisition is thus a difficult one. But it is not a hopeless one. A variety of procedures have been developed in an attempt to assess the effects of drugs on learning and memory independently of other effects on performance.

1. *Pentobarbital*

A large number of studies have shown that central nervous system (CNS) depressants impair performance in acquisition tasks (see Section I,A,2). Some attempts have been made to demonstrate that the performance impairment found with depressants may be due to decreased efficiency of neprophysiological processes involved in learning or memory storage. In an early study, for example, Headlee and Kellogg (1941) showed that pentobarbital in mildly hypnotic doses (0.08 gr/lb) retarded conditioned response learning in dogs. Conditioning was obtained but it was less efficient than that found under control (i.e., nondrug) conditions. Retention tests given a week later without pentobarbital indicated that some learning had occurred but that the performance of the dogs was very poor in comparison with what would have been predicted if the pentobarbital merely interfered with the animals' ability to perform the response. The findings appeared to justify the authors' conclusion that ". . . the decrease in learning ability was of neural origin" (p. 336). Similarly Rosenzweig *et al.* (1956), and Moroz (1959) demonstrated that small doses of pentobarbital (10 mg/kg) retard problem-solving behavior in rats without seriously affecting the performance of learned responses. It seems clear from these, as well as from other studies discussed earlier in this review, that learning is retarded by CNS depressants. Possibly, however, the impairment observed is due to depression of sensory processes rather than (or in addition to) impairment of memory storage processes. Reduced attention or vigilance, or decreased receptor sensitivity are alternative interpretations of the learning impairment. Although these latter interpretations are weakened by the fact that pentobarbital in small doses did not affect the performance of a learned response, they are still relevant, because attention and vigilance are particularly critical during the early stages of learning. Electrophysiological correlates of arousal (e.g., desynchronization or alpha block) are generally less extensive after a response is well learned (Galambos, 1961; Morrell, 1961b).

2. *Anticholinergics*

There is increasing evidence (Rosenzweig *et al.*, 1960; Carlton, 1963) that the acetylcholine–acetylcholinesterase system is critically involved in learning and memory. A number of recent studies have shown that atropine impairs learning and performance in experimental animals. These findings are of interest because of the anticholinergic action of atropine and also because of the effect of atropine on EEG activity. Atropine induces a slow wave, high-voltage EEG pattern somewhat resembling that of sleep even in doses that do not produce behavioral evidence of drowsiness or sleep. Whitehouse (1964) has shown that atropine (2 mg/kg) impairs successive discrimination learning in rats. Aniimals in his study were given 10 trials a day beginning 60 minutes after atropine injections. After 7 days of training, the injections were discontinued and training was continued. The performance of the animals that had received atropine prior to each previous training session remained inferior to that of control subjects for several days after withdrawal of the drug. These findings are consistent with the interpretation that the performance impairment during the initial training was due to less efficient learning rather than to simple depression of performance. As in the pentobarbital studies discussed above, however, the view that learning impairment was due to sensory or attentional influences cannot be ruled out. Also the question of the duration of action of atropine on various physiological systems is not considered.

Additional evidence of learning impairment with atropine was presented in a recent study by Burešová *et al.* (1964). In their study, rats failed to learn to avoid entering a small compartment where they received punishing foot shocks if the trials were begun 20 minutes after injections of atropine (6 mg/kg). EEG changes produced by atropine were found to be maximal 20 minutes after injection. Injections administered only 10 minutes prior to training failed to affect learning. Furthermore, atropine injected 1 day after the learning trial but 1 day before a retention test, had no influence on retention. Retention was impaired by atropine administered 20 minutes before the retention test if the response was not well learned. Impairment of retention was not found in rats given two treatments of punishing shock on the initial day of training. One possible interpretation of these findings is that the impairment was due to interference with attention.

The findings of Herz (1959) are consistent with the above. He found that atropine (10 mg/kg) and scopolamine (1 mg/kg) depressed rats' performances of learned avoidance responses only in the early stages of training. No effects were found if the avoidance responses were well established. Scopolamine impaired auditory discrimination learning only during the initial stages of training. Similar results were reported by Michelson (1961). Carlton has shown that atropine and scopolamine disrupt rats' performances of a learned alternation response as well as their learning of a complex multiple choice discrimination. On the basis of these, as well as other related findings (e.g., Hearst, 1959), Carlton suggested that the behavioral effects of anticholinergics may be due, at least in part, to blocking of a cholinergic system concerned with behavioral inhibition. This interpretation is consistent with the findings of Burešová *et al.* that atropine-injected rats failed to avoid entering a place where they had previously been punished. In more recent work, Carlton (1964) reported evidence more consistent with the view that anticholinergics interfere with perceptual or attentional processes. In a variety of situations, rats failed to habituate to stimuli presented after injections of scopolamine.

The performance impairment found with these anticholinergics is most likely due to effects on the central nervous system, for peripherally acting quaternary compounds such as methylscopolamine and methylatropine have not been found to impair either learning or performance (Herz, 1959; Carlton, 1964; Michelson, 1961).

B. Drug Impairment of Memory Storage

It is difficult to draw conclusions about the effects of drugs on memory storage on the basis of their effects on either acquisition or performance of learned responses. This problem has led to the development of alternative experimental procedures for assessing drug effects on memory storage. During the past two decades an increasing amount of evidence has supported the view, originally proposed by Mueller and Pilzecker in 1900, that memory storage involves the perseveration of neural processes for some time after the termination of training. The evidence, as reviewed by Glickman (1961) and Deutsch (1962) indicates that retention of learned responses is impaired if animals are subjected shortly after training to treatments interfering with CNS activity. Amnesia produced in this way (termed retrograde amnesia) is greatest if short intervals elapse between training and treatment. All the following can produce retrograde amnesia: concussion, temperature changes, electroconvulsive shock (ECS), subcortical brain stimulation, hypoxia, spreading depression of electrical activity, and, of particular significance for this review, depressant drugs. A methodological issue should be mentioned here. Since the treatments are generally administered shortly after training, it has been suggested that at least a part of the impairment may be due to punishing effects of the treatments. This criticism is particularly relevant to ECS as a treatment (Coons and Miller, 1960), but is applicable to the other treatments as well. Control studies have shown that, although ECS is punishing when administered repeatedly, amnesia is obtained without punishment when only one ECS treatment is given after a single learning trial (Madsen and McGaugh, 1961; McGaugh and Madsen, 1964).

1. *Depressants*

The procedure of administering drugs *after* training rather than *before* training has been adopted by a number of investigators as a means of assessing memory storage effects independently of other possible effects of drugs. This technique is primarily suitable for drugs which are maximally effective within seconds or minutes and which are metabolized prior to retention tests. By using this procedure, Leukel (1957) found that thiopental injected into rats 1 minute after each daily trial in a water maze retarded their rate of learning. No impairment was found in rats injected 30 minutes after each trial. A plausible interpretation is that the drug interfered with the storage of information acquired on each trial if given immediately after the trial. It should be noted that the animals were repeatedly dosed, and that the injections may have been painful. Thus the possibility that the drug was punishing cannot be completely excluded. In order to avoid the complications arising from repeated drug administration, Jarvik and Essman and their associates have developed a variety of single-trial learning tasks which have proved suitable for studies of memory storage (e.g., Jarvik and Essman, 1960; Essman and Alpern, 1964; Jarvik, 1964). In one study (Pearlman *et al.*, 1961), rats were first trained to press a lever for food reward and then were given a single shock delivered through the lever or drinking tube. When tested 24 hours later, these animals exhibited a markedly depressed rate of lever pressing. However, for animals similarly trained but anesthetized with ether or pentobarbital (30 mg/kg iv) within a few minutes after receiving the punishing shock, the rates of lever pressing were less markedly affected. This could be interpreted as an effect on memory. The degree of this effect was directly related to the length of the interval between punishment and drug administration. Other subjects were treated with convulsant doses of pentylenetetrazole (20 mg/kg iv). Evidence of amnesia was found after pentylenetetrazole even when the convulsions were induced as long as 4 *days* after training. This latter finding is both interesting and perplexing, since retrograde amnesia is rarely found if training–treatment intervals are greater than 1 or 2 hours. In several subsequent studies using even simpler single-trial learning tasks, Jarvik and his associates found additional evidence of the amnesic effect of CNS depressants (Essman and Jarvik, 1960; Abt *et al.*, 1961). In one study, naïve mice anesthetized with ether within a few minutes after receiving a foot shock upon stepping from a small platform, tended to step readily from the platform when placed on it again 24 hours later. Control mice which were shocked but not anesthetized tended to avoid stepping from the platform. In recent work, Jarvik (1964) has reported that amnesia is obtained with ether anesthesia only when the room temperature is warm (above 80°F). The significance of this curious finding is unknown.

It is difficult to explain these findings in other terms than impairment of memory storage. An explanation based on punishment is unsupported by these studies, because the effectiveness of the drugs is indicated by an increased tendency of animals to perform responses punished by shock.

The findings of other recent studies using posttraining administration of depressants have been similar to those of Jarvik *et al.* Paré (1961) found that secobarbital (35 mg/kg) impaired rats' retention of a visual discrimination if injections were administered within 2 minutes after massed training trials. The retention test was given 48 hours after the training and injections. Recently Doty and Doty (1964) studied the effect of daily posttraining injections of chlorpromazine (2 mg/kg) on avoidance learning in rats of varying ages. In all groups (30–600 days) the rate of learning was lowest in the groups dosed immediately after each trial. In the young and old groups, performance was impaired even with injections administered 2 hours after each trial. They concluded that the ". . . similarity of effects produced by the tranquilizer and certain CNS depressants in impeding the acquisition of avoidance responses, suggests that chlorpromazine may exert its effects on fear-motivated learning, not by reducing fear, but by interfering with memory consolidation" (p. 333). The evidence from this study is consistent with that from other work (Thompson, 1957; McGaugh and Cole, 1965) indicating that memory storage efficiency varies with age. Gutekunst and Youniss (1963) reported that imprinting in chicks was impaired if the chicks were anesthetized with ether immediately after an imprinting "training" session. Imprinting was not affected if anesthetization was administered 15 or 30 minutes after the imprinting.

2. *Topical Application of Drugs*

Impairment of learning and memory storage has also been found in several experiments in which drugs have been applied directly to the cerebral cortex of animals. Aluminum hydroxide cream has been used in several experiments. This substance elicits chronic seizure discharges similar to those recorded from epileptic foci. Several investigators have shown that different types of learning deficits are found with different sites of application. In monkeys, occipital applications impair visual discrimination learning (Kraft *et al.*, 1960), whereas bilateral applications to the frontal lobes impair learning of a delayed alternation task (Stamm and Pribram, 1960). However, this treatment did not affect the performance of a response that had been learned prior to the operation. The deficit seemed to be specific to learning, not retention. This effect is similar to that found with posttrial ECS and subcortical brain stimulation. Wyers (1963) has reported that retrograde amnesia can be produced by a single shock delivered to the caudate nucleus immediately after training. It seems reasonable to conjecture that the performance effects found with aluminum hydroxide may be based on interference with memory storage resulting from the chronic abnormal tissue discharges.

The phenomenon of "spreading depression" has provided a rather unique method for investigating brain functioning. Application of mechanical, electrical, or chemical stimuli directly to the cortex can produce a depression of electrical activity which spreads concentrically through the gray matter at a uniform rate of from 3 to 6 mm/minute and which lasts for several hours. In a series of excellent studies, Burés and Burešová and their associates have used spreading depression induced by topical application of potassium chloride (25% solution) as a means of producing temporary "decortication" of rats (Bureš, 1959). Most of their research has been concerned with the problem of localization of brain processes mediating memory. In recent work, they (Bureś and Burešová, 1963) and others (Pearlman and Jarvik, 1961; Ray and Emley, 1964) have shown that memory storage is impaired by KCl-induced spreading depression. In a very ingenious study (Ray and Emley, 1964), rats with unilateral KCl-induced spreading depression were trained on a visual discrimination task. No evidence of memory was found when they were then tested following depression of the opposite hemisphere. Apparently memory storage had been restricted to the untreated hemisphere. They were then given a single trial with neither cortex depressed. Then, either 15 seconds or 10 minutes later, KCl was applied to the cortex which was not depressed throughout the original training. Thirty minutes later, they were given four test trials in the discrimination task. On these trials, the performances of the animals treated 10 minutes after the single trial with both hemispheres functioning, were perfect, that is they made no errors, whereas that of the rats treated only 15 seconds after the trial revealed no evidence of any learning. This study confirms earlier work showing that a single experience is sufficient for the bilateral replication of memory storage processes originally located unilaterally, and also indicates that this process, like that involved in original learning, is time-dependent. The time course found with KCl is comparable to that found with posttraining ether anesthetization (Pearlman *et al.*, 1961).

3. *Drugs Influencing Ribonucleic Acid and Protein Synthesis*

a. Ribonucleic Acid Synthesis. A number of investigators have proposed that memory storage may involve ribonucleic acid (RNA) and protein synthesis (Hydén, 1959; Morrell, 1961a) which are known to vary with neuronal activity (Hydén, 1959). Hydén has suggested that memory storage may be based on specific alterations in RNA composition (perhaps base sequences) produced by the specific CNS activity occurring during learning. The lasting change in protein formation which would follow the alteration of RNA could, according to Hydén, provide a stable intraneuronal basis for memory. In support of this general hypothesis, Hydén and Egyhazi (1962, 1963) have reported that base ratios of neuronal and glial RNA in rats' vestibular Deiter's nuclei are altered by training the rats in a task requiring balancing. In both types of cells, the adenine–uracil ratio was increased. In the glial cells, there was also a decrease in cytosine. Since base ratio changes were not observed in rats given vestibular stimulation by rotation but not trained in the balancing task, the alterations appear not to be due merely to an increase in the vestibular stimulation. Furthermore, changes were not found if the RNA analyses were made 24 hours after the training was terminated.

Although a number of questions might be raised concerning the adequacy of the learning task as well as the appropriateness of the control stimulation, the results clearly justify the further investigation of possible relationships between RNA and learning.

Other investigators have attempted to elucidate the role in learning of RNA synthesis by injecting compounds known to interfere with RNA synthesis. Dingman and Sporn (1961) reported that intracerebral injections of the antimetabolite, 8-azaguanine, which is readily incorporated into brain RNA, impaired the ability of rats to learn a maze without significantly affecting the rats' performances of a previously well-learned maze. The training and retention tests were given 15 minutes after the injections. These findings are consistent with the hypothesis that 8-azaguanine interfered with learning by interfering with brain RNA metabolism. However, the data do not eliminate the possibilities that 8-azaguanine may interfere with other aspects of brain metabolism necessary for memory but unrelated to RNA metabolism or that the impairment may be due to interference with attentional processes which are critical in the early stages of learning in complex tasks. Gerard and his coworkers (Chamberlain *et al.*, 1963a,b) reported no significant effects of intraperitoneal injections of 8-azaguanine (50 mg/kg) on either maze learning or avoidance conditioning. In other work, however, these investigators have found that 8-azaguanine (50–200 mg/kg ip) retards the rate of development of hindlimb postural asymmetry produced by cerebellar lesions. Rats were subjected to cerebellar lesions first; then their spinal cords were transected at different intervals following the cerebellar lesions. In control (non-drug) rats, the postural asymmetries persisted if 45 minutes lapsed between the lesion and transection. In rats injected with 8-azaguanine, the asymmetry persisted following spinal transection only when 70 minutes or longer elapsed between the lesion and transection. Gerard (1963) suggested that these findings, based on "fixation" of postural asymmetry, are analogous to those obtained in more conventional studies of memory storage. Whether the mechanism of fixation in the spinal cord is identical or similar to that at higher CNS levels, is, of course, not known. These interesting results suggest that the whole question of the degree of plasticity at the spinal level needs to be re-examined.

More recently, Barondes and Jarvik (1964) reported that intracerebral injections of actinomycin D did not affect one-trial learning in mice. The animals were injected with a dose of actinomycin sufficient to produce an 83% inhibition of brain RNA synthesis during the 4–5 hour interval after the injection. Four hours after injection, the mice were given a single shock in a small activity-exploration apparatus. On a retention test given 3 hours later, the amount of reduction in exploratory activity (which is taken as an index of memory of the shock) was comparable in experimental and control mice. As Barondes and Jarvik pointed out, these data are not completely inconsistent with the hypothesis that memory storage involves RNA synthesis, because the residual RNA synthesis (17%) might have been sufficient to mediate memory storage. In a similar study, Appel (1964) found no effect of intracerebral injections of actinomycin D either on learning or on memory in mice. The amount of the drug injected was sufficient to stop all RNA synthesis by the time of each animal's death. Thus, the findings of studies using intracerebral injections of actinomycin D seem to pose serious questions for theories of memory storage that rely heavily upon RNA synthesis mechanisms.

Other efforts to link RNA synthesis with memory storage have been based on studies using planaria. Several studies have shown that when planaria are trained to respond to a light paired with a shock and then are cut in half and allowed to regenerate, retention of the response is subsequently found in animals regenerated from either head or tail sections (McConnell *et al.*, 1959). Corning and John (1961) trained planaria, cut them in half and allowed them to regenerate in either pond water or pond water containing ribonuclease (0.07–0.10 mg/ml). This experiment was conducted to examine the possibility that RNA might be involved in the transmission of an acquired structural configuration from the trained portion of the animal to the regenerating tissue. According to this assumption, tails regenerated in the ribonuclease solution would be expected to have anterior portions with altered RNA and, as a consequence, to have "naïve" dominant heads. The regenerated planaria were tested for 3 days to see if they retained the response learned prior to transection and then were retrained to the original learning criterion of 34 conditioned responses per daily session of 40 trials. Animals regenerated from heads in ribonuclease were superior to those regenerated in pond water, whereas animals regenerated from tails in ribonuclease were inferior to those regenerated in pond water. This interaction was not found with the *relearning* scores, however. Regenerated heads relearned faster than regenerated tails, and the sections regenerated in pond water relearned faster than those regenerated in the enzyme. The difference in relearning trials for heads and tails regenerated in the enzyme was very similar to the difference between heads and tails regenerated in pond water. These results are comparable to those obtained with animals that were cut, regenerated, and then trained for the first time. Regenerated heads learned faster than regenerated tails and animals regenerated in pond water learned faster than animals regenerated in ribonuclease. Thus, considered together, these results indicate that (1) both learning and relearning were poor in animals regenerated in ribonuclease, (2) regenerated heads learned and relearned faster than regenerated tails, (3) at least some degree of savings was obtained in *both heads and tails* regenerated in the ribonuclease solution. The relearning scores of the head and tail sections regenerated in ribonuclease were lower than the original learning scores. They were also lower than those of planaria trained for the first time after being regenerated in either ribonuclease or pond water. As Corning and John (1961, p. 1364) pointed out, the relearning scores ". . . suggest that the tails treated with ribonuclease may retain some residual effects of experience, although they are unable to transmit the effects to the regenerating tissue. A clearer understanding of these findings seems to require a more intimate understanding of the mechanism of information transfer." We heartily concur.

We are forced to conclude that studies using compounds designed to alter RNA synthesis have not yet provided clear evidence concerning the role of RNA synthesis in memory storage processes. One view is that of Dingman and Sporn (1964) who have asserted that it would be surprising to find that RNA and protein synthesis are *not* involved in memory storage.

b. Protein Synthesis. Recently Flexner *et al.* (1962, 1963) investigated in mice the effects of inhibition of brain protein synthesis on learning and memory. In the first of two studies, they found that subcutaneous injections of the antibiotic, puromycin, in doses (0.42 mg/gm) sufficient to produce an 83% inhibition of protein synthesis lasting 2–8 hours failed to affect either avoidance learning or simple maze learning. More complete inhibition (95%) produced by a combination of subcutaneous and intraventricular injections produced severe behavioral disorientation. The effect of intraventricular injection itself was an uncontrolled variable.

In a second study, Flexner *et al.* (1963) reported evidence that memory storage was impaired by intracerebral injections of puromycin (0.03–0.09 mg). Bilateral temporal injections of the smaller doses were given 1 day after training; retention was impaired on tests given 3 days later. Memory loss was also found with injections given 18–43 days after the original training (but 3 days before the retention tests) if the mice were given combined bilateral, frontal, temporal, and ventricular injections. A single bilateral temporal injection of 0.09 mg of puromycin was found to impair memory only if the injections were given within 5 days after training. The greatest impairment was found with injections given within 2 or 3 days after training. Mice given bilateral temporal injections 1 day after position-reversal learning in a Y-maze, but 3 weeks after original position learning, reverted to the originally learned response on retention tests given 3 days after the injection. The amnesic effects of puromycin appear to be similar to those found with pentylenetetrazole (Pearlman *et al.*, 1961), but the extent of the retrograde amnesic effects is greater than that found with any other amnesic treatment. Retrograde amnesia is rarely reported if the time lapse between training and treatment is greater than a few hours. The findings of studies of pentylenetetrazole and puromycin suggest that the processes underlying memory storage retain some degree of lability long after they have become resistant to electroconvulsive shock and depressant drugs. The differential effectiveness of various amnesic agents is consistent with the view that memory storage involves a sequence of steps and that protein synthesis may be one essential part of the sequence. As Flexner *et al.* indicate, the loss of memory following intracerebral injections could be due to effects unrelated to protein synthesis. Although most animals dosed with puromycin were able to relearn after the loss of memory, the relearning after the injections was inferior to the original learning. This effect would not be expected according to the view that the sole effect of puromycin is that of interfering with memory storage processes initiated by previous training. It suggests that at least part of the impairment might be due to impairment of either performance or memory storage at the time of *relearning.* Another possible interpretation is that puromycin may produce long-lasting but reversible damage or disturbance to cells which have recently been involved in memory storage. This view would be consistent with the finding that recent memory is more susceptible to interference than is older memory when a constant time (3 days) elapses between injections and retraining. It would, however, lead to the prediction that the amnesia might disappear with longer intervals between injections and retention testing. Shrinking of the interval for which the patient has amnesia as time passes is a common observation in clinical cases of amnesia following brain concussion.

The studies of Flexner *et al.* (1962, 1963) are of interest and importance because they provide very suggestive evidence of a link between memory storage and a biochemical process which might reasonably be expected to be involved in memory. In addition, they are to some degree consistent with other work which has shown that memory storage is time-dependent.

C. Drug Facilitation of Learning

Most psychopharmacological investigations of learning and memory have focused on the deleterious effects of drugs. The findings of such studies have contributed both to our knowledge of drug action and to our thinking about the nature of the neurophysiological and biochemical bases of behavior. Biochemical "lesions" (Russell, 1960) have become part of the methodological armamentarium of researchers concerned with brain function. The assumption, long supported by lesion studies, that controlled impairment of brain function can increase our understanding of the brain functions underlying behavior has received support from drug studies such as those cited in the previous section.

Over the past several years, an increasing number of studies have indicated that it is possible to enhance performance with drugs. Until fairly recently, many studies of drug facilitation have been motivated by an interest in compounds which might be of value in the treatment of mental retardation. The research with glutamic acid and thiamine discussed above are examples of such research. Other studies of drug facilitation have been concerned primarily with the beneficial effects of drugs on the performance of learned responses. In these studies, the focus is usually on motivational or perceptual effects of the compounds, rather than on problems of learning and memory. In a recent paper, for example, Hearst and Whalen (1963) found that rats' performances on a task which required them to press a lever upon presentation of a signal in order to avoid a shock was improved by injections of amphetamine (3 mg/kg). The improvement was only temporary, however. Performance returned to the pre-experimental level on subsequent tests without the drug. Hearst and Whalen suggested that the improvement may have been due to an interference with "freezing" behavior typically displayed by rats in this task. Increased alertness or attention is another possible basis of the effect. These findings are, of course, in contrast with the findings of the effects of amphetamine on performance cited earlier. However, the findings of those earlier studies are also unsupported by the more recent studies of the effect of amphetamine on learning which are reviewed below.

Other evidence that rats' performances can be improved by influencing their motivation, has been reported by Gonzales and Ross (1961). These investigators found that chlorpromazine (1.0–4.0 mg/kg) improved discrimination-reversal learning in rats. They suggested that the drug may have alleviated the emotional consequences of the lack of reward during the first few trials. Thus the drug prevented the fixation of position responses found with control rats. If their suggested interpretation is correct, improvement in learning was an indirect effect of the tranquilizing effect of chlorpromazine rather than a direct effect of the drug on associational mechanisms. These findings are difficult to reconcile with other evidence (Doty and Doty, 1964) that chlorpromazine interferes with memory consolidation.

Studies of drug effects on performance are always somewhat subject to interpretations which stress the motivational and/or perceptual effects of the drugs. However, a number of investigations of drug facilitation of learning are more difficult to interpret in such terms. This section will review studies of facilitating effects of drugs on learning and memory storage, with particular emphasis on the hypothesis that drugs may facilitate acquisition, performance, and retention by potentiating the neurophysiological processes underlying memory storage. Clear evidence of drug facilitation of memory storage, together with the knowledge of the mechanisms of drug action, could provide some leads concerning the nature of the processes involved in storing information in the central nervous system. Results of some of the studies reviewed below provide a preliminary step in this direction.

1. *Amphetamine*

As indicated above, a number of studies have reported that learning is either impaired or unaffected by amphetamine. These findings are somewhat surprising, since it might be expected that at least some improvement in performance would result from increased alertness or increased activity level. Recent evidence supports this common sense expectation. Kelemen and Bovet (1961) found that small doses of amphetamine (0.3–1.0 mg/kg sc) facilitated rats' escape and avoidance learning. The rats were placed on a hotplate (60°C) and allowed to escape by jumping up onto the rim of a cylinder. On the first trial, the latency of the jumping response was shorter in amphetamine-injected rats than in control rats. With additional trials given at 30-second intervals, the latencies of the amphetamine animals remained well below those of control animals. Since amphetamine increases activity (Dews, 1953), this could be interpreted as indicating merely that amphetamine facilitated performance by increasing the probability of occurrence of the correct response. However, with the lower dose (0.3 mg/kg), amphetamine facilitated learning on the successive trials but did not affect the latency of the correct response on the first trial. Learning of this problem was impaired by chlorpromazine (1.0 mg/kg). Other recent evidence indicates that small doses of methamphetamine (0.5 mg/kg) facilitate discrimination learning in hamsters (Rahmann, 1961; Rensch and Rahmann, 1960). This is difficult to explain solely in terms of the effect of the drug on activity level, since accuracy of choice rather than latency of response was used as the learning measure. Learning was impaired by a dose (2.0 mg/kg) which produced a high activity level. Rensch and Rahmann suggest that the improvement in performance was due to increased attention and motivation. The effects were not temporary, however, because retention of the amphetamine-injected subjects tested over a 3-month period was superior to that of controls.

Considered together, these recent studies indicate that learning is facilitated by small doses of amphetamine and that the facilitation is probably not due solely to any temporary effect of the drug on performance. Whether the effect is due to increased attention, to a more direct facilitation of processes involved in memory storage, or both is at present an open question. It is not readily apparent why the findings of these recent studies are different from those of the earlier studies. Additional research is needed to gain understanding of the bases of the difference between the earlier and the more recent research with amphetamine.

2. *Nicotine*

For obvious social and medical reasons, nicotine is one of the common drugs of which the effects on learning and performance have been studied in a number of laboratories. Interest in nicotine has, to a large degree, centered on the effects on performance of long-term repeated administration. Some impairment of rats' performances of learned responses have been found after even a single injection of nicotine (e.g., Macht and Bloom, 1921). Daily administration of nicotine, either by fuming rats with large amounts of tobacco smoke or by injecting them with nicotine, has been found to produce serious impairment of performance when the drug is repeatedly administered over long periods of time (Peckstein and Reynolds, 1937; Essenberg, 1954). Smaller doses of nicotine have been found to have either no effect (Phillips, 1937) or facilitating effects on learning in rats. Peckstein and Reynolds (1937) reported that rats fumed daily with a limited amount of tobacco smoke were superior to all control groups in maze learning.

More recent studies which have not been concerned with the

long-term effects of nicotine have obtained similar results. Lucomskaja (1957) found that nicotine (0.05–0.2 mg/kg sc) facilitated avoidance learning in mice. Similar results were obtained with the cholinesterase inhibitor, diethyl *p*-nitrophenyl phosphate (0.1 mg/kg sc), and the cholinergic compound, arecoline (0.1 mg/kg). As mentioned earlier, Lucomskaja (1957) found that avoidance learning was impaired by atropine in doses which did not affect the performance of well-learned responses. In other recent work, Bovet and his associates have reported that small doses of nicotine (0.2 mg/kg ip) facilitated maze learning (Robustelli, 1963) as well as avoidance learning (Bovet *et al.*, 1963). Facilitation of maze learning by nicotine was found with water motivation but not with food motivation. This differential effect may have been due to a depressing effect of nicotine on appetite. The fact that facilitation by nicotine was found with the two diverse learning tasks, maze learning and avoidance learning, is particularly important in view of the lack of a significant correlation between learning in these two tasks (Robustelli *et al.*, 1963). The basis of the facilitating effect of nicotine on learning is not clear from the studies published to date. In the avoidance-learning study (Bovet *et al.*, 1963), all animals were given 50 trials per day for 6 days in an automated shuttle box. On each of the first 3 days, the experimental rats were given drug injections before the day's series of trials. Control injections were then given to these animals on the next 3 days. During this time, the performance of the animals was considerably below that of the last day with drug. The drop was greatest in the group which had been given the largest dose of nicotine (1.0 mg/kg). The group's performance on the last 3 days was comparable to that of the control rats on the first 3 days of training. This finding suggests either that the facilitation was due to some temporary effect of the drug on performance or that the learning with large doses of nicotine was state-dependent. Domino (1964) has found that smaller doses of nicotine (40–80 μg/kg sc) have a slight facilitating effect on avoidance learning in rats, whereas larger doses (80–320 μg/kg sc) impair avoidance learning. These findings are somewhat in agreement with those reported by Bovet *et al.*, but since the experimental animals were not tested without the drug, the findings offer no additional evidence concerning the basis of the effect of nicotine on learning.

The findings in the study of Bovet *et al.* are strikingly similar to those obtained by Sachs *et al.* (1962) with chlordiazepoxide. This drug, in a dose of 15 mg/kg was found to facilitate rats' learning of a simple hurdle-jump avoidance response. It is possible that this effect may have been due in part to the relaxation produced by chlordiazepoxide since the tendency of the rats to freeze when shocked was reduced. The learning of this task was impaired, however, by chlorpromazine (0.25–2.0 mg/kg). As discussed above, chlordiazepoxide and chlorpromazine produce the phenomenon of dissociation. Since Bovet *et al.* did not study the effect of nicotine on the performance of trained saline-control rats, it is not possible, on the basis of their data, to compare the effects of nicotine with other compounds that produce dissociation. Subsequent studies of nicotine should take into account the possibility that dissociation may occur with this compound.

3. *Cations*

In a very interesting and careful study, Sachs (1962) investigated the effects of intraventricular injections of calcium (22.5 μequiv $CaCl_2$, 0.25% solution) and potassium (25 μequiv KCl, 0.375%) on avoidance learning in cats. One group of control cats was treated with injections of comparable doses of saline, and two control groups were not treated at all. On each experimental day, the cats were given 20 training trials in a shuttle box 10 minutes after the injections. The cats were trained to jump from one compartment to another at the onset of a flashing light. Failures to respond within 15 seconds, as well as responses in the absence of the flashing light, were punished with shock. The training sessions were spaced 4 days apart and training was continued to a criterion of 18 out of 20 correct responses. The rate of learning of the animals treated with KCl was superior to that of the combined control groups, whereas the rate of learning of the animals treated with $CaCl_2$ was inferior to that of the controls. There was no overlap in the scores of the $CaCl_2$ and KCl groups. Although the KCl animals were superior to the saline groups, the difference was not statistically significant. The KCl group did differ significantly from the two untreated groups, however. In the control groups, the most rapid learners were those animals who had the greatest initial tendencies to jump, as measured by spontaneous shuttling during the earlier trials. Although the KCl injections produced clear behavioral signs of increased alertness and arousal, this change was not associated with increased spontaneous crossing. This indicates that the enhanced learning rate was not a simple consequence of a drug effect on activity level. Further analyses indicated that, in comparison with the controls, the KCl animals learned very rapidly following the initial successful performance of the avoidance response. Although the KCl cats made about as many errors as the control cats prior to making three correct responses, they made significantly fewer errors thereafter. Sachs suggested that the facilitating effects of KCl and the depressing effect of $CaCl_2$ on learning are due to the excitatory and depressing effects of these substances on the activity of neural structures adjacent to the ventricles, in particular the hippocampus. Additional research is needed to investigate the possibility that the improved performance was due to increased attention rather than (or perhaps in addition to) improved memory storage processes. Nevertheless, the evidence clearly provides no support for the interpretation that KCl improves performance merely by increasing the probability of occurrence of the response independently of its effects on learning and memory.

4. *Strychnine*

Strychnine has been studied for many years in various aspects of neuropharmacological research. Until recently, however, behavioral research with strychnine has been limited primarily to studies of its convulsive effect. There have been some exceptions to this. In an early study, Lashley (1917) reported that small doses of strychnine by injection (0.05 or 0.10 mg per rat) facilitated rats' maze learning. The rats in his study were dosed each day 10 minutes before the first of 5 daily trials in a Watson maze. Although the smaller dose did not affect learning significantly, the performances of the animals given the larger dose were superior to those of the controls, despite slight tremors. The strychnine animals ran more slowly than controls but made fewer errors. Less enhancement of learning was found when the experiment was repeated with heavier animals.

In other early work, Miles (1929) found that strychnine did not affect rats' performances of well-learned maze habits. Zalmanson (1929) reported, however, that topical application of a 0.5% solution of strychnine enhanced dogs' performances of a conditioned withdrawal response. Ward and Kennard (1942) found that daily administration of strychnine facilitated recovery of motor function following the removal of the cortex in monkeys. Although there was no evidence that the enhanced rate of recovery was due to learning, the finding is worth noting and could be of significance for hypotheses concerning the basis of strychnine effects.

More recent studies have provided additional evidence that learning can be enhanced with small doses of strychnine sulfate and other convulsants in subconvulsant doses. McGaugh and Petrinovich (1959) reported that rats treated daily with small doses of strychnine sulfate (0.33, 0.66, or 1.0 mg/kg ip), 10 minutes before 5 massed trials on a Lashley III alley maze, made fewer errors than control subjects in attaining a criterion of 5 out of 6 errorless trials. Hunger motivation and food reward were used. The strychnine and control rats did not differ significantly in running speeds or weight loss. Thus the enhanced learning with strychnine could not be interpreted readily in terms of perceptual or motivational effects of strychnine. In a subsequent study, McGaugh (1961) found both facilitative and disruptive effects of strychnine learning by rats of a 14-unit alley maze. With a small dose (0.33 mg/kg), the best strychnine-treated rats (those below the group's median in total errors) made significantly fewer errors than the best control animals. With a larger dose (1.0 mg/kg), the worst strychnine animals made significantly more errors than the worst controls. Evidence for a disruptive effect of strychnine in the performance of some animals has been found in several subsequent studies (Petrinovich, 1963; Prien *et al.*, 1963; Calhoun, 1964). Evidence that strychnine facilitates learning has also been found with tasks other than maze learning. McGaugh and Thompson (1962) found that strychnine facilitated learning by rats of a simultaneous visual discrimination task. Experimental rats from two strains (S_1 and S_3 descendants of the Tryon maze-bright and maze-dull strains) were dosed with strychnine sulfate (0.33 mg/kg ip) 6 minutes prior to massed training trials on a problem requiring discrimination between horizontal-stripe vs. vertical-stripe stimuli. Controls were dosed with saline injections. Avoidance of shock was used as motivation. Table I shows the trials required and errors made by the rats in attaining the criterion. As can be seen, the strychnine animals were superior to the control animals. With the exception of one subgroup (S_3 females), the trial and error scores of the strychnine animals were lower than those of the control subgroups of the same sex and strain. Petrinovich (1963) obtained further evidence of the

TABLE I

TRIALS AND ERRORS TO A CRITERION OF 9 OUT OF 10 CORRECT RESPONSES IN THE LEARNING OF A HORIZONTAL VS. VERTICAL STRIPE DISCRIMINATION PROBLEM[a]

	Strychnine (0.33 mg/kg ip)				Saline (0.9%)			
	S_1		S_3		S_1		S_3	
	♂	♀	♂	♀	♂	♀	♂	♀
Trials to criterion	30	16	14	17	16	32	35	25
	35	21	62	32	152	50	123	27
	57	29	76	50	215	67	149	51
	117	31	149	86	215[b]	215[b]	215[b]	96
Median	46.0	25.0	69.0	41.0	183.5	58.5	136.0	39.0
Errors to criterion	10	3	5	5	6	13	10	6
	15	4	25	9	63	17	56	8
	20	10	28	18	108	36	73	21
	55	11	53	24	114[b]	114[b]	106[b]	45
Median	17.5	7.0	27.0	13.5	85.5	26.5	64.5	14.5

[a] From McGaugh and Thomson (1962).
[b] These did not reach criterion within 215 trials.

generality of the effects of strychnine on learning. Male rats of the S_1 and S_3 strains were dosed with strychnine sulfate (1.0 mg/kg) 10 minutes before daily massed training trials on a visual successive-discrimination problem. One group of control rats received saline injections and another group was not dosed. The rats had been deprived of food and were rewarded with wet mash. The relevant cue in the problem was the brightness of the gray doors in a 6-unit apparatus. Half of the rats had to learn to choose the right door if both doors were light gray, or the left door if both doors were dark gray. The position and brightness cues were reversed for the other half of the animals. The mean number of trials made by rats of the two strains in reaching a criterion of 16 out of 18 correct choices is shown in Table II. In both strains, the trial scores of the strychnine animals were lower than those of either of the control groups. Furthermore, the mean trial scores of the two control groups were similar. There was some evidence that strychnine affected motivation. In a test given before the training, the

TABLE II
MEAN AND STANDARD DEVIATIONS OF TRIALS TO CRITERION (16 OUT OF 18) IN A SUCCESSIVE DISCRIMINATION TASK[a]

		Groups		
Strain		Strychnine (1.0 mg/kg)	Saline controls	Noninjected controls
S_1	M	272.7	364.2	398.0
S_1	SD	48.6	75.6	86.0
S_3	M	320.7	385.2	378.0
S_3	SD	97.0	95.9	107.3

[a] From Petrinovich (1963).

strychnine rats ate slightly less than the controls. They also took slightly longer to leave the starting point of the apparatus during the preliminary training trials. Rats of the S_1 strain given strychnine also ran more slowly than controls of this strain during the training trials. Strychnine and control S_3 rats, however, did not differ in running times. Thus, although strychnine affected the rats' performances as measured by the amount eaten and latencies in running, it would be difficult to account for the enhanced learning in terms of these motivational factors. Another finding was that the strychnine-injected rats with above-median trial scores also made more errors than did the animals with above-median trial scores in either of the control groups. As indicated above, similar effects were obtained by McGaugh (1961) and Prien *et al.* (1963).

5. *Diphenyldiazadamantanol*

Learning facilitation has also been found with a synthetic strychnine-like compound, 5,7-diphenyl-1,3-diazadamantan-6-ol (1757 I.S.). Longo and his associates (Longo, 1961, 1962; Longo *et al.*, 1959) have shown that this compound, which is structurally unlike strychnine, has effects on CNS activity which are strikingly similar to those of strychnine. In one study (McGaugh *et al.*, 1961), rats of the S_1 and S_3 strains, as well as first generation S_1 by S_3 crosses, were given injections on each of three days, 10 minutes before 5 massed trials on a Lashley III maze. The animals had been deprived of food and wet mash was given as a reward. Experimental animals of each strain were given injections of 1757 I.S. (1.0 mg/kg ip).

Controls received a citric acid solution. Table III shows the mean number of errors made by experimental and control rats of each strain on trials 2 through 15. In the control groups, the S_1 mean was lowest, the S_3 mean was highest, and the F_1 mean was intermediate. There was no significant difference, however, among the means of the groups injected with 1757 I.S. Furthermore, the means

TABLE III
MEAN NUMBER OF ERRORS MADE BY EXPERIMENTAL AND CONTROL S_1, S_3, AND F_1 Ss ON TRIALS 2–15 IN A LASHLEY III MAZE[a]

	Control groups (1.0 ml/kg citric acid)			Experimental groups (1.0 mg/kg 1757 I.S.)		
Strain	N	M	SD	N	M	SD
S_1	7	12.86	4.64	7	15.71	8.94
F_1 cross	12	23.75	7.12	11	17.27	7.44
S_3	13	33.15	18.12	12	17.33	10.30

[a] From McGaugh *et al.* (1961).

of the three drug groups were almost as low as that of the control S_1 rats. No facilitation of learning was found with the animals of the S_1 strain. McGaugh *et al.* suggested that 1757 I.S. affects learning by enhancing intertrial memory storage processes. However, alternative interpretations stressing attentional as well as motivational effects of 1757 I.S. were not precluded. Other data discussed below provide additional support for the interpretation that the 1757 I.S. acts by affecting memory storage. In other work, Kelemen and Bovet (1961) found that 1757 I.S. (0.6 mg/kg) and strychnine sulfate (0.3 mg/kg) had facilitated avoidance learning in a way similar to that of amphetamine. Unlike the results obtained with larger doses of amphetamine, however, strychnine and 1757 I.S. did not affect the latency of the initial successful jumping response. Facilitation was found only in the rate of improvement of responding from trial to trial. Thus the effects seem to be due to enhanced learning rather than to enhanced motor activity.

D. Drug Facilitation of Memory Storage

The results of the studies discussed in the preceding section provide strong evidence that learning, as measured by improvement in performance, can be facilitated by several CNS stimulants. The difficulty with all these studies is that, since the animals were trained shortly after receiving the drug injections, drug effects on learning are difficult to distinguish from drug effects on other processes affecting performance. Even in those studies in which the results strongly support the view that the drug facilitates performance by enhancing learning, the methods used have not provided evidence that could allow for a distinction to be made between learning improvement due to enhanced arousal and/or attention and learning improvement due to potentiation of the processes involved in storing information in the CNS. This difficulty is, of course, common to all studies of drug effects on performance.

A number of recent studies have shown that learning can be facilitated by dosing rats with CNS stimulants within a short period of time *after* training trials. These results are more difficult to interpret in terms of motivational, perceptual, or attentional hypotheses since the animals are neither trained nor tested while under the immediate influence of the drug. By excluding at least some drug effects, the posttrial injection studies have provided clear evidence in support of the hypothesis that some of the learning enhancement found with CNS stimulants is due to a potentiation of perseverating processes underlying memory storage.

1. *Strychnine*

In an initial study using posttrial injections, McGaugh (1959) found that rats given injections of strychnine (0.33–1.5 mg/kg) after each daily trial in a Lashley III maze made fewer errors than did rats given saline after each trial. In a more extensive study (McGaugh *et al.*, 1962a), rats of the S_1 and S_3 strains were given daily injections of strychnine (1.0 mg/kg ip) either 6 minutes before each daily trial in a Lashley III maze or at one of the following intervals after each daily trial: 1, 15, 30, or 90 minutes. As Table IV indicates, the animals that were dosed within 15 minutes after each trial made fewer errors than those that received the drug 90 minutes after each trial. This finding of "retrograde facilitation" is consistent with the findings of drug and ECS-induced retrograde amnesia. The magnitude of the effect is inversely related to the time interval between training and treatment.

These findings are evidence against the view that the drug effects are due to an influence on performance in the trial given 24

TABLE IV

MEANS AND STANDARD DEVIATIONS (WITHIN PARENTHESES) OF THE ERRORS MADE BY SUBJECTS IN EACH SEX, STRAIN, AND INJECTION-TIME SUBGROUP ON TRIALS 2–8 IN THE LASHLEY III MAZE[a]

	Injection time				
Strain	6 min before	1 min after	15 min after	30 min after	90 min after
S_1	16.3(7.0)	12.5(3.8)	12.6(4.8)	13.6(6.7)	18.5(10.1)
S_3	11.8(3.2)	12.3(3.9)	13.3(7.1)	25.3(12.2)	18.3(8.5)

[a] From McGaugh *et al.* (1962a).

hours after each injection. In view of these findings, the report (Cooper and Krass, 1963) that rats' maze learning was facilitated by a single injection of strychnine given several days before training, is difficult to interpret. In a more recent study, Greenough failed to find evidence for the long-term strychnine effects reported by Cooper and Krass (McGaugh, 1965a).

In other recent work, Hudspeth (1964) reported that posttrial injections of strychnine sulfate (0.20 mg/kg ip) facilitated rats' learning of visual discrimination, discrimination reversal, and oddity discrimination learning tasks. Rats were first taught to avoid a shock by entering one of three doors which differed in brightness from the other two (i.e., one black door and two white doors). After all animals had attained a learning criterion, the significance of the brightness cues was reversed, and the rats had to learn to use a door which was previously incorrect but which differed in brightness from the other two doors (i.e., one white door and two black doors). After the rats had learned the reversal, they were then rewarded only for choosing a door which differed from the other two. On some trials, the choice was between two white doors and one black door; on other trials, there were two black doors and one white door. Throughout the training, injections were given each day immediately after completion of the day's blocks of trials. Ten trials were given each day during the discrimination learning and reversal learning, and 12 trials were given each day during the oddity training. On all three problems, the learning of the strychnine animals was superior to that of the controls. Furthermore, the strychnine animals learned the oddity problem whereas the controls showed no evidence of learning, even though all rats were given

300 trials. Unfortunately, training was terminated at this point. It would be interesting to know whether or not this problem is beyond the capacity of the control rats of the strain used. Other research with strychnine has provided additional evidence that facilitation is not limited to tasks requiring fixed response patterns from trial to trial. In one study (Petrinovich, Bradford, and McGaugh, 1965), rats from two strains were first trained to alternate choice of goal boxes on an elevated T-maze on successive trials. This procedure was similar to that used by Petrinovich and Bolles (1957). The animals were thirsty and were rewarded with water. After they had learned this task, the intertrial intervals were gradually increased from ½ to 8 hours. On half of the trials, the animals were dosed with strychnine within a minute after reaching the goal box. On the remaining trials they were dosed with saline. At intertrial intervals up to 3½ hours, the rats performed the delayed alternation response equally well on trials that followed either strychnine or saline injections. At the longer intervals, however, the rats made a significantly greater number of correct responses on the trials that followed the strychnine injections. Since there were no differential external cues available to the rats at the choice point, these data suggest that strychnine facilitates performance by enhancing the rat's memory rather than by merely strengthening specific response tendencies.

2. *Diphenyldiazadamantanol*

Evidence of learning facilitation using posttrial injections has also been found with the strychnine-like compound, 1757 I.S. (McGaugh *et al.*, 1962b; Hudspeth and Thomson, 1962; Westbrook and McGaugh, 1964). In one of these recent studies (Westbrook and McGaugh, 1964), rats of the S_1 and S_3 strains were dosed with injections of either 1757 I.S. (1.0 mg/kg ip) or a control solution each day for 5 days within 1 minute after each training trial on a 6-unit alley U-maze. All animals were both hungry and thirsty. Half of the animals in each group were rewarded in the goal box with wet mash, and half were not. On the fifth trial, and on 5 succeeding trials, all animals were rewarded in the goal box. No further drug injections were given; instead, all animals were given injections of a control solution after each trial. As Table V shows, on the first 5 trials, there was no difference in the performance of the nonrewarded, drug and control groups; neither group improved.

TABLE V

MEANS AND STANDARD DEVIATIONS (IN PARENTHESES) OF INITIAL ERRORS MADE IN A 6-UNIT ALLEY MAZE BY SUBJECTS IN EACH SUBGROUP ON TRIALS 2–5 (PRIOR TO REWARD INTRODUCTION) AND TRIALS 6–10 (AFTER REWARD INTRODUCTION)[a]

		Trials 2–5[b]				Trials 6–10[b]			
Strain	Sex	RC	RE	NRC	NRE	RC	RE	NRC	NRE
S_1	♂	14.5(4.3)	13.0(1.5)	15.2(1.2)	14.8(1.9)	12.3(4.0)	11.7(2.1)	13.8(1.7)	9.0(2.2)
S_1	♀	13.3(1.8)	11.0(1.7)	15.7(2.7)	17.7(1.1)	12.7(3.4)	8.7(2.1)	14.7(2.9)	11.8(2.4)
S_3	♂	13.8(1.9)	13.7(2.4)	15.0(2.1)	16.7(2.5)	12.3(2.6)	9.2(2.7)	12.2(2.0)	9.0(3.2)
S_3	♀	15.3(2.0)	12.7(2.3)	17.5(3.0)	15.8(1.6)	15.7(3.2)	8.7(2.5)	12.2(2.3)	11.0(2.1)
Combined mean		14.2	12.6	15.8	15.5	13.2	9.5	13.2	10.2

[a] From Westbrook and McGaugh (1964).

[b] R, reward; NR, nonreward on trials 1–4; C, control injections; E, 1757 I.S. (1.0 mg/kg).

The rewarded groups did improve, as was expected, and the mean number of errors made by the 1757 I.S. animals was less than that of the controls. On trials 6 through 10, all subjects were treated alike but did not behave alike. The two groups previously given posttrial injections of 1757 I.S. made significantly fewer errors than did the two control groups. These data indicate that 1757 I.S. facilitates "latent" learning as well as conventional maze learning. Furthermore, they indicate that the posttrial facilitation is not due to a rewarding effect of the drug since there was no difference between the 1757 I.S. and control animals during the nonrewarded trials. These findings provide strong evidence that memory storage is facilitated by strychnine and 1757 I.S.

3. *Other Compounds Affecting CNS Activity*

Although the most extensive work has been done with strychnine and 1757 I.S., there is evidence that comparable effects can be obtained with other CNS stimulants. Breen and McGaugh (1961) reported that small doses of picrotoxin (0.75–1.25 mg/kg ip) injected after each trial facilitated the learning of a 14-unit alley maze by rats. As Table VI indicates, the degree of facilitation was

TABLE VI
MEANS AND STANDARD DEVIATIONS OF ERRORS MADE ON TRIALS 2–7 IN A 14-UNIT ALLEY MAZE[a]

	Control group (0.9% saline)			Low dose (0.75 mg/kg)			Medium dose (1.0 mg/kg)			High dose (1.25 mg/kg)		
Strain	N	M	SD	N	M	SD	N	M	SD	N	M	SD
S_1	10	26.5	4.5	10	25.6	8.7	10	25.9	5.9	12	20.2	5.4
S_3	10	22.2	3.0	10	16.6	9.4	11	14.5	7.3	11	13.8	4.6

[a] From Breen and McGaugh (1961).

greater with the larger doses and with the rats of the S_3 strain. Prien *et al.* (1963) interpreted their results as indicating that rats' learning of a 32-unit elevated maze was unaffected by posttrial injections of either strychnine or picrotoxin. However, a careful reanalysis of their original data indicated that the combined strychnine and picrotoxin groups made fewer errors than the controls (McGaugh, 1965a; McGaugh and Petrinovich, 1963b). Of particular interest was the finding that almost a third of the experimental animals had error scores less than that of the best control animal. In addition, some of the drug animals had the greatest error scores. As we indicated earlier, this effect has been obtained in several studies (e.g., McGaugh, 1961; Petrinovich, 1963; Calhoun, 1964). The fact that the animals treated with strychnine had increased variability in their learning scores suggests that analyses based solely on group means may fail to reveal important drug effects.

Recently Hunt and Krivanek (1964) reported that rats' learning is facilitated by small doses of pentylenetetrazole (10.0–25.0 mg/kg ip). This finding is interesting in view of the similarity of the CNS effects of picrotoxin and pentylenetetrazole. In a series of experiments, rats were trained daily, 15 minutes after injections. The animals treated with drug were superior to the controls in their rates of learning a variety of tasks, including both successive and simultaneous visual-discrimination learning as well as position-discrimination learning. The drugged animals also acted more slowly at the choice points of the discrimination tasks. The effects were both large and consistent. Although Hunt and Krivanek interpret their results in terms of possible effects of pentylenetetrazole on the subjects' ability to respond to stimulus cues, their methods did not provide any evidence which would distinguish the effects of the drug on attention from those on memory storage. Preliminary analyses of more recent research (Hunt and Krivanek, 1965) indicate that discrimination learning in rats is also facilitated by posttrial injections of pentylenetetrazol. This finding strengthens the interpretation that the drug enhances memory storage. The finding does not, however, rule out the possibility that facilitation found with pre-trial injections is due at least in part to effects on attentional processes. In very recent research with mice we have obtained additional evidence that maze and discrimination learning can be facilitated with posttrial injections of pentylenetetrazole (McGaugh, 1965b).

Recently Rahmann (1963) studied the effects of caffeine on discrimination learning and transposition by hamsters. Learning and retention were facilitated by pretrial injections of 0.5 mg/kg (sc) and impaired with larger doses (1.0–10.0 mg/kg). The larger doses also caused increases in motility. Rahmann suggested that the effects on learning could have been due to either enhanced attention or enhanced memory storage. The latter interpretation is supported by Paré's (1961) finding that visual-discrimination learning by rats was facilitated by posttrial injections of caffeine. Rats were given a single injection of caffeine (30.0 mg/kg) either 5 seconds, 2 minutes, or 1 hour after massed training trials on a horizontal-stripe vs. vertical-stripe discrimination problem. On relearning trials 2 days later, the animals dosed with caffeine 5 seconds after training made fewer errors than the animals given saline. No facilitation was found when the injections were given 2 minutes or 1 hour after the training. Although these findings are consistent with those of Rahmann, it should be noted that the dose used by Paré was considerably greater than that found by Rahmann to be optimal for facilitation of learning by hamsters. Furthermore, it is not clear why the facilitation was found only with the 5-second posttrial injections. In the same paper, Paré reported that retention was impaired by secobarbital (35 mg/kg) injected 2 minutes after the training trials, and in a number of other studies, evidences of facilitation (as well as impairment) of memory have been found even with considerably longer training–treatment intervals.

Most of the studies of facilitation of learning have used compounds classed variously as CNS stimulants, analeptics, or convulsants. Unfortunately, we do not yet know a great deal about the mechanisms of effects of these compounds on CNS activity. Thus is it difficult at this time to make any precise guesses concerning the basis of drug effects on memory storage. Another experimental approach in several studies has been that of employing drugs to produce relatively specific biochemical "lesions" of which the effects on learning might be understandable in terms of the knowledge of the particular drug's mechanism of action. For example, a number of studies have investigated the effects on learning of compounds affecting acetylcholine (ACh) and acetylcholinesterase (AChE). As we have seen earlier, the anticholinergic compounds, atropine and scopolamine, impair learning. This is, of course, not surprising in view of the evidence that ACh is involved in synaptic transmission. Recently, several studies have indicated that learning is facilitated by small doses of the reversible anticholinesterase compound, physostigmine. Bureš *et al.* (1962) reported that the learning of a one-trial avoidance problem by rats was facilitated by small doses (0.5 to 1.0 mg/kg) of physostigmine administered a few minutes before the training trials. Learning was impaired with larger doses. Similar findings were also reported by Cardo (1959). The effect is not limited to avoidance learning. Stratton and Petrinovich (1963) treated rats of the S_1 and S_3 strains with small doses of physostigmine 30 seconds after each daily trial in a Lashley III maze. The optimal dose for facilitation of learning was 0.50 mg/kg for the S_1 strain and 0.75 mg/kg for the S_3 strain. In both strains, impairment occurred with larger doses. Since the electrophysiological effects of physostigmine (e.g., production of hippocampal theta activity) persists only for about an hour after injection and since there is no evidence that physostigmine can accumulate in the system with repeated injections, these findings suggest that physostigmine improves performance by facilitating memory storage. Furthermore, they provide additional evidence that learning efficiency depends upon levels of ACh and AChE: learning is impaired by drugs that block ACh and is facilitated by a drug that inhibits AChE. These findings are particularly interesting in view of other evidence that learning efficiency in rats is related to normal variations in levels of ACh and AChE (Rosenzweig *et al.*, 1960).

The hypothesis that RNA synthesis is involved in memory storage has stimulated a number of experimental investigations of the effects on learning and memory of drugs known to affect RNA synthesis. Some of the evidence reviewed earlier indicates that memory storage may be impaired by compounds that interfere with RNA synthesis. Gerard and his associates (Chamberlain *et al.*, 1963b) studied the effects of the compound 1,1,3-tricyano-2-amino-1-propene (U-9189) on avoidance learning and spinal cord "fixation" in rats. This drug was chosen for investigation because of evidence that it stimulates RNA synthesis. In the avoidance-learning experiment, rats were injected with U-9189 (15 mg/kg) 45 minutes prior to the training trials. The subjects learned to press a lever during a 10-second signal in order to avoid a shock. The drug was only injected on the first day of training. On this day, the drugged animals did not differ from controls. On two subsequent days, however, the performance of the drugged group was superior to that of controls. Furthermore, injections of U-9189 were found to enhance the rate of "fixation" of the hindlimb postural asymmetry produced by cerebellar lesions. "Fixation time" was increased by 8-azaguanine. As Chamberlain *et al.* pointed out, these findings do not prove that RNA is as essential link in memory storage. They are, however, consistent with the hypothesis.

In other recent work, Cook *et al.* (1963) found that rats given daily injections of RNA (160 mg/kg) performed significantly better than controls in acquisition of an avoidance response. As these investigators pointed out, it would be premature to conclude, on the basis of these findings, that RNA directly affects the processes involved in memory storage. The findings do, however, add to the steadily increasing evidence that RNA is in some way involved with learning and memory.

IV. Discussion

The studies reviewed in this paper provide clear evidence that drugs can influence learning. The results of the studies using posttrial injections indicate that many of the compounds influence learning by affecting the processes involved in memory storage. Other compounds seem to affect performance by modifying attentional, perceptual, or motivational processes. An understanding of the bases of the effects of several of the compounds (e.g., amphetamine and nicotine) will require additional research using such procedures as posttrial injections. This will provide clearer distinctions between drug influences on memory storage and drug influences on attentional, perceptual, and motivational processes.

A. Bases of the Effects of Posttrial Drug Administration

Since the drugs that influence learning are known to affect the CNS, it seems reasonable to assume that their effects on learning are due to their effects on CNS processes. The strongest support for this hypothesis is provided by the experiments which used posttrial injections. Since most of the drugs investigated in these studies are readily metabolized prior to the time at which retention tests are given, it is likely that the effects on behavior are due to some effects produced shortly after the training. It may be that some of the effects of posttrial injections are due to some influence(s) other than those on CNS activity, but as yet there is no evidence to support this view. For example, Thiessen *et al.* (1961) suggested that strychnine may enhance learning by decreasing locomotor activity, thus decreasing the amount of potentially interfering stimulation occurring after training. As we have pointed out elsewhere (McGaugh and Petrinovich, 1963a), this hypothesis does not explain very well the facilitating effects of pretrial injections of strychnine when massed training trials are used (e.g., McGaugh and Thomson, 1962). It also does not account for the fact that learning can be facilitated by compounds known to increase activity levels (e.g., Paré, 1961). Furthermore, in a recent study,

Calhoun (1964) found maximum facilitation of learning by post-trial injections of strychnine when the animals (mice) were placed in a darkened, sound-dampened box immediately after the injections. No facilitation was found if the drugged animals were stimulated by sound, light, and rotation after the training. These findings are contrary to the interpretation of strychnine effects offered by Thiessen *et al.* Another possibility would be that the punishing and rewarding effects of the drug injections account for the impairing and facilitating effects found in the posttrial injection studies. This also is unsupported by the evidence. One-trial passive-avoidance learning is impaired by posttrial injections of CNS depressants (Jarvik, 1964). According to a punishment interpretation, the additional punishment provided by the drug injection would be expected to summate with the other punishment and facilitate rather than retard the avoidance learning. On the other hand, there is no evidence that posttrial injections of CNS stimulants are rewarding. Posttrial injections of 1757 I.S., for example, did not enhance the maze performance of otherwise unrewarded, sub-unrewarded subjects (Westbrook and McGaugh, 1964). Facilitating effects of the drug on learning were evidenced by superior performance of the drug-treated animals only after the reward was introduced. Although there may be additional alternative interpretations of the posttrial drug studies, the available evidence indicates that the behavioral effects are most probably due to the actions of the drugs in the CNS.

B. Implications for Hypotheses of Memory Storage Mechanisms

At a very general level, the evidence provided by studies of drug effects on learning is consistent with other evidence (Glickman, 1961) that memory storage involves processes which are active for some time after the termination of an experience. A number of attempts have been made to measure the time required for memory storage by finding the shortest training–treatment interval for which there is no significant effect of the treatment on subsequent performance. This procedure is based on the assumptions that all the treatments affect the process of memory storage and that if a treatment has no effect on memory then this is evidence that memory storage was complete at the time when the treatment was administered. Memory storage time, as measured in this way, has been found to depend upon a variety of conditions including the age, sex, strain, and species, as well as the specific training procedures (Glickman, 1961). More important, however, is the fact that the "memory storage time" varies with the specific treatment used to impair memory storage. For example, memory storage is impaired by topical application of KCl only when the treatment is administered within a few minutes after training. Under some conditions, other treatments, such as ECS and depressant drugs, affect memory storage even if they are administered an hour or longer after training. Studies using pentylenetetrazole and puromycin indicate that memory storage is not complete for several days after training. These results suggest that memory storage involves sequences of processes and that various drugs and other treatments affect these sequences differentially. The process of memory storage is, in all probability, *at least* as complicated as other basic biological processes such as photosynthesis and carbohydrate metabolism.

A common assumption in current hypotheses about memory storage (e.g., Hebb, 1949) is that short-term memory is based on transient neuronal processes, such as graded dc potentials or reverberations in networks of cells stimulated by an experience, and that more lasting memory is based on further changes initiated or produced by these transient neuronal processes. It seems likely that some of the effects of drugs on learning depend upon the drugs' effects on these transient posttrial neuronal processes. Differential effects would be expected with stimulants and depressants. Furthermore, different effects would be expected with different stimulants and depressants, because of different mechanisms of action, absorption rate, and toxicity. Strychnine, 1757 I.S., picrotoxin, caffeine, pentylenetetrazole, amphetamine, and physostigmine all have excitatory effects on CNS activity but have different patterns of CNS effects and different mechanisms of action (Longo, 1962; Washizu *et al.*, 1961; Chang, 1951; Bremer, 1953).

Another way in which drugs might affect learning is by directly modifying the specific processes involved in the formation of "permanent" traces. For example, a drug might have no striking effect on transient neuronal activity but still impair or retard by disrupting the biochemical processes underlying memory storage. Although the evidence is far from conclusive, the results of some of the studies reviewed in this paper provide fairly strong support for the hypothesis that memory storage involves RNA and protein synthesis and is ultimately based on changes in enzyme concentrations in brain cells (Smith, 1962; Briggs and Kitto, 1962).

According to this hypothesis, the sequence of memory storage is somewhat as follows: Increased activity in neurons increases the amount of transmitter substance released by the cells. The increased utilization of transmitter substance causes an increase (enzyme induction) of the enzymes involved in the manufacture of the transmitter substance. This, in turn, would lead to far-reaching intracellular changes. Thus, ". . . it becomes clear that an increased amount of transmitter substance released by any axon following repeated stimulation could be the major factor in establishing and maintaining the particular mechanisms of memory . . ." (Briggs and Kitto, 1962, p. 539). The recent evidence (Bennett *et al.*, 1964) the brain AChE activity in rats is affected by environmental stimulation and training provides additional support for this general hypothesis.

There are, of course, numerous other ways in which neuronal activity might be modified to produce stable processes underlying memory. Even within the general scheme outlined here, there are other ways in which drugs might affect storage mechanisms. For example, drugs might interfere with synaptic processes or with the axoplasmic transport of newly synthesized proteins to synaptic terminals (Dingman and Sporn, 1964). Nevertheless, whatever the nature of the processes involved in the storage of information in the nervous system, drugs will undoubtedly continue to be important tools in research leading to the discovery of the nature of the processes.

References

Abt, J. P., Essman, W. B., and Jarvik, M. E. (1961). *Science* **133**, 1477.

Albert, K., and Warden, C. (1944). *Science* **100**, 476.

Alexander, I. E., and Siegel, P. S. (1947). *Am. Psychologist* **2**, 400.

Alpern, E. B., Finkelstein, N., and Gantt, W. H. (1943). *Bull. Johns Hopkins Hosp.* **73**, 287–299.

Appel, S. (1964). Unpublished observations.

Armitage, S. G. (1952). *J. Comp. Physiol. Psychol.* **45**, 146–152.

Astin, A. W., and Ross, S. (1960). *Psychol. Bull.* **57**, 429–434.

Barondes, S. H., and Jarvik, M. E. (1964). *J. Neurochem.* **11**, 187.

Bennett, E. L., Diamond, M. C., Krech, D., and Rosenzweig, M. R. (1964). *Science* **146**, 610.

Bernhardt, K. S. (1936a). *J. Comp. Psychol.* **22**, 273–276.

Bernhardt, K. S. (1936b). *J. Comp. Psychol.* **22**, 277–278.

Biel, W. C., and Wickens, D. D. (1941). *J. Comp. Psychol.* **32**, 329–340.

Black, A. H. (1958). *J. Comp. Physiol. Psychol.* **51**, 519–524.

Black, A. H., and Lang, W. M. (1964). *Psychol. Rev.* **71**, 80–85.

Black, A. H., Carlson, N. J., and Solomon, R. L. (1962). *Psychol. Monographs* **76** (29, Whole No. 548).

Blodgett, H. C. (1929). *Univ. Calif. Publ. Psychol.* **4**, 113–134.
Boughton, L. L. (1942). *J. Am. Pharm. Assoc.* **31**, 240–244.
Bovet, D., Bignami, G., and Robustelli, F. (1963). *Compt. Rend. Acad. Sci.* **276**, 778.
Breen, R. A., and McGaugh, J. L. (1961). *J. Comp. Physiol. Psychol.* **54**, 498.
Bremer, F. (1953). *Ciba Found. Symp. Spinal Cord*, p. 78. Churchill, London.
Bridgman, P. W. (1928). "The Logic of Modern Physics." Macmillan, New York.
Briggs, M. H., and Kitto, G. B. (1962). *Psychol. Rev.* **69**, 537.
Brown, C. W., and Searle, L. V. (1938). *J. Exptl. Psychol.* **22**, 555–563.
Bureš, J. (1959). "The Central Nervous System and Behavior" (M. A. B. Brazier, ed.), *2nd Conf. Macy Foundation, Josiah Macy Foundation, New York.*
Bureš, J., and Burešová, O. (1963). *J. Comp. Physiol. Psychol.* **56**, 268.
Bureš, J., Bohdanecký, Z., and Weiss, T. (1962). *Psychopharmacologia* **3**, 254.
Burešová, O., Bureš, J., Bohdanecký, Z., and Weiss, T. (1964). *Psychopharmacologia* **5**, 255.
Calhoun, W. H., Jr. (1964). The effects of strychnine sulfate on behavior and oxygen consumption of 3 inbred strains of mice. Unpublished doctoral dissertation. University of California, Berkeley, California.
Cardo, B. (1959). *J. Physiol.* (Paris) **5**, 845.
Carlton, P. L. (1963). *Psychol. Rev.* **70**, 19–39.
Carlton, P. L. (1964). *Brain Chem. Behavior Res. Project Newsletter* **9**, 2.
Chamberlain, T. J., Halick, P., and Gerard, R. W. (1963a). *J. Neurophysiol.* **26**, 662.
Chamberlain, T. J., Rothschild, G. H., and Gerard, R. W. (1963b). *Proc. Natl. Acad. Sci. U. S.* **49**, 918.
Chang, H. T. (1951). *J. Neurophysiol.* **14**, 23.
Cook, L., and Kelleher, R. T. (1963). *Am. J. Pharmacol.* **3**, 205.
Cook, L., Davidson, A. B., Davis, D. J., Green, H., and Fellows, E. J. (1963). *Science* **141**, 268.
Coons, E. E., and Miller, N. E. (1960). *J. Comp. Physiol. Psychol.* **53**, 524.
Cooper, R. M., and Krass, M. (1963). *Psychopharmacologia* **4**, 472.
Corning, W. C., and John, E. R. (1961). *Science* **134**, 1363.
Deutsch, J. A. (1962). *Ann. Rev. Physiol.* **24**, 259.
Dews, P. B. (1953). *Brit. J. Pharmacol.* **8**, 46.
Dews, P. B. (1955a). *J. Pharmacol. Exptl. Therap.* **113**, 393–401.
Dews, P. B. (1955b). *J. Pharmacol. Exptl. Therap.* **115**, 380–389.
Dingman, W., and Sporn, M. B. (1961). *J. Psychiat. Res.* **1**, 1.
Dingman, W., and Sporn, M. B. (1964). *Science* **144**, 26.
Dispensa, J., and Barrett, M. E. (1941). *J. Psychol.* **1**, 397–410.
Domino, E. F. (1964). Unpublished paper.
Doty, B. A., and Doty, L. A. (1964). *J. Comp. Physiol. Psychol.* **57**, 331.
Epstein, W. (1964). *Psychol. Bull.* **61**, 115–128.
Essenberg, J. M. (1954). *J. Psychol.* **37**, 291.
Essman, W. B., and Alpern, H. (1964). *Psychol. Rep.* **14**, 731.
Essman, W. B., and Jarvik, M. E. (1960). *Psychopharmacologia* **2**, 172.
Ewing, P. L., Moore, B. M., and Moore, W. T. (1952). *J. Pharmacol. Exptl. Therap.* **105**, 343–348.

Fields, P. E. (1928). *J. Comp. Psychol.* **8,** 143–158.
Flexner, J. B., Flexner, L. B., Stellar, E., De la Haba, G., and Roberts, R. B. (1962). *J. Neurochem.* **9,** 595.
Flexner, J. B., Flexner, L. B., and Stellar, E. (1963). *Science* **141,** 57.
Fuller, J. L., and Thompson, W. R. (1960). "Behavior Genetics." Wiley, New York.
Galambos, R. (1961). *In* "Brain Mechanisms and Learning" (J. F. Delafresnaye, ed.). Blackwell, Oxford.
Gerard, R. W. (1963). *J. Verb. Learn. Verb. Behav.* **2,** 22.
Girden, E. (1940). *Am. J. Psychol.* **53,** 397–406.
Girden, E. (1942). *J. Exp. Psychol.* **31,** 322.
Girden, E. (1947). *Am. J. Psychol.* **60,** 571–587.
Girden, E., and Culler, E. (1937). *J. Comp. Psychol.* **23,** 261–274.
Glickman, S. E. (1961). *Psychol. Bull.* **58,** 218.
Gonzalez, R. C., and Ross, S. (1961). *J. Comp. Physiol. Psychol.* **54,** 645.
Gutekunst, R., and Youniss, J. (1963). *Perceptual Motor Skills* **16,** 348.
Hamilton, H. C., and Maher, E. (1947). *J. Comp. Physiol. Psychol.* **40,** 463.
Harlow, H. F., and Stagner, R. (1933). *J. Exptl. Psychol.* **16,** 283–294.
Headlee, C. R., and Kellogg, W. N. (1941). *Am. J. Psychol.* **54,** 353.
Hearst, E. (1959). *J. Pharmacol. Exptl. Therap.* **126,** 349.
Hearst, E., and Whalen, R. E. (1963). *J. Comp. Physiol. Psychol.* **56,** 124.
Hebb, D. O. (1949). "The Organization of Behavior." Saunders, Philadelphia, Pennsylvania.
Herz, A. (1959). *Arch. Exptl. Pathol. Pharmakol.* **236,** 110.
Herz, A. (1960). *Intern. Rev. Neurobiol.* **2,** 229.
Himwich, H. E. (1951). "Brain Metabolism and Cerebral Disorders." Williams & Wilkins, Baltimore, Maryland.
Himwich, W. A., and Petersen, J. C. (1958). *Diseases Nervous System* **19,** 104–107.
Hudspeth, W. J. (1964). *Science* **145,** 1331.
Hudspeth, W. J., and Thomson, C. W. (1962). *Psychol. Rep.* **10,** 222.
Hughes, K. R., and Zubek, J. P. (1956). *Can. J. Psychol.* **10,** 132–138.
Hughes, K. R., and Zubek, J. P. (1957). *Can. J. Psychol.* **11,** 182–184.
Hughes, K. R., Cooper, R. M., and Zubek, J. P. (1957). *Can. J. Psychol.* **11,** 253–255.
Hunt, E., and Krivanek, J. (1964). Unpublished paper.
Hunt, E., and Krivanek, J. (1965). Personal communications.
Hydén, H. (1959). *Proc. 4th Intern. Congr. Biochem. Vienna* ("Biochemistry of the Central Nervous System"), Vol. 3, p. 64. Macmillan (Pergamon), New York.
Hydén, H., and Egyhazi, E. (1962). *Proc. Natl. Acad. Sci. U. S.* **48,** 1366.
Hydén, H., and Egyhazi, E. (1963). *Proc. Natl. Acad. Sci. U. S.* **49,** 618.
Jarvik, M. E. (1964). *Ciba Found. Symp. Animal Pharmacologia and Drug Action,* p. 44. Little, Brown, Boston, Massachusetts.
Jarvik, M. E., and Essman, W. B. (1960). *Psychol. Rep.* **6,** 290.
Jones, M. R. (1943). *J. Comp. Psychol.* **35,** 1–10.
Jones, M. R., and Jones, C. E. (1943). *J. Comp. Psychol.* **36,** 133–142.

Kelemen, K., and Bovet, D. (1961). *Acta Physiol. Acad. Sci. Hung.* **19,** 143.
Kraft, M. S., Obrist, W. D., and Pribram, K. H. (1960). *J. Comp. Physiol. Psychol.* **53,** 109.
Lashley, K. S. (1917). *Psychobiol.* **1,** 141.
Lashley, K. S. (1930). *J. Genet. Psychol.* **37,** 453–460.
Lauer, D. W. (1951). Unpublished Ph.D. Thesis, University of Michigan.
Leeper, R. (1932). *Genet. Psychol. Monographs* **11,** 141–245.
Leukel, F. (1957). *J. Comp. Physiol. Psychol.* **50,** 300.
Longo, V. G. (1961). *J. Pharmacol. Exptl. Therap.* **132,** 240.
Longo, V. G. (1962). "Electroencephalographic Atlas for Pharmacological Research." Elsevier, Amsterdam.
Longo, V. G., Silvestrini, B., and Bovet, D. (1959). *J. Pharmacol. Exptl. Therap.* **126,** 41.
Lucomskaja, N. J. (1957). *In* "Physiologitscheskaja Rol Acetylcholina I Isyskanije Novych Lekarstvennych Veschestv" (M. J. Michelson, ed.), p. 73. Leningrad.
McConnell, J., Jacobson, A. L., and Kimble, D. P. (1959). *J. Comp. Physiol. Psychol.* **52,** 1.
McGaugh, J. L. (1959). Some neurochemical factors in learning. Unpublished doctoral dissertation. University of California, Berkeley, California.
McGaugh, J. L. (1961). *Psychol. Rep.* **8,** 99.
McGaugh, J. L. (1965a). *In* "The Anatomy of Memory" (D. P. Kimble, ed.). Science and Behavior Books, Palo Alto, California.
McGaugh, J. L. (1965b). Unpublished findings.
McGaugh, J. L., and Cole, J. O. (1965). *Psychon. Sci.* **2,** 253.
McGaugh, J. L., and Madsen, M. C. (1964). *Science* **144,** 182.
McGaugh, J. L., and Petrinovich, L. (1959). *Am. J. Psychol.* **72,** 99.
McGaugh, J. L., and Petrinovich, L. (1963a). *Psychol. Rep.* **12,** 211–214.
McGaugh, J. L., and Petrinovich, L. (1963b). Unpublished paper.
McGaugh, J. L., and Thomson, C. W. (1962). *Psychopharmacologia* **3,** 166.
McGaugh, J. L., Westbrook, W. H., and Burt, G. (1961). *J. Comp. Physiol. Psychol.* **54,** 502.
McGaugh, J. L., Thomson, C. W., Westbrook, W. H., and Hudspeth, W. J. (1962a). *Psychopharmacologia* **3,** 352.
McGaugh, J. L., Westbrook, W. H., and Thomson, C. W. (1962b). *J. Comp. Physiol. Psychol.* **55,** 710.
Macht, D. I., and Bloom, W. (1921). *Proc. Soc. Exptl. Biol. Med.* **18,** 99.
Macht, D. I., and Leach, M. C. (1929). *Proc. Soc. Exptl. Biol. Med.* **26,** 4.
McIlwain, H. (1955). "Biochemistry and the Central Nervous System." Little, Brown, Boston, Massachusetts.
Madsen, M. C., and McGaugh, J. L. (1961). *J. Comp. Physiol. Psychol.* **54,** 522–523.
Marx, M. H. (1948a). *J. Comp. Physiol. Psychol.* **41,** 82–92.
Marx, M. H. (1948b). *J. Comp. Physiol. Psychol.* **41,** 364–371.
Marx, M. H. (1949). *J. Comp. Physiol. Psychol.* **42,** 313–319.
Marx, M. H., and Ederstrom, H. E. (1950). *J. Comp. Physiol. Psychol.* **43,** 428–435.
Maurer, S. (1935). *J. Comp. Psychol.* **20,** 385–387.
Mendenhall, M. C. (1940). *J. Comp. Psychol.* **29,** 257–276.

Michelson, M. J. (1961). *Activatis Nervosa Super.* 3, 140.
Miles, W. R. (1929). *Am. J. Physiol.* **90**, 451.
Miller, N. E., and Barry, H. III (1960). *Psychopharmacologia* **1**, 169–199.
Miller, N. E., Bailey, C. J., and Stevenson, J. A. F. (1950). *Science* **112**, 256–259.
Minkowsky, W. L. (1939). *J. Comp. Psychol.* **28**, 349–360.
Moroz, M. (1959). *J. Comp. Physiol. Psychol.* **52**, 172.
Morrell, F. (1961a). *In* "Brain Mechanisms and Learning" (J. F. Delafresnaye, ed.), p. 375. Blackwell, Oxford.
Morrell, F. (1961b). *Physiol. Rev.* **41**, 443.
Mueller, G. E., and Pilzecker, A. (1900). *Z. Psychol.* **1**, 1–300.
O'Kelley, L. I., and Weiss, H. H. (1955). *J. Comp. Physiol. Psychol.* **48**, 123–125.
Omwake, L. (1933). *J. Comp. Psychol.* **16**, 317–325.
O'Neill, P. H. (1949). *J. Genet. Psychol.* **74**, 85–95.
Otis, L. S. (1964). *Science* **143**, 1347.
Overton, D. A. (1964). *J. Comp. Physiol. Psychol.* **57**, 3–12.
Paré, W. (1961). *J. Comp. Physiol. Psychol.* **54**, 506.
Pearlman, C., Sharpless, S. K., and Jarvik, M. E. (1961). *J. Comp. Physiol. Psychol.* **54**, 109.
Pearlman, C. A., Jr., and Jarvik, M. E. (1961). *Federation Proc.* **20**, 340.
Peckstein, I. A., and Reynolds, W. R. (1937). *J. Comp. Psychol.* **24**, 459.
Petrinovich, L. (1963). *Psychopharmacologia* **4**, 103.
Petrinovich, L., and Bolles, R. (1957). *J. Comp. Physiol. Psychol.* **50**, 363.
Petrinovich, L., Bradford, D., and McGaugh, J. L. (1965). *Psychon. Sci.* **2**, 191.
Phillips, H. C. (1937). *J. Comp. Psychol.* **24**, 471.
Pilgrim, F. J., Zabarenko, L. M., and Patton, R. A. (1951). *J. Comp. Physiol. Psychol.* **44**, 26–36.
Poe, C. F., Poe, E., and Muenzinger, K. F. (1937). *J. Comp. Psychol.* **23**, 67.
Poe, E., Poe, C. F., and Muenzinger, K. F. (1939). *J. Comp. Psychol.* **27**, 211.
Popper, K. C. (1959). "The Logic of Scientific Discovery." Basic Books, New York.
Porter, P. B., and Griffin, A. C. (1950). *J. Comp. Physiol. Psychol.* **43**, 1.
Porter, P. B., Griffin, A. C., and Stone, C. P. (1951). *J. Comp. Physiol. Psychol.* **44**, 543–550.
Prien, R. F., Wayner, M. J., Jr., and Kahan, S. (1963). *Am. J. Physiol.* **204**, 488.
Rahmann, H. (1961). *Arch. Ges. Physiol.* **273**, 247.
Rahmann, H. (1963). *Arch. Ges. Physiol.* **276**, 384.
Ray, O. S., and Emley, G. (1964). *Science* **144**, 76.
Rensch, R., and Rahmann, H. (1960). *Arch. Ges. Physiol.* **271**, 693.
Robustelli, F. (1963). *Atti Accademia Nazl. Lincei Mem. Classe Sci. Fis. Mat. Nat.* **34**, 703.
Robustelli, F., McGaugh, J. L., and Bovet, D. (1963). *Psychol. Rep.* **13**, 103.
Rosenzweig, M. R., Krech, D., and Bennett, E. L. (1956). *Science* **123**, 371.
Rosenzweig, M. R., Krech, D., and Bennett, E. L. (1960). *Psychol. Bull.* **57**, 476.
Ross, S., and Cole, J. O. (1960). *Ann. Rev. Psychol.* **11**, 415.

Russell, R. W. (1960). *In* "Drugs and Behavior" (L. Uhl and J. G. Miller, eds.). Wiley, New York.

Russell, R. W. (1964). *Ann. Rev. Psychol.* **15,** 87.

Sachs, E. (1962). The role of brain electrolytes in learning and retention. Unpublished doctoral dissertation. University of Rochester, Rochester, New York.

Sachs, E., Weingarten, M., and Klein, N. W., Jr. (1962). Unpublished paper.

Schmidt, H., Jr. (1958). *J. Comp. Physiol. Psychol.* **51,** 26–28.

Smith, C. E. (1962). *Science* **138,** 889.

Smith, K. (1964). *Psychol. Rev.* **71,** 77–79.

Smith, S. M., Brown, H. O., Toman, J., and Goodman, L. S. (1947). *Anesthesiology* **8,** 1–14.

Solomon, R. L., and Turner, L. H. (1962). *Psychol. Rev.* **69,** 202–219.

Stamm, J. S., and Pribram, K. H. (1960). *J. Neurophysiol.* **23,** 552.

Stellar, E., and McElroy, W. D. (1948). *Science* **108,** 281–283.

Stevens, H. (1937). *J. Comp. Psychol.* **24,** 441–458.

Stratton, L. O., and Petrinovich, L. (1963). *Psychopharmacologia* **5,** 47.

Sweet, A. L. (1951). *Am. Psychologist* **6,** 280.

Terrace, H. S. (1963a). *J. Exptl. Anal. Behavior* **6,** 1–27.

Terrace, H. S. (1963b). *Science* **140,** 318.

Thiessen, D. D., Schlesinger, K., and Calhoun, W. H. (1961). *Psychol. Rep.* **9,** 493.

Thistlethwaite, D. L. (1951). *Psychol. Bull.* **48,** 97–129.

Thompson, R. (1957). *J. Comp. Physiol. Psychol.* **50,** 644.

Tolman, E. C., and Honzik, C. H. (1930). *Univ. Calif. Publ. Psychol.* **4,** 257–275.

Verplanck, W. S., and Hayes, J. R. (1953). *J. Comp. Physiol. Psychol.* **46,** 327–333.

Waelsch, H. B. (1952). *In* "The Biology of Mental Health and Disease," p. 106. Harper (Hoeber), New York.

Waelsch, H. B. (1955). *In* "Neurochemistry" (K. A. Elliott, I. H. Page, and J. H. Quastel, eds.), p. 173. Thomas, Springfield, Illinois.

Ward, A. A., Jr., and Kennard, M. A. (1942). *Yale J. Biol. Med.* **15,** 189.

Washizu, Y., Bonewell, G. W., and Terzuolo, C. A. (1961). *Science* **133,** 333.

Westbrook, W. H., and McGaugh, J. L. (1964). *Psychopharmacologia* **5,** 440.

Whitehouse, J. (1964). *J. Comp. Physiol. Psychol.* **57,** 13.

Williams, G., and O'Brien, C. (1937). *J. Comp. Psychol.* **23,** 457–474.

Wyers, E. (1963). Unpublished symposium paper presented at the American Psychological Association Meeting, Philadelphia.

Zabarenko, L. M., Pilgrim, F. J., and Patton, R. A. (1951). *J. Comp. Physiol. Psychol.* **44,** 126–133.

Zalmanson, A. N. (1929). *Vyschaya Nervnaya Deyatl'nost, Moscow Giz.,* 39.

Zieve, L. (1937). *Psychol. Rec.* **23,** 393–396.

Zimmerman, F. T., and Ross, S. (1944). *A.M.A. Arch. Neurol. Psychiat.* **51,** 446–451.

BIOGENIC AMINES IN MENTAL ILLNESS

By Günter G. Brune

Neurologische Universitatsklinik und -Poliklinik, Hamburg, Germany

I. Introduction

During recent years many investigations pertaining to the question of a biochemical lesion in mental diseases have focused attention on the metabolism of biogenic amines.

This article will review some of the work on the metabolism of indoleamines and catecholamines in relation to mental illness. It will include a brief presentation of biochemical patterns observed in syndromes of inborn errors of metabolism. In addition, investigations of tryptophan and catecholamine metabolism in relation to schizophrenia and various other neurological and psychiatric disorders will be discussed.

II. Metabolism of Biogenic Amines in Inborn Errors of Metabolism Associated with Mental Disorders

The study of inborn errors of metabolism can be traced back to Garrod (1902) who discovered that alkaptonuria represents a metabolic anomaly recessively inherited owing to the effect of a single abnormal gene. Since that time various other inborn errors of metabolism including those resulting in mental symptoms have been described. Usually these syndromes were named after the most prominent biochemical lesion detected. This, however, does not imply that these particular metabolic disturbances bear a causal relationship to the clinical symptomatology. In recent years derangements of various metabolic pathways have been described in some syndromes, and it may well be that these and not the most prominent metabolic lesions are involved as biochemical factors in the clinical symptomatology.

In the relationship between amine metabolism and mental illness it is of interest that in at least four different inborn errors of metabolism abnormalities in indole and/or catechol metabolism have been reported, i.e., in phenylpyruvic oligophrenia, Hartnup disease, maple syrup disease, and hepatolenticular degeneration. All these syndromes are associated with mental disorders and, therefore, the biochemical results obtained in these relatively well-defined syndromes may also be of significance in regard to other mental diseases.

A. Phenylpyruvic Oligophrenia

Phenylketonuria, first described by *Fölling* in 1934, is an inborn error of phenylalanine metabolism. Genetic studies indicate that the condition is transmitted by a single autosomal recessive gene. The parents of almost all patients are heterozygous for the gene and show no clinical symptoms of the illness (Penrose, 1935; Jervis, 1937, 1939). The most important clinical manifestations of the disease is mental deficiency. About 25% of the patients have epileptic seizures. In addition minor neurological symptoms, such as hypertonicity of muscles, tremors, and ataxia, have been observed. Marked behavioral deviations in form of hyperactivity, destructiveness, and rage have been reported in more severely affected individuals. Physical features include reduction of structure and head measurements, the hair is often blond, the eyes blue, and the skin lightly pigmented, not infrequently showing eczematous lesions.

Fundamentally, the biochemical disorder is represented by a failure of hydroxylation of phenylalanine to tyrosine in the liver (Jervis, 1953; Udenfriend and Bessman, 1953; Armstrong and Shaw, 1955) due to the lack of the hydroxylating enzyme (Mitoma *et al.*,

1957). This defect results in a high plasma concentration of phenylalanine and the presence of various abnormal metabolites in the urine of which phenylpyruvic acid is the most prominent.

Although no correlations between the intelligence quotient and either phenylalanine blood levels or urinary excretion of phenylpyruvic acid have been established (Borek *et al.*, 1950; Jervis, 1950), various investigators have treated phenylpyruvic children with a phenylalanine low diet and some improvement of both mental as well as physical conditions have been reported (Bickel *et al.*, 1953; Armstrong and Tyler, 1955; Woolf *et al.*, 1955).

In 1954, Armstrong and Robinson offered evidence of an abnormal indole metabolism in phenylpyruvic oligophrenia including increased urinary excretion of indole-3-acetic acid and decreased urinary levels of 5-hydroxyindoleacetic acid. Brune and Himwich (1960) using quantitative methods determined total indole-3-acetic acid and tryptamine in two phenylketonuric siblings. Urinary total indole-3-acetic acid was found to be elevated in both patients, whereas urinary tryptamine was in the lower range of normal for the less severely affected boy and at or below the lower borderline of normal for the other boy who showed marked mental deficiency and behavioral deviations. Pare and his associates (1957, 1958) found decreased serotonin levels as well as decreased urinary output of 5-hydroxyindoleacetic acid and claimed a decreased 5-hydroxytryptophandecarboxylase activity in phenylketonuria. Tada and Bessman (1960) reported disturbances of the kynurenine as well as of the indole pathway of tryptophan metabolism in phenylketonuric children. Urinary output of kynurenic acid, xanthurenic acid, *N*-methylnicotinamide, and 5-hydroxyindoleacetic acid was found to be decreased, whereas indole-3-acetic acid and indican were increased. Because the abnormalities of indole metabolism tended to disappear under a low phenylalanine diet (Armstrong and Tyler, 1955; Tada and Bessman, 1960), it was generally assumed that the derangement of tryptophan metabolism in phenylketonuria may be secondary to the impairment of phenylalanine metabolism. On the hypothesis that the mental disorders observed in phenylpyruvic oligophrenia may be related to an impaired formation of serotonin, Woolley and Van der Hoeven (1964a,b) studied the effects of serotonin congeners, such as 5-hydroxytryptophan and melatonin, on the maze-learning ability of mice made phenylketonuric by the administration of phenylalanine plus tyrosine. It was found that phenylketonuric mice had a subnormal maze-learning ability which was largely prevented when, from birth on to maturity, serotonin congeners were administered continuously. These results were interpreted to mean that the mental failure in experimental phenylpyruvic oligophrenia is attributable to the serotonin deficiency imposed in infancy. On the other hand, similar to the observations on blood phenylalanine levels and urinary phenylpyruvic acid, no correlations were found between intelligence quotients and levels of urinary 5-hydroxyindoleacetic acid (Pare *et al.*, 1959).

Bergsman (1959) determined urinary adrenaline and noradrenaline in two phenylpyruvic oligophrenics and found no appreciable differences compared to control groups. At one time an elevation was found in one patient who reacted strongly with anxiety and dysphoria to the catheterization. Weil-Malherbe (1955) reported low catecholamine levels in phenylpyruvic oligophrenia.

B. Hartnup Disease

This syndrome was first described by Baron *et al.* (1956). The heredity basis of this disease is almost certainly recessive, and no relevant anomalies have been observed in heterozygous carriers. The clinical manifestations of Hartnup disease appear irregularly. These include a photosensitive pellagra-like rash and episodes of ataxia. In addition, mental impairment and behavioral disorders including psychotic states (Hersov, 1955) have been described. The disease occurs in childhood, and in contrast to most other hereditary metabolic conditions tends to improve with increasing age (Milne *et al.*, 1960).

The most characteristic and constant biochemical abnormalities were found to be a generalized aminoaciduria, not being associated with increases of plasma amino acids. In addition large quantities of indole-3-acetic acid, indole-3-acetylglutamine, and indican were found in the urine, whereas formylkynurenine was reduced. This was thought to indicate either a deficiency of tryptophan pyrrolase or reduced transport of substrate to the enzyme (Nemeth and Nachmias, 1958; Milne *et al.*, 1960). Jepson (1956) reporting on two patients found indole-3-acetic acid and indole-3-acetylglutamine considerably increased in the urine, but a later examination by Milne *et al.* (1960) revealed normal excretion patterns and only after the tryptophan loading test did lesions in tryptophan metabolism become evident.

This discrepancy was probably explained by the fact that the patients when studied at the later date were in a more quiescent period of the disease.

C. Maple Syrup Disease

In 1954, Menkes *et al.* described maple syrup disease as a new syndrome. The heredity patterns indicate that maple syrup disease is probably due to a simple autosomal recessive gene. Lonsdale *et al.* (1963) suggested that parents of affected children are phenotypically normal carriers. Maple syrup disease occurs in infancy and the clinical manifestations include symptoms of central nervous system disturbances characterized by vomiting, poor feeding, muscular hypertonicity, and severe cerebral degeneration. Mental retardation rapidly becomes evident.

The primary genetic lesion appears to be a metabolic defect characterized by an accumulation of the three keto acids corresponding to the partial breakdown of the three branched-chain amino acids—leucine, isoleucine, and valine. These substances were found to occur in excess in urine, blood, and other body fluids (Menkes, 1959). Woody and Hancock (1963) reported that the branched-chain ketoaciduria in an infant with maple syrup disease was brought to normal by means of a formula restricted in its content of valine, leucine, and isoleucine. With a reduced intake of these amino acids the corresponding keto acids returned to normal. Clinical improvement followed the decrease in the urinary levels of keto acids and convulsions ceased, hypertonicity and paralyses abated, and the EEG became normal.

Markedly increased urinary levels of indole-3-acetic acid in maple syrup disease were reported by Mackenzie and Woolf (1959).

D. Hepatolenticular Degeneration (Wilson's Disease)

The condition was first described by Wilson in 1912. Analysis of family data gave evidence that the disease is recessively inherited (Bearn, 1960). The possibility was considered that more than one type of defect is involved (Bearn, 1959). Although one form of the disease becomes evident in the third or fourth decade of life, frequently the clinical manifestations of the illness occur in late childhood or early adolescence. The main clinical features are represented by cirrhosis of the liver and progressive damage to the nervous system, resulting in such symptoms as tremor, rigidity, dystonia, pseudobulbar symptoms, mental retardation, and behavioral deviations, the latter including psychotic states (Filimonoff, 1928; Stutte, 1960). The Kayser-Fleischer ring is characteristic of the disease but is a constant finding only in the more chronic states.

Disturbances of copper and amino acid metabolism are the predominant biochemical lesions in Wilson's disease. Consistently high urinary levels of copper and amino acids are found and, in addition, there is an increased copper deposition in all organs (Uzman and Denny-Brown, 1948; Zimdahl *et al.,* 1953).

Derangements in indole and catecholamine metabolism in Wilson's disease have been reported recently. Sunderman (1963) observed an increased urinary excretion of the serotonin metabolite, 5-hydroxyindoleacetic acid, whereas Barbeau and Sourkes (1961) found increased urinary amounts of adrenaline and dopamine.

It is evident from this brief presentation that amino acid metabolism was studied most intensively in phenylpyruvic oligophrenia and that, as in the other syndromes, abnormalities of indole metabolism were observed. Thus, beside disturbances of other metabolic pathways, lesions of tryptophan metabolism will become evident in these syndromes either in infancy or early childhood. These lesions appear to be marked and permanent in the various syndromes with the exception of Hartnup disease, in which clinical improvement together with normalization of tryptophan metabolism has been reported. The recent findings of a disturbed catecholamine metabolism in hepatolenticular degeneration emphasizes the need for further systematic investigations of amine metabolism in the syndromes of inborn errors of metabolism.

III. Metabolism of Biogenic Amines in Schizophrenia

A single biochemical concept of schizophrenia is impossible in that this diagnosis is not clearly defined, and, therefore, it may cover a variety of different pathogenic conditions. The difficulty of biochemical research in schizophrenia is further enhanced by the variability of the symptomatology even in individual patients. Remissions or partial remissions may alternate with severe psychotic states or dementia may be the most prominent clinical feature. In addition, personality factors and anxiety may help to shape the clinical picture. Biochemical studies have been performed in relation to the diagnosis of schizophrenia as well as in relation to the actual clinical psychopathology observed in schizophrenic patients. In the following, investigations relevant to the question of a role of indole and catechol metabolism in schizophrenia and its various mental states will be discussed.

A. Urinary Excretions of Indoles and Catechols in Schizophrenic Patients

Many investigations on indole metabolism in schizophrenic patients have centered around the urinary excretion of tryptamines and their metabolic products, especially indole-3-acetic acid and 5-hydroxyindoleacetic acid. So far no unique excretion patterns could be established for these substances in relation to the diagnostic category of schizophrenia. In the case of urinary tryptamine other than a greater variability no consistent abnormalities could be detected in the schizophrenic group (Brune and Himwich, 1960; Rodnight, 1961). Ross (1913a,b) and more recently Sherwood (1957) and Masuda *et al.* (1960) reported increased urinary levels of indole-3-acetic acid, but Banerjee and Agarwal (1958) and Rodnight and Aves (1958) could not confirm these results. No consistent abnormality in urinary, total indole-3-acetic acid was found by Brune and Himwich (1960) in a group of schizophrenic patients. Similar discrepancies in results were also obtained for 5-hydroxyindoleacetic acid. Lauer *et al.* (1958) found an increase in the urinary excretion of 5-hydroxyindoleacetic acid in their control group after giving tryptophan but not in schizophrenics. Banerjee and Agarwal (1958) reported exactly the opposite results, while Kopin (1959) found no differences between the normal and the schizophrenic groups after a tryptophan loading test. Leyton (1958) reported decreased urinary excretion of this serotonin metabolite in schizophrenic patients. In contrast, Masuda *et al.* (1960) and Villar Palasi and Solduga (1963) observed an increased urinary output of 5-hydroxyindoleacetic acid, whereas normal values including a greater variation in the schizophrenic group were reported from various laboratories (Buscaino and Stefanachi, 1958a,b; Feldstein *et al.*, 1958, 1959; Haverback *et al.*, 1956; Riegelhaupt, 1958; Robins *et al.*, 1956; Sano *et al.*, 1957; Brune and Pscheidt, 1961).

These differences in excretion patterns may be due in part to various factors unrelated or not directly related to the psychosis. Several investigations have shown that factors such as diet (Waalkes *et al.*, 1958; Anderson *et al.*, 1958; Sjoerdsma *et al.*, 1959; Sjoerdsma,

1959; Weissbach *et al.*, 1959), drug treatment (Sjoerdsma, 1956; Valcourt, 1959), metabolism of intestinal bacteria (Jepson, 1956; Armstrong *et al.*, 1958), and the function of the intestine itself (Sjoerdsma, 1959) may influence urinary excretion patterns.

Considering these interfering factors and excluding them as far as possible, Brune and Himwich (1960) and Brune and Pscheidt (1961) determined urinary levels of tryptamine, total indole-3-acetic acid, and 5-hydroxyindoleacetic acid in relation to the actual psychopathology of schizophrenic patients. These investigations showed that associated with the intensification of the psychosis there occurs a continuous and significant increase in the excretion levels of all three indoles. Except for total indole-3-acetic acid, which was slightly elevated, tryptamine and 5-hydroxyindoleacetic acid were in the range of normal when the psychosis was apparently inactive, but abnormally high values were found with psychosis, and especially with the paranoid hallucinatory type of psychosis. Tryptamine, which chiefly represents tissue metabolism (Sjoerdsma *et al.*, 1959), showed the most pronounced changes in relation to the alterations of the psychopathology, followed by total indole-3-acetic acid, and 5-hydroxyindoleacetic acid in decreasing order. Further investigations confirmed these findings (Brune and Himwich, 1963; Berlet *et al.*, 1964).

Because of their hallucinogenic properties, tryptamine congeners, especially *N,N*-dimethylated tryptamines have received much research attention. Several laboratories attempted to isolate *N,N*-dimethylated tryptamines from the urine of normal persons and psychotic patients. Bumpus and Page (1955) using bioassay and paper chromatography reported the presence of *N,N*-dimethyl-5-hydroxytryptamine (bufotenin) in the human urine. Rodnight (1961) could not detect this compound. Fischer *et al.* (1961) found with the paper chromatographic methods a spot characteristic of bufotenin in 25 out of 26 hallucinating schizophrenic patients, and this compound was not found in the urine of 15 nonschizophrenic patients. Brune *et al.* (1963a) obtained similar results. Sprince *et al.* (1963), however, did not detect this compound in the urine of psychotic patients.

The kynurenine pathway of tryptophan metabolism was investigated by Price *et al.* (1959) in some schizophrenic patients. In studying a total number of 19 schizophrenics these authors found abnormal tryptophan metabolism in 6 patients, whereas the other

13 metabolized the amino acid in a normal manner. Both these groups of schizophrenic patients excreted significantly less of pyridone before or after tryptophan ingestion, compared with the controls. The patients with abnormal metabolism excreted significantly more kynurenic acid, *o*-aminohippuric acid, acetylkynurenine, kynurenine, and hydroxykynurenine after administration of tryptophan than did the controls. The other group of schizophrenic patients excreted significantly less kynurenic acid and *o*-aminohippuric acid before or after tryptophan supplementation and less kynurenine after tryptophan as compared with the controls. Thus the "normal" response to tryptophan in the group of 13 patients was actually subnormal in that they excreted significantly less of some of the metabolites than did the controls. Four of the 6 subjects of the abnormal group and 5 of the 13 individuals of the "normal" group were considered to be acutely ill in that their admissions represented the first hospitalization for schizophrenia. The remaining subjects had been treated on one or several occasions for their schizophrenic psychoses. Brown *et al.* (1960) did not confirm this but observed that their patients excreted less of a nicotinamide metabolite in comparison with the control group. The difference was abolished after tryptophan supplementation.

As with indoleamine metabolism, the possibility that disturbances of catecholamine metabolism may be involved as a biochemical factor in schizophrenia has been widely discussed. In regard to the urinary excretion of adrenaline and noradrenaline in schizophrenic patients, various excretion patterns were observed. Gaddum *et al.* (1958) found elevated values for adrenaline but not for noradrenaline in schizophrenic patients. Bergsman (1959) reported normal excretion values for both amines in chronic schizophrenics, and thus found no evidence of a relationship between schizophrenia and the production and excretion of catecholamines. In acute schizophrenia, as well as in mania, increased urinary levels of adrenaline were observed. Based on these and other studies Bergsman concluded that irritation, anxiety, and dysphoria seem to increase the excretion of noradrenaline in the urine. Elmadjian *et al.* (1958) came to the conclusion that active, aggressive, emotional display is related to increased excretion of noradrenaline, whereas tense, anxious, but passive emotional displays are related to increased excretions of adrenaline in association with normal excretion of norepinephrine. Determination of total catecholamines (adrenaline and noradrenaline) in schizophrenic patients revealed a correlation between the urinary levels of these amines with the degree of anxiety, but there was no correlation with the severity of psychotic behavior (Pscheidt *et al.*, 1960; Brune and Pscheidt, 1961). Similar results were also obtained for urinary catecholamine metabolites (Berlet *et al.*, 1964). Curtis *et al.* (1960) stated that despite the different secretion of adrenaline and noradrenaline the amounts excreted into the urine are correlated significantly in mental patients under special stress, just as in normals. Von Euler and Lundberg (1953) determined urinary adrenaline and noradrenaline in air force pilots during flight and found an elevation of adrenaline output in both groups, which they attributed to the stress present during flight. Urinary noradrenaline was normal in the passengers who served as controls. During strenuous muscular work Von Euler and Hellner (1952) observed an increase in the urinary excretions of both adrenaline as well as noradrenaline. In professional hockey players Elmadjian *et al.* (1958) compared urinary adrenaline and noradrenaline formed during the contest with that of the pregame control period. They reported a sixfold increase in norepinephrine excretion over the control level with a moderate increase of adrenaline excretion.

In summary, investigations on urinary indoles and catechols indicate that there are no consistent correlations between biochemical patterns and the diagnosis of schizophrenia. Correlations were, however, found between the intensity of the psychoses and especially the paranoid hallucinatory type of psychoses and indole metabolism on one hand, and between urinary catechols and various kinds of stress including anxiety, on the other.

B. Effects of Psychotropic Drugs, Biogenic Amines, and Amino Acids on the Behavior of Animals and Man, Including Schizophrenics

A further biochemical approach to mental illness is represented by the study of the effects of psychoactive drugs, biogenic amines, and amino acids on the behavior of animals, healthy people, and mentally ill patients. The interest in these investigations may be attributed to various discoveries. It was observed that some drugs used in the treatment of mental patients interfere with the metabolism of amines. In addition, it was found that the highest levels of indole- and catecholamines are located in those areas of the brain that, according to current concept, include the anatomical substrate of emotion (Papez, 1958; McLean, 1958).

Raab (1943) obtained evidence for the presence of catecholamines in the brain, and in 1953, Twarog and Page detected serotonin in that organ. Since that time the distribution of these amines in the brain has been carefully studied in several species, including man (Vogt, 1954; Amin *et al.*, 1954; Kuntzman *et al.*, 1961; W. A. Himwich and Costa, 1960; Pscheidt and Himwich, 1963). The highest amounts of serotonin and norepinephrine were found in the midbrain hypothalamus, thalamus, and pons medulla; relatively high amounts were also found in the caudate nucleus and the hippocampus, but only low levels were found in the cortex. Recently, large amounts of serotonin were also detected in pineal gland of both animal and man (Giarman *et al.*, 1960).

Reserpine, a tranquilizing and antipsychotic drug, as well as the antidepressant, monoamine oxidase inhibitors were observed to alter the level of biogenic amines in the brain. When it was observed that the reserpine-induced behavioral effects persisted long after the drug had disappeared from the body and that the drug-induced decrease of brain serotonin also persisted for days, the hypothesis was advanced that the change in brain amines was related to the central action of the drug. Reserpine, however, decreases not only serotonin but brain norepinephrine as well and, thus, the question arose whether this change was also important in reserpine action (Brodie *et al.*, 1958). Further studies with the synthetic amino acid α-methyl-*m*-tyrosine suggest that the reserpine-induced tranquilization is associated with changes of brain serotonin and not with brain norepinephrine (Brodie *et al.*, 1961). In regard to the action of monoamine oxidase inhibitors, it has been claimed that the excitatory effects of these substances is the result of an elevation of cerebral biogenic amines evoked by the action of these drugs (Spector *et al.*, 1958; Shore, 1958).

Considering the mechanisms of action of these compounds on serotonin metabolism it may be concluded that the highest levels of free serotonin occur in the initial phase of reserpine administration and in the latter phase of treatment with monoamine oxidase inhibitors, while a slight elevation of free serotonin may be present in the initial phase of treatment with a monoamine oxidase inhibitor and during the latter phase of reserpine administration.

Clinical observations show relationships to those biochemical patterns. Both reserpine as well as the monoamine oxidase inhibitors can induce excitement in animals and man as well as recurrences and activation of the psychoses in schizophrenic patients. These effects will occur mainly during the initial phase of reserpine treatment and during the latter phase of treatment with monoamine oxidase inhibitors. The calming and antipsychotic action of these drugs, however, becomes evident after prolonged reserpine administration and during the initial phase of treatment with monoamine oxidase inhibitors (Barsa and Kline, 1955/56; Kline *et al.*, 1957; Ayd, 1959; Voelkel, 1959; Brune and Himwich, 1961).

In order to study the relationship between indoleamine metabolism and behavior, indoleamine precursors as well as indoleamines were administered to both animals and man, singly and in combination with a monoamine oxidase inhibitor. In animal experiments it was observed that moderate doses of 5-hydroxytryptophan had a calming action on the animals, whereas with higher doses excitement and disturbed behavior became evident (Bogdanski *et al.*, 1958; W. A. Himwich and Costa, 1960).

5-Hydroxytryptophan was also given to humans, but on account of severe peripheral side effects, only low doses could be employed (Pare and Sandler, 1959; Pollin *et al.*, 1961), and no clear-cut mental changes were observed. Nevertheless, Klee *et al.* (1960) reported reactivation of the psychosis in one schizophrenic patient during infusion of 5-hydroxytryptophan.

Sjoerdsma *et al.* (1959) administered tryptophan in combination with a monoamine oxidase inhibitor to healthy humans and observed behavioral alterations similar to alcoholic intoxication. When tryptophan was given alone, no behavioral changes were observed. Lauer *et al.* (1958) and Pollin *et al.* (1961) found behavioral alterations in schizophrenic patients after administration of tryptophan in combination with a monoamine oxidase inhibitor. Shaw *et al.* (1959) gave tryptophan alone to schizophrenic children and to controls and reported bizarre and exaggerated behavior in the schizophrenic group, whereas the behavioral effects in the control group were less pronounced. Brune and Himwich (1961) observed an accentuation of the psychopathology in 2 out of 7 schizophrenic patients receiving 2 gm of L-tryptophan for 2 days, whereas the other 5 patients who were either in full or partial remission showed no behavioral effects.

In contrast to 5-hydroxytryptophan, serotonin passes the blood-brain barrier only to a limited extent (McIsaac and Page, 1959). Even when blood serotonin is high as is the case in carcinoid syndrome, no appreciable changes in behavior have been observed, suggesting either that little penetration occurs or that the brain has adapted to higher concentrations and no longer reacts (Schneckloth *et al.*, 1959). Tryptamine, in contrast, appears to penetrate the blood-brain barrier more readily (Green and Sawyer, 1960). B. Brown (1960) observed sedation in mice after administration of tryptamine. Effects of tryptamine on the central nervous system were also described by Tedeschi *et al.* (1959). Therefore, it may be concluded that serotonin, tryptamine, and other indoleamines may affect the function of the central nervous system.

The above presented investigations indicate that both drugs, reserpine as well as the monoamine oxidase inhibitors, may induce sedation as well as excitation in animals and humans, and that they may evoke recurrences and intensification of the psychoses in schizophrenic patients. However, no clear-cut evidence exists that these drugs may induce a schizophrenia-like psychosis in mentally healthy humans. This also appears to be true for the indoleamine precursors.

As judged from behavioral observations, these studies with psychotropic drugs and indoleamine precursors may suggest latent metabolic lesions in some schizophrenic patients which may become activated during administration of these compounds. In interpreting the behavioral effects of psychotropic drugs in biochemical terms it is, however, necessary to consider that these drugs not only affect the metabolism of biogenic amines but also various other biochemical parameters.

In contrast to serotonin, tryptamine, and indoleamine precursors, administration of even relatively small amounts of *N,N*-dimethylated tryptamines evoke psychosis-like states in mentally healthy human beings. *N,N*-Dimethyltryptamine was found by Szara (1956) and Boszormenyi and Szara (1958) to produce psychotic behavior in humans. The psychotropic principle of *Psilocybe mexicana* Heim, psilocybin, was isolated by Hofman *et al.* (1958) and has been identified as the phosphoric ester of *N,N*-dimethyl-4-hydroxytryptamine. The nonphosphorylated analog, psilocin, was observed to possess identical properties (Hofman and Troxler, 1959). Administration of 10 mg of psilocybin to humans resulted in marked behavioral alterations including hallucinations (Weidmann *et al.*,

1958). *N,N*-Dimethyl-5-hydroxytryptamine or bufotenin is another tryptamine congener which has hallucinogenic properties (Fabing *et al.*, 1956; Fabing and Hawkins, 1956). Recently, Axelrod (1961) demonstrated that *N,N*-dimethyltryptamine as well as bufotenin can be formed in the mammalian organism. These observations indicate that *N,N*-dimethylation changes tryptamines to hallucinogenic compounds and that such compounds may be formed in mammals. The *N,N*-dimethyl configuration was also found to be of importance for the pharmacological effects of chlorpromazine (Brune *et al.*, 1963b).

These investigations point to the possibility that transmethylation processes may be involved in psychotic behavior. In 1952, Osmond and Smythies discussed this possibility in regard to the formation of a mescaline-like compound in schizophrenic patients.

C. Effects of Methyl Donors on the Behavior of Schizophrenic Patients

In order to further elucidate the role of transmethylation processes in relation to psychotic behavior, various investigations were tried. Hoffer *et al.* (1957) treated schizophrenic patients with nicotinic acid and nicotinamide on the hypothesis that these substances may compete for methyl groups and in this way may reduce the amount of methylated psychoactive compounds. Berlet *et al.* (1964) reduced methionine in the diet but observed no improvement in the symptomatology of chronic schizophrenic patients. These authors felt, however, that they could not use dietary exclusion to extremes for fear of affecting adversely the health of the patients and that, therefore, transmethylation may not have been severely affected. Pollin *et al.* (1961), on the other hand, administered the methyl donor, methionine, in combination with a monoamine oxidase inhibitor to schizophrenic patients and observed in a number of these patients a general activation, with increased anxiety, rising flood of associations, and extreme garrulousness as well as exacerbations of psychotic behavior. The observed behavioral effects did not seem to be clearly related to the dose of the monoamine oxidase inhibitor. With the exception of tryptophan and methionine no other amino acids were observed to have an effect on the behavior of schizophrenic patients. Brune and Himwich (1962, 1963) administered methionine singly and in combination with a monoamine oxidase inhibitor to schizophrenic patients. The sole administration of methionine was found to have little effect on behavior. In 2 out of 5 patients a slight increase of psychotic activity was observed. When methionine was administered in combination with a monoamine oxidase inhibitor marked behavioral effects became evident. The main characteristics of the observed behavioral alterations were described in terms of two behavioral components: the first one being characterized by symptoms commonly observed during alcohol intoxication as, for example, euphoria, sleepiness, and confusion, whereas the other component appeared to be an intensification of individual psychotic behavior. After cessation of methionine, the behavior returned to premedication levels or was even improved in comparison to baseline behavior. Similar observations were reported by Sprince *et al.* (1963).

With betaine in combination with a monoamine oxidase inhibitor, similar effects on the behavior of schizophrenics were observed as with the combination of methionine and monoamine oxidase inhibitors (Brune and Himwich, 1963). In contrast to methionine, however, the behavioral changes (including accentuation of psychotic behavior) appeared more slowly and were constantly accompanied by an elevation of mood, a reduction of anxiety, and simultaneously by a decrease of urinary catecholamines.

The behavioral effects observed in schizophrenic patients during the administration of methionine and betaine in combination with a monoamine oxidase inhibitor thus show similarities but also dissimilarities to spontaneously occurring psychoses because in the latter euphoria, sleepiness, and confusion were not observed. Possibly these symptoms represent side effects due to the relatively high doses of methyl donors and the monoamine oxidase inhibitors. The existence of these effects, however, has to be considered in interpreting the actions of methyl donors and monoamine oxidase inhibitors in relation to psychotic behavior. Psychotic states in connection with the administration of methionine and a monoamine oxidase inhibitor were not only observed in schizophrenia but also in other conditions. Sprince *et al.* (1963) reported that administration of these compounds to psychoneurotic patients provoked rises of indole metabolites in the urine as well as hallucinations and delusions. Summerskill *et al.* (1956) found that administration of methionine to patients with hepatic diseases either reproduced or accentuated neuropsychiatric symptoms while at the same time blood ammonia levels remained unaltered.

Although many questions on the relationship between indole

metabolism and psychotic behavior remain to be answered, on the whole, the presented data on urinary indoles as well as the studies with psychotropic drugs, indoleamine precursors, indoleamines, and methyl donors, are compatible with the hypothesis that an increase of indoleamines and/or a facilitation of transmethylation processes may lead to high levels of highly psychoactive compounds in the brain and that this mechanism may act as a biochemical factor in psychotic behavior. A disturbed balance of biogenic amines in the brain is another factor to be considered in this connection.

Furthermore, the findings of normal urinary levels of indole metabolites during periods of relatively undisturbed behavior alternating with abnormally high urinary levels of indoles during psychotic behavior suggest a latent lesion of tryptophan metabolism in some schizophrenic patients. These lesions may have many causes and may become activated or aggravated by various factors. Increased levels of amino acids owing to an increased breakdown of muscle protein may act as endogenous factors, as was proposed by Berlet *et al.* (1964), whereas the administration of some psychotropic drugs, amino acids, or amines may represent exogenous factors.

It should be emphasized that these hypothetical biochemical mechanisms are discussed in relation to psychotic behavior and especially to the paranoid hallucinatory psychoses and not to the diagnostic term of schizophrenia. This suggests that similar biochemical mechanisms may operate in psychoses of a different clinical nature. This concept is in agreement with the well-recognized fact that psychotropic drugs which either lower the level of biogenic amines in the brain or interfere with their actions, have their most beneficial effects on the symptoms of various psychoses, but that they do not cure the underlying diseases.

IV. Metabolism of Biogenic Amines in Various Clinical States Associated with Psychotic Behavior

This section will include a number of studies in which the kynurenine pathway but not the indole pathway of tryptophan metabolism was investigated.

Price *et al.* (1959) reported lesions in the kynurenine pathway in a variety of psychoses including reactive depression, involutional depression, postpartum psychoses, and toxic psychoses. In addition marked disturbances in this metabolic pathway were observed in hepatic porphyria, and some of these patients had previously been considered schizophrenic on account of the clinical symptomatology. In one patient who appeared to be a paraporphyric patient (Peters *et al.*, 1958) it was observed that the metabolic disturbance was paralleled by psychosis. Exaggeration of psychotic symptoms was noted with iproniazid therapy. Lesions in the kynurenine pathway were also observed in a second patient with acute porphyria who showed tetraplegia due to peripheral neuropathy. Beside aberrations in tryptophan metabolism, a disturbed balance of polyvalent cations was observed, and the possibility was discussed that the clinical and biochemical manifestations of porphyria might be related to that disturbed balance of polyvalent cations. Porphyria has generally been defined in the past as an "inborn error of metabolism," but also the existence of acquired forms has been considered (Watson, 1960).

Nutritional disorders as exemplified by pellagra may be associated with a variety of neuropsychiatric symptoms including paranoid hallucinatory psychoses. This deficiency disease which shows many similarities to the genetically determined Hartnup disease has been linked in man to a lack of tryptophan and nicotinic acid. The deficiency of the latter may be enhanced by a food containing large amounts of leucine (Gopalan and Srikantia, 1960). Beside the lack of nicotinic acid there may also be a deficiency of various other vitamins, i.e., vitamin B_6 (György, 1934), which may help further to impair a normal tryptophan metabolism. Lesions of indole metabolism, which have been established in Hartnup disease, are suggested by the work of Sullivan (1922) who isolated tryptamine from the urine of pellagrins.

Soon after the introduction of the antituberculous drug, isoniazid, a variety of neuropsychiatric disorders including peripheral neuropathy (Jones and Jones, 1953; Lubing, 1953; Biehl and Vilter, 1954) and psychotic states were reported to occur in patients treated with that drug. Stucki (1961) described three cases of severe psychosis from large doses of cycloserine and/or isoniazid. The patients became manic, agitated, and unable to control affectivity. Unlike the usual symptom patterns encountered in the toxic psychoses, there appeared to be no clouding of consciousness or temporal–spatial disorientation. The patients were aggressive and inaccessible, with paranoid ideation and schizoform delusions and/or hallucinations. Treatment with chlorpromazine resulted in prompt remission of the symptoms.

The influence of isoniazid and deoxypyridoxine on urinary excretion of tryptophan metabolites in tuberculous patients was studied by Price *et al.* (1957). All had an essentially normal tryptophan metabolism prior to treatment with these drugs. During treatment with isoniazid or deoxypyridoxine, abnormally large amounts of kynurenine, *N*-acetylkynurenine, and xanthurenic acid were found in the urine. Pyridoxine administration resulted in a return to normal tryptophan metabolism even when the ingestion of isoniazid or deoxypyridoxine was continued.

Another condition which may be associated with behavioral deviations is represented by chronic alcoholism. Price *et al.* (1959) observed in one patient with alcoholic hallucinosis a low-normal response to tryptophan administration in terms of excretion rates of kynurenine metabolites. Olson *et al.* (1960) noted normal excretion patterns for xanthurenic acid and *N*-methylnicotinamide before and after a tryptophan load. These authors, however, reported low urinary levels of 5-hydroxyindoleacetic acid and suggested conversion of tryptophan to 5-hydroxyindoleacetic acid might be preferentially depressed in chronic alcoholism.

V. Conclusion

It was the purpose of this article to review some of the work relevant to the question of the role of various biogenic amines in mental illness and especially in psychotic behavior.

From the work presented it is evident that there is no final answer to that question at the present time. Despite an element of controversy, many investigations are, however, consistent with the hypothesis that biogenic amines may be involved as biochemical factors in some forms of mental illness and psychotic states.

In regard to indoleamines it is of interest that disorders in tryptophan metabolism, including the indole as well as the kynurenine pathway, have been observed in various clinical conditions associated with mental symptoms, i.e., in syndromes of inborn errors of metabolism, in nutritional disorders, during drug treatments, and alcoholism, as well as in schizophrenic patients.

In the case of inborn errors of metabolism the various metabolic lesions as well as the clinical symptoms usually become evident in infancy or early childhood, and these disorders appear to be permanent. Hartnup disease appears to be an exception because normalization of tryptophan metabolism together with clinical improvement has been observed. In other syndromes of inborn errors of metabolism, i.e., in phenylpyruvic oligophrenia, lesions in tryptophan metabolism may be corrected by therapeutic means either by a low phenylalanine diet or, as is suggested by animal experiments, by application of serotonin precursors. Therapeutic success has been claimed when the treatment was started shortly after birth. Lesions of tryptophan metabolism that occur in the nutritional disorder pellagra appear to be primarily due to a nutritional deficiency of tryptophan and various vitamins. These metabolic lesions will disappear after correction of the diet and, except for permanent damage during the deficiency state, clinical recovery will be achieved.

Similarly, derangements of tryptophan metabolism as well as mental symptoms can be induced by pharmacologically active agents such as isoniazid, and both may disappear after cessation of the treatment.

In all these relatively well-defined syndromes, lesions of tryptophan metabolism may be related to either endogenous or exogenous causes.

In schizophrenic patients, on the other hand, in whom lesions of tryptophan metabolism were observed during active psychoses no definite statement as to the etiology can be made at the present time. The studies on urinary indoles, which showed normal patterns during remissions but abnormal patterns during psychotic states, as well as the studies on the behavioral effects of psychotropic drugs, indoleamines, and amino acids suggest latent lesions of tryptophan metabolism in some schizophrenics which may become activated or aggravated by various factors, both endogenous and exogenous.

On the whole, the investigations point to the possibility that lesions of tryptophan metabolism of various origin may be associated with similar clinical symptoms. In addition, the time of the manifestation of the metabolic lesion, whether in infancy or adult life, as well as the duration, the location, and the range of these metabolic lesions may represent metabolic factors in the sometimes complex clinical symptomatology.

In order to elucidate further the role of indoles in mental illness it would be helpful to investigate systematically the indole, as well as the kynurenine, pathway of tryptophan metabolism in close association with clinical psychiatry in order to define more clearly the metabolic lesions in relation to the various clinical syndromes and to the actual clinical symptomatology.

In regard to catecholamine metabolism, it appears that variations of the level of urinary catecholamines reflect the degree of various kinds of stress including anxiety in healthy people as well as in mentally ill patients. This, however, does not exclude the possibility that an aberrant catecholamine metabolism may be involved in some forms of mental disease.

Finally, it should be mentioned that in this article only a few metabolic pathways were traced and discussed in relation to mental illness. The possibility exists that other biogenic amines as well as other metabolic disturbances may be involved in mental disorders.

References

Amin, A. H., and Crawford, T. B. B. (1954). *J. Physiol. (London)* **126,** 596.

Anderson, J. A., Ziegler, M. R., and Doeden, D. (1958). *Science* **127,** 236.

Armstrong, M. D., and Robinson, K. S. (1954). *Arch. Biochem. Biophys.* **52,** 287.

Armstrong, M. D., and Shaw, K. N. F. (1955). *J. Biol. Chem.* **213,** 805.

Armstrong, M. D., and Tyler, F. H. (1955). *J. Clin. Invest.* **34,** 565.

Armstrong, M. D., Shaw, K. N. F., Gortatowski, M. J., and Singer, H. J. (1958). *J. Biol. Chem.* **232,** 17.

Axelrod, J. (1961). *Science* **134,** 343.

Ayd, F. J., Jr. (1959). *Ann. N. Y. Acad. Sci.* **80,** 734.

Banerjee, S., and Agarwal, P. S. (1958). *Proc. Soc. Exptl. Biol. Med.* **97,** 657.

Barbeau, A., and Sourkes, T. L. (1961). *In* "Extrapyramidal System and Neuroleptics" (J. M. Bordeleau, ed.), pp. 101–107. Editions Psychiatriques, Montreal.

Baron, D. N., Dent, C. E., Harris, H., Hart, E. W., and Jepson, J. B. (1956). Lancet **II,** 421.

Barsa, J. A., and Kline, N. S. (1955/56). *Am. J. Psychiat.* **112,** 684.

Bearn, A. G. (1959). *Proc. Roy. Soc. Med.* **52,** 61.

Bearn, A. G. (1960). *Ann. Human Genet. (London)* **24,** 33.

Bergsman, A. (1959). The urinary excretion of adrenaline and noradrenaline in some mental diseases, *Acta Psychiat. Neurol. Scand.* Suppl. 133.

Berlet, H. H., Bull, C., Himwich, H. E., Kohl, H. H., Matsumoto, K., Pscheidt, G. R., Spaide, J., Tourlentes, T. T., and Valverde, J. M. (1964). *Science* **144,** 311.

Bickel, H., Gerrard, J., and Hickmans, E. M. (1953). Lancet **II,** 812.

Biehl, J. P., and Vilter, R. W. (1954). *Proc. Soc. Exptl. Biol. Med.* **85,** 389.

Bogdanski, D. F., Weissbach, H., and Udenfriend, S. (1958). *J. Pharmacol. Exptl. Therap.* **122,** 182.

Borek, E., Brecher, A., Jervis, G. A., and Waelsch, H. B. (1950). *Proc. Soc. Exptl. Biol. Med.* **75,** 86.

Boszormenyi, Z., and Szara, St. (1958). *J. Mental Sci.* **104,** 445.

Brodie, B. B., Prockop, D. J., and Shore, P. A. (1958). *Postgrad. Med.* **24,** 296.

Brodie, B. B., Sulser, F., and Costa, E. (1961). *In* "Extrapyramidal System

and Neuroleptics" (J. M. Bordeleau, ed.), pp. 183–189. Editions Psychiatriques, Montreal.
Brown, B. B. (1960). *Arch. Intern. Pharmacodyn.* **128,** 391.
Brown, F. C., White, J. B., Jr., Kennedy, J. J. (1960). *Am. J. Psychiat.* **117,** 63.
Brune, G. G., and Himwich, H. E. (1960). *Acta Intern. Meeting Techniques for the Study of Psychotropic Drugs, Bologna, 1960, Società Tipografica Modenese.*
Brune, G. G., and Himwich, H. E. (1961). *Science* **133,** 190.
Brune, G. G., and Himwich, H. E. (1962). *J. Nervous Mental Disease* **134,** 447.
Brune, G. G., and Himwich, H. E. (1963). *Recent Advan. Biol. Psychiat.* **5,** 144.
Brune, G. G., and Pscheidt, G. R. (1961). *Federation Proc.* **20,** S889.
Brune, G. G., Kohl, H. H., and Himwich, H. E. (1963a). *J. Neuropsychiat.* **5,** 14.
Brune, G. G., Kohl, H. H., Steiner, W. G., and Himwich, H. E. (1963b). *Biochem. Pharmacol.* **12,** 679.
Bumpus, F. M., and Page, I. H. (1955). *J. Biol. Chem.* **212,** 111.
Buscaino, G. A., and Stefanachi, L. (1958a). *Confinia Neurol.* **18,** 188.
Buscaino, G. A., and Stefanachi, L. (1958b). *A.M.A. Arch. Neurol. Psychiat.* **80,** 78.
Curtis, G. C., Cleghorn, R. A., and Sourkes, T. L. (1960). *J. Psychosomatic Res.* **4,** 176.
Elmadjian, F., Hope, J. M., and Lamson, E. T. (1958). *Recent Progr. Hormone Res.* **14,** 513–545.
Fabing, H. B., and Hawkins, J. R. (1956). *Science* **123,** 886.
Fabing, H. B., Kropa, E. L., Hawkins, J. R., and Leake, C. D. (1956). *Federation Proc.* **15,** 421.
Feldstein, A., Hoagland, H., and Freeman, H. (1958). *Science* **128,** 358.
Feldstein, A., Hoagland, H., and Freeman, H. (1959). *J. Nervous Mental Disease* **129,** 62.
Filimonoff, J. N. (1928). *Z. Ges. Neurol. Psychiat.* **115,** 27.
Fischer, E., Lagravere, T. A. F., Vasquez, A. J., and DiStefano, A. O. (1961). *J. Nervous Mental Disease* **133,** 441.
Fölling, A. (1934). *Z. Physiol. Chem. Hoppe-Seyler's* **227,** 169.
Gaddum, J. H., Krivoy, W. A., and Laverty, G. (1958). *J. Neurochem.* **2,** 249.
Garrod, A. E. (1902). *Lancet* **II,** 1616.
Giarman, N. J., Freedman, D. X., and Picard-Ami, L. (1960). *Nature* **186,** 480.
Gopalan, C., and Srikantia, S. G. (1960). *Lancet* **I,** 954.
Green, H., and Sawyer, J. L. (1960). *Proc. Soc. Exptl. Biol. Med.* **104,** 153.
György, P. (1934). *Nature* **133,** 498.
Haverback, B. J., Sjoerdsma, A., and Terry, T. L. (1956). *New Engl. J. Med.* **255,** 270.
Hersov, L. A. (1955). *J. Mental Sci.* **101,** 878.
Himwich, W. A., and Costa, E. (1960). *Federation Proc.* **19,** S838.
Hoffer, A., Osmond, H., Callbeck, M. J., and Kahan, I. (1957). *J. Clin. Exptl. Psychopathol. & Quart. Rev. Psychiat. Neurol.* **18,** 131.
Hofman, A., and Troxler, F. (1959). *Experientia* **15,** 101.

Hofman, A., Heim, R., Brack, A., and Kobel, H. (1958). *Experientia* **14,** 107.
Jepson, J. B. (1956). *Biochem. J.* **64,** 14P.
Jervis, G. A. (1937). *A.M.A. Arch. Neurol. Psychiat.* **38,** 944.
Jervis, G. A. (1939). *J. Mental Sci.* **85,** 719.
Jervis, G. A. (1950). *Proc. Soc. Exptl. Biol. Med.* **75,** 83.
Jervis, G. A. (1953). *Proc. Soc. Exptl. Biol. Med.* **82,** 514.
Jones, W. A., and Jones, G. P. (1953). Lancet **I,** 1073.
Klee, G. D., Bertino, J., Goodman, A., and Aronson, H. (1960). *J. Mental Sci.* **106,** 309.
Kline, N. S., Barsa, J. A., and Gosline, E. (1957). *In* "Tranquilizing Drugs" (H. E. Himwich, ed.), p. 149, Am. Assoc. Advance. Sci., Washington, D. C.
Kopin, I. J. (1959). *Science* **129,** 835.
Kuntzman, R., Shore, P. A., Bogdanski, D. F., and Brodie, B. B. (1961). *J. Neurochem.* **6,** 226.
Lauer, J. W., Inskip, W. M., Bernsohn, J., and Zeller, E. A. (1958). *A.M.A. Arch. Neurol. Psychiat.* **80,** 122.
Leyton, G. B. (1958). *Brit. Med. J.* **2,** 1136.
Lonsdale, D., Mercer, R. D., and Faulkner, W. R. (1963). *Am. J. Diseases Children* **106,** 258.
Lubing, H. N. (1953). *Am. J. Tuberc.* **68,** 458.
McIsaac, W. M., and Page, I. H. (1959). *J. Biol. Chem.* **234,** 858.
Mackenzie, D. Y., and Woolf, L. I. (1959). *Brit. Med. J.* **1,** 90.
McLean, P. D. (1958). *Am. J. Med.* **25,** 611.
Masuda, M., Stonecker, J. S., and Dorpat, T. L. (1960). *J. Nervous Mental Disease* **130,** 125.
Menkes, J. H., Hurst, P. L., and Craig, J. M. (1954). *Pediatrics* **14,** 462.
Menkes, J. H. (1959). *Pediatrics* **23,** 348.
Milne, M. D., Crawford, M. A., Girao, C. B., and Loughridge, L. W. (1960). *Quart. J. Med.* **29,** 407.
Mitoma, C., Auld, R. M., and Udenfriend, S. (1957). *Proc. Soc. Exptl. Biol. Med.* **94,** 634.
Nemeth, A. M., and Nachmias, V. T. (1958). *Science* **128,** 1085.
Olson, R. E., Gursey, D., and Vester, J. W. (1960). *New Engl. J. Med.* **263,** 1169.
Osmond, H., and Smythies, J. R. (1952). *J. Mental Sci.* **98,** 309.
Papez, J. W. (1958). *In* "Reticular Formation of the Brain" (Jasper, H. H., ed.), p. 591. Little, Brown, Boston, Massachusetts.
Pare, C. M. B., and Sandler, M. (1959). *J. Neurol. Neurosurg. Psychiat.* **22,** 247.
Pare, C. M. B., Sandler, M., and Stacey, R. S. (1957). *Lancet* **II,** 551.
Pare, C. M. B., Sandler, M., and Stacey, R. S. (1958). *Lancet* **II,** 1099.
Pare, C. M. B., Sandler, M., and Stacey, R. S. (1959). *Arch. Disease Childhood* **34,** 422.
Penrose, L. S. (1935). *Lancet* **II,** 192.
Peters, H. A., Eichman, P. L., and Reese, H. H. (1958). *Neurology* **8,** 621.
Pollin, W., Cardon, W. P. V., and Kety, S. S. (1961). *Science* **133,** 104.
Price, J. M., Brown, R. R., and Larson, F. C. (1957). *J. Clin. Invest.* **36,** 1600.
Price, J. M., Brown, R. R., and Peters, H. A. (1959). *Neurology* **9,** 456.

Pscheidt, G. R., and Himwich, H. E. (1963). *Biochem. Pharmacol.* **12,** 65.

Pscheidt, G. R., Brune, G. G., and Himwich, H. E. (1960). *Physiologist* **3,** 126.

Raab, W. (1943). *Biochem. J.* **37,** 471.

Riegelhaupt, L. M. (1958). *J. Nervous Mental Disease* **127,** 228.

Robins, E., Lowe, I. P., and Havner, N. M. (1956). *Clin. Res. Proc.* **4,** 149.

Rodnight, R. (1961). *Intern. Rev. Neurobiol.* **3,** 251–292.

Rodnight, R., and Aves, E. K. (1958). *J. Mental Sci.* **104,** 1149.

Ross, E. L. (1913a). *Arch. Internal Med.* **12,** 112.

Ross, E. L. (1913b). *Arch. Internal Med.* **12,** 231.

Sano, I., Kakimoto, Y., Okamoto, T., Nakajima, H., and Kudo, Y. (1957). *Schweiz. Med. Wochschr.* **87,** 214.

Schneckloth, R. E., Page, I. H., and Corcoran, A. C. (1959). *Circulation* **19,** 766.

Shaw, C. R., Lucas, J., and Rabinovitch, R. D. (1959). *Arch. Gen. Psychiat.* **1,** 366.

Sherwood, W. K. (1957). "Biochemistry of Mental Illness," Biol. Sci. Series No. 4, p. 30. Univ. of British Columbia Publications, Vancouver, British Columbia.

Shore, P. A. (1958). *J. Clin. Exptl. Psychopathol.* **19,** Suppl. 1, 56.

Sjoerdsma, A. (1956). *Proc. Soc. Exptl. Biol. Med.* **93,** xix.

Sjoerdsma, A. (1959). *New Engl. J. Med.* **261,** 181.

Sjoerdsma, A., Oates, J. A., Zaltsman, P., and Udenfriend, S. (1959). *J. Pharmacol. Exptl. Therap.* **126,** 217.

Spector, S., Prockop, D., Jr., Shore, P. A., and Brodie, B. B. (1958). *Science* **127,** 704.

Sprince, H., Parker, C. M., Jameson, D., and Alexander, F. (1963). *J. Nervous Mental Disease* **137,** 246.

Stucki, A. (1961). *Praxis (Bern)* **50,** 592.

Stutte, H. (1960). *In* "Psychiatrie der Gegenwart, II. Klinische Psychiatrie," p. 1025. Springer, Berlin.

Sullivan, M. X. (1922). *J. Biol. Chem.* **50,** 39.

Summerskill, W. H. J., Davidson, E. A., Sherlock, S., and Steiner, R. E. (1956). *Quart. J. Med.* **49,** 245.

Sunderman, F. W. (1963). *Am. J. Med. Sci.* **246,** 165.

Szara, St. (1956). *Experientia* **12,** 441.

Tada, K., and Bessman, S. P. (1960). *Paediat. Japonica* 3 (5), 41.

Tedeschi, D. H., Tedeschi, R. E., and Fellows, E. J. (1959). *J. Pharmacol. Exptl. Therap.* **126,** 223.

Twarog, B. M., and Page, I. H. (1953). *Am. J. Physiol.* **175,** 157.

Udenfriend, S., and Bessman, S. P. (1953). *J. Biol. Chem.* **203,** 961.

Uzman, L. L., and Denny-Brown, D. (1948). *Am. J. Med. Sci.* **215,** 599.

Valcourt, A. J. (1959). *A.M.A. Arch. Neurol. Psychiat.* **81,** 292.

Villar Palasi, V., and Solduga, J. (1961). Abstracts of Communications, *Proc. 5th Intern. Congr. Biochem., Moscow, 1961,* p. 360. Macmillan (Pergamon), New York.

Voelkel, A. (1959). *Ann. N. Y. Acad. Sci.* **80,** 680.

Vogt, M. (1954). *J. Physiol. (London)* **123,** 451.

von Euler, U. S., and Hellner, S. (1952). *Acta Physiol. Scand.* **26,** 183.

von Euler, U. S., and Lundberg, U. (1953/54). *J. Appl. Physiol.* 6, 551.
Waalkes, T. P., Sjoerdsma, A., Creveling, C. R., Weissbach, H., and Udenfriend, S. (1958). *Science* **127,** 648.
Watson, C. J. (1960). *New Engl. J. Med.* **263,** 1205.
Weidmann, H., Tacschler, M., and Korzett, H. (1958). *Experientia* **14,** 378.
Weil-Malherbe, H. (1955). *J. Mental Sci.* **101,** 733.
Weissbach, H., King, W., Sjoerdsma, A., and Udenfriend, S. (1959). *J. Biol. Chem.* **234,** 81.
Wilson, S. A. K. (1912). *Brain* **34,** 295.
Woody, N. C., and Hancock, C. D. (1963). *Am. J. Diseases Children* **106,** 578.
Woolf, L. I., Griffith, R., and Moncrieff, A. (1955). *Brit. Med. J.* **1,** 57.
Woolley, D. W., and Van der Hoeven, Th. (1964a). *Science* **144,** 883.
Woolley, D. W., and Van der Hoeven, Th. (1964b). *Science* **144,** 1593.
Zimdahl, W. T., Hyman, I., and Cook, E. D. (1953). *Neurology* **3,** 569.

THE EVOLUTION OF THE BUTYROPHENONES, HALOPERIDOL AND TRIFLUPERIDOL, FROM MEPERIDINE-LIKE 4-PHENYLPIPERIDINES

By Paul A. J. Janssen

Janssen Pharmaceutica, Research Laboratoria, Beerse, Belgium

I. Introduction

For many years we have been using in this laboratory a modification of Eddy's hot plate screening method in mice (Jageneau and Janssen, 1956; Janssen, 1960, 1961a; Janssen and Eddy, 1960; Janssen and Jageneau, 1956, 1957, 1958; Janssen *et al.*, 1958, 1959a,b,c, 1960a,b). A newly synthesized compound is given subcutaneously and at various time intervals thereafter the general behavior of the animal is recorded, its pupil diameter is measured, and the reaction time of a typical licking reflex, elicited by dropping the mouse onto a 55°C hot plate is determined. Using profit analysis, median effective dose levels for "hot plate activity" (AD_{50} in micromoles per kilogram) and for "mydriatic activity" (MD_{50} in micromoles per kilogram) are calculated. The most striking gross behavioral effects observed at the lowest of these two ED_{50}'s are described in standardized terms such as excitement, Straub phenomenon, cataleptic immobility, palpebral ptosis, loss of righting reflex, and ataxia.

This simple screening procedure distinguishes easily between morphine-like analgesics, atropine-like anticholinergics, chlorpromazine-like neuroleptics, and barbiturate-like hypnotics. This statement is supported by the data in Table I.

The ratio AD_{50}/MD_{50} is not significantly different from unity for all of the more than 50 classical morphine-like analgesics

TABLE I

Drug	μMoles/kg (subc.) AD₅₀	MD₅₀	Gross behavior at AD₅₀ or MD₅₀
Morphine	30	40	Excitement and Straub phenomenon
Meperidine	81	81	
Atropine	>100	0.34	Normal
Scopolamine	>100	0.055	
Chlorpromazine	4.8	>100	Cataleptic immobility and palpebral ptosis
Reserpine	4.1	>100	
Phenobarbital	264	>100	Ataxia and loss of righting reflex
Pentobarbital	140	>100	

studied and a typical state of excitement with Straub tail reaction is observed at these atoxic dose levels with all of these drugs (Janssen and Jageneau, 1956).

II. Chemistry and Screening

In 1954 we were studying an extensive series of 4-phenylpiperidines related to meperidine. One of the ideas was to try to increase morphine-like potency by replacing the *N*-methyl group of meperidine by other chemical moieties. This turned out to be easy: a Mannich reaction with normeperidine and acetophenone yielded the propiophenone derivative, R 951 (Table II), which was found to be about one hundred times more potent as a morphine-like drug than meperidine itself (Janssen *et al.*, 1958, 1959b). This interesting result, contradicting the classical belief that the *N*-methyl group was "optimal" for morphine-like activity (Eddy, 1959; Janssen 1962a,b), led to further experiments in this newly opened chemical field. Lengthening the ethylene side chain of R 951 to a propylene chain produced the butyrophenone derivative of normeperidine, R 1187 (Janssen *et al.*, 1960a). The first screening results of the hot plate method clearly indicated that this compound possesses highly unusual properties, the induced effects being both morphine-like and chlorpromazine-like (Table II). The ratio $AD_{50}/MD_{50} = 6.7/38 = 0.18$ was found to be significantly lower than unity and lower, therefore, than is commonly found with typical morphine-like drugs. At the AD_{50} dose level a moderate degree of morphine-like excitement was followed by a longer lasting state of chlor-

TABLE II

Hot Plate Activity (AD_{50} in μg/kg and Mydriatic Activity (MD_{50} in μg/kg) in Mice (Subcutaneous Injection of 4-Phenylpiperidines of Type I)

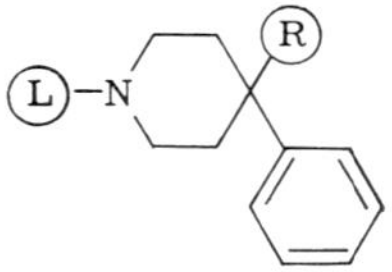

I

Substituent (L)		Substituent (R): Carbalkoxy esters: Carbethoxy ($COOC_2H_5$)	Carbalkoxy esters: Carbomethoxy ($COOCH_3$)	Tertiary alcohol: Hydroxy (OH)
CH_3	#	Meperidine	R 1137	R 1139
	AD_{50}	81	319	> 526
	MD_{50}	81	267	> 526
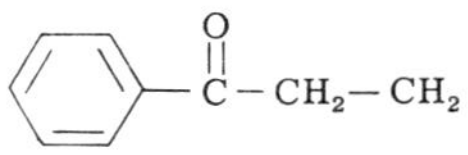	#	R 951	R 993	R 1106
	AD_{50}	1.1	2.4	110
	MD_{50}	1.9	5.4	150
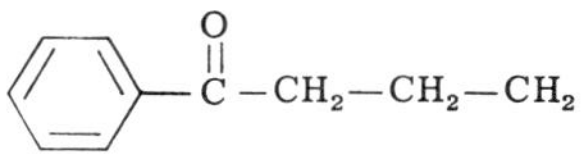	#	R 1187	R 1338	R 1472
	AD_{50}	6.7	6.2	6.1
	MD_{50}	38	140	> 111
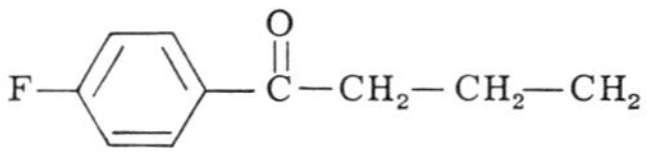	#	R 1823	R 1830	R 1589
	AL_{50}	4.4	3.8	2.9
	MD_{50}	≥ 92	> 100	> 100
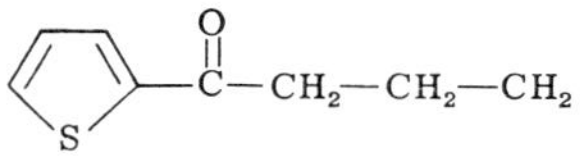	#	R 1822	R 1829	R 1546
	AD_{50}	4.5	5.6	14
	MD_{50}	12	98	> 120

promazine-like immobility and palpebral ptosis, the Straub phenomenon being observed in a few animals only. Administration of a mixture of morphine and chlorpromazine induces similar behavioral changes in mice.

Subsequent studies revealed the fact that it is possible by "molecular manipulation" of R 1187, to increase its chlorpromazine-like potency while decreasing the intensity of its morphine-like effects (Table II), e.g., by replacement of $COOC_2H_5$ by $COOCH_3$ or, preferably, by OH; by substituting the ketonic phenyl ring with fluorine in para position (the isosteric butyrothienones are as a rule slightly less potent) (Janssen *et al.*, 1959c, 1960a).

The 4-fluorobutyrophenone derivative of 4-phenylpiperidin-4-ol, R 1589, is a typical chlorpromazine-like neuroleptic, completely devoid of morphine-like properties. In mice this compound is slightly more potent than chlorpromazine or reserpine, but it is shorter acting (Janssen *et al.*, 1959c). It was finally found that several aromatic substituents on the phenyl ring attached to the piperidine nucleus produce more potent and longer acting neuroleptic drugs (Table III).

Most of the piperidines mentioned above were screened in mice, rats, and dogs. In the course of these studies many screening methods were explored and subsequently rejected. The following ones, however, are still being used today and considered reliable, simple, efficient, and useful for the evaluation of neuroleptic drugs:

1. The hot plate method in mice, described above.

2. The catalepsy-ptosis method in rats (Janssen, 1961a,b; Janssen *et al.*, 1963b). All neuroleptic drugs induce a state of typical cataleptic immobility. Handled animals show a certain degree of palpebral ptosis. Both phenomena are measured quantitatively.

3. The jumping box method in rats (Janssen, 1961a, 1962c; Janssen and Niemegeers, 1961a; Janssen *et al.*, 1963a,b) or in dogs (Janssen, 1961a; Janssen, 1962c; Janssen *et al.*, 1963b; Niemegeers and Janssen, 1960a). The animals are trained to jump over a hurdle in order to avoid punishment. A buzzer serves as the warning signal and failing to make the avoidance response within 15 seconds is punished with electrical foot shock. A typical neuroleptic produces avoidance loss in fully trained animals at dose levels that are devoid of obvious behavioral effects.

4. The antiamphetamine method in rats (Janssen, 1961a; Janssen, 1962c; Janssen *et al.*, 1963b) consists in determining the dose

TABLE III

The Effect of Various Aromatic Substituents on Neuroleptic Potency in Mice (hot plate method), in Rats, (ΔW-test), and in Dogs (Antiapomorphine Test) of Butyrophenones (II), Derived from 4-Phenylpiperidin-4-ol (ED_{50} in $\mu g/kg$ Subc.)

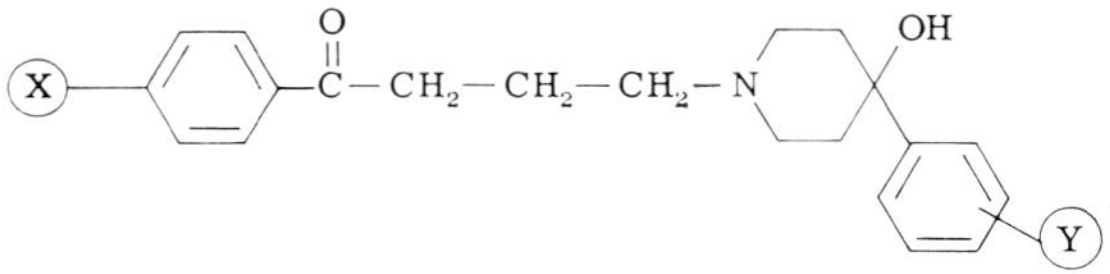

II

Y	X = H			X = F		
	Mice	Rats	Dogs	Mice	Rats	Dogs
H	6.1	7.2	1.1	2.9	2.6	0.30
2 CH_3	18	12	1.5	4.8	5.0	0.50
3 CH_3	4.5	3.3	0.20	1.8	1.5	0.080
4 CH_3	6.2	1.6	0.13	2.0	0.46	0.080 (M)[a]
3 C_2H_5	3.9	3.1	0.30	1.2	1.2	0.070
4 C_2H_5	—	—	—	16	0.73	0.095
3 F	3.4	5.8	0.30	2.0	1.3	0.10
4 F	9.0	6.4	0.53	2.0	1.0	0.20
3 Cl	—	—	—	1.7	0.90	0.10
4 Cl	6.2	1.3	0.17	1.2	0.56	0.058 (H)[b]
3 CF_3	2.1	0.47	0.035	0.70	0.18	0.030 (T)[c]
2 OCH_3	21	12	5.1	7.8	8.8	1.0
4 OCH_3	6.5	6.4	0.17	4.0	2.2	0.080

[a] (M), Methylperidol, moperone (R 1658).
[b] (H), Haloperidol (R 1625).
[c] (T), Trifluperidol, triperidol (R 2498).

needed for blocking the compulsory gnawing movements induced by a high intravenous dose of amphetamine. Most neuroleptics are effective amphetamine antagonists at very low dose levels, but reserpine is inactive in this test.

5. The antiapomorphine method in rats (Janssen, 1961a, 1962c; Janssen *et al.*, 1960c, 1963b) is a similar procedure. Apomorphine also produces compulsory gnawing in rats and this is blocked by many neuroleptics at low, moderate, or relatively high dose levels.

6. The ΔW-test in rats (Janssen, 1961a, 1962c; Janssen *et al.*, 1963b). Rats are trained to consume their daily ration of standard pellets on a 22-hour food deprivation schedule. After about 3 weeks of training these animals show a highly predictable weight increase (ΔW in grams) during the 2-hour feeding period. Many drugs, including neuroleptics, anticholinergics, morphine-like narcotics, and amphetamine-like stimulants depress food consumption and weight increase in these trained rats.

7. The open field test in rats (Janssen, 1961a, 1962c; Janssen *et al.*, 1960d, 1963b) consists in measuring exploratory ambulation, rearing, preening, and "emotional defecation" in naive rats. Neuroleptics inhibit the motor phenomena at low dose levels. Emotional defecation is specifically blocked by a few neuroleptics only.

8. The antiepinephrine and antinorepinephrine tests in rats (Janssen, 1961a, 1962c; Janssen *et al.*, 1963b) consists in determining the ED_{50} that will protect rats against the lethal effects of both catecholamines.

9. The antitryptamine test in rats (Janssen, 1961a, 1962c; Janssen *et al.*, 1963b) consists in determining the ED_{50} that will protect rats against the clonic seizures of the forepaws induced by tryptamine. Most neuroleptics, except reserpine, are active blockers of norepinephrine, epinephrine, and tryptamine at low, moderate, or relatively high dose levels.

10. The Noble and Collip drumming procedure (Janssen, 1961a, 1962c; Janssen *et al.*, 1963b) is a convenient method for producing traumatic shock in rats. Many vasodilating drugs, including all known neuroleptics, protect the animals against shock-induced mortality.

11. The antiapomorphine test in dogs (Janssen, 1961a, 1962c; Janssen and Niemegeers, 1961b; Janssen *et al.*, 1960e, 1963b) consists in determining the median effective antiemetic dose. The dog is pretreated with the drug under investigation and challenged ½,

TABLE IV

COMPARATIVE SCREENING DATA (ED_{50} IN MG/KG) IN MICE, RATS, AND DOGS FOR HALOPERIDOL, TRIFLUPERIDOL, AND A FEW STANDARD NEUROLEPTIC DRUGS

Screening method	Species	Route	Haloperidol[a]	Trifluperidol[a]	Fluphenazine[a]	Perphenazine[a]	Prochlorperazine[a]	Chlorpromazine[a]	Promazine[a]	Reserpine[a]	Thioridazine[a]
Hot plate	Mice	Subc.	0.46	0.32	1.2	1.3	3.7	1.7	5.8	7.0	9.0
Mydriasis	Mice	Subc.	∞	∞	∞	∞	∞	∞	∞	∞	∞
Catalepsy (CD_3)	Rats	Subc.	0.20	0.16	0.16	0.31	4.0	7.5	40	0.90	13
Ptosis (PD_4)	Rats	Subc.	1.2	1.2	1.2	1.8	10	10	30	0.45	5.0
Antiamphetamine	Rats	Subc.	0.038	0.025	0.10	0.16	0.47	1.1	32	>10	7.1
Antiapomorphine	Rats	Subc.	0.20	0.030	0.13	0.32	2.0	6.5	>80	>10	>160
Antinorepinephrine	Rats	Subc.	2.1	0.30	0.93	0.50	7.0	0.52	0.70	>10	0.55
Antitryptamine	Rats	Subc.	1.7	0.63	2.5	1.1	2.3	1.3	20	>10	16
Antishock	Rats	Subc.	2.0	0.60	1.0	3.0	6.0	0.80	0.50	0.65	0.50
Inhibition of ambulation	Rats	Subc.	0.21	0.090	0.10	0.22	1.6	4.5	50	1.2	12
Inhibition of rearing	Rats	Subc.	0.13	0.050	0.14	0.15	1.3	3.7	25	1.0	30
ΔW-test	Rats	Subc.	0.21	0.080	0.27	0.18	3.2	2.3	15	1.5	36
Jumping box	Rats	Subc.	0.058	0.025	0.025	0.10	0.80	0.93	10	0.20	20
Jumping box	Rats	Oral	0.14	0.63	0.43	1.6	3.8	7.0	35	>10	13
Jumping box	Dogs	Subc.	0.065	0.060	0.060	0.16	3.0	2.3	25	Toxic	20
Jump ng box	Dogs	Oral	0.10	0.13	0.50	0.90	2.5	4.6	25	Toxic	14
Antiapomorphine	Dogs	Subc.	0.020	0.0065	0.0065	0.025	0.40	1.0	15	Toxic	3.6
Antiapomorphine	Dogs	Oral	0.025	0.050	0.070	0.40	1.3	4.0	>40 (Vomit.)	Toxic	3.0
Acute toxicity	Mice	Subc.	60	100		150	270	63	110		
Acute toxicity	Rats	Iv.	19	14		58	80	30	29		
Acute toxicity	Rats	Subc.	63	70	≥640	>640	>320	137	300		

[a] Subtoxic dose levels, ∞.

2, 4, 8, 16, or 32 hours thereafter with a 100% emetic dose of apomorphine (0.31 mg/kg subcutaneously). ED_{50} values may be computed for each time interval; ED_{50} vs. time curves are used for evaluating onset, peak, and duration of action.

On the basis of the results obtained in this battery of screening tests (Table IV), it was concluded that haloperidol and trifluperidol possess a series of pharmacological properties that are quite comparable to the properties of several neuroleptics or major tranquilizers derived from phenothiazine (Boissier and Pagny, 1960; Boissier and Simon, 1963, 1964a,b; Boissier *et al.*, 1960, 1961, 1964; Carlsson and Lindqvist, 1963; Frommel and Chmouliovsky, 1964; Frommel and Joye, 1963; Frommel *et al.*, 1960; Gözsy and Kato, 1962; Janssen, 1961a, 1962c; Janssen and Niemegeers, 1959, 1961a; Janssen *et al.*, 1959c, 1960b,c,d, 1963a; Niemegeers, 1960; Niemegeers and Janssen, 1960a; Randrup *et al.*, 1963; Raynaud and Valette, 1963; Revol, 1961; Schaper *et al.*, 1960a; Van Nueten, 1962; Weaver *et al.*, 1964).

Graphical representation of the median effective dose levels (listed in Table IV) is attempted in Figs. 1a–i and 2a–h. Figure 1a–i contains nine so-called "neuroleptic activity spectra" for rats (Janssen *et al.*, 1965), and Fig. 2a–h contains eight "neuroleptic activity spectra" for dogs (reserpine is quite toxic in dogs and cannot be adequately studied in this species).

From these and similar data the following conclusions were drawn:

1. All neuroleptic drugs induce a relative long lasting state of

TABLE V

Drug	Potency ratio for mean catalepsy scores: 1	3	6
1. Trifluperidol	75	45	20
2. Fluphenazine	45	45	20
3. Haloperidol	30	40	20
4. Perphenazine	25	25	10
5. Reserpine	4.5	8	10
6. Prochlorperazine	2.5	2	1.5
7. Chlorpromazine	①	①	①
8. Thioridazine	1	$\frac{1}{2}$	$\frac{1}{6}$
9. Promazine	$\frac{1}{4}$	$\frac{1}{5}$	∞ [a]

[a] Catalepsy scores 6 cannot be obtained with any dose of promazine.

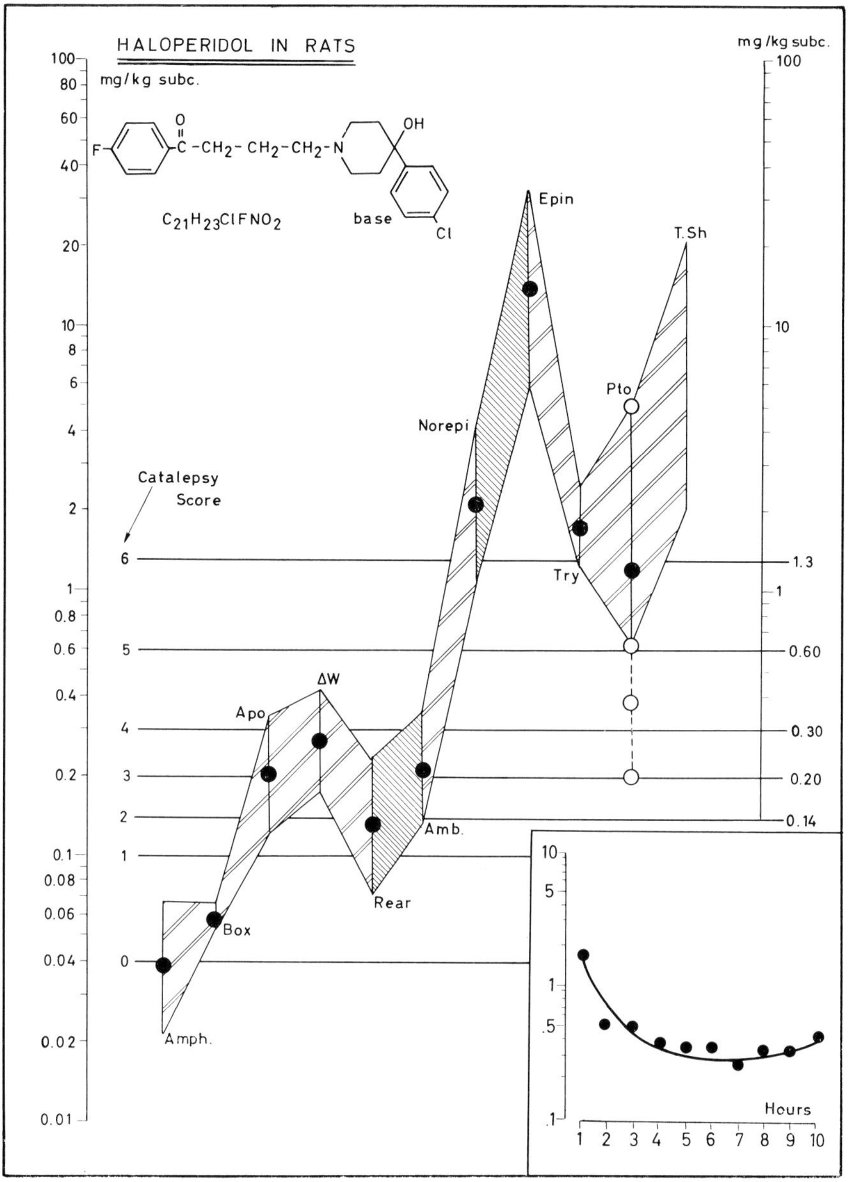

FIG. 1a. Activity spectrum of haloperidol in rats.

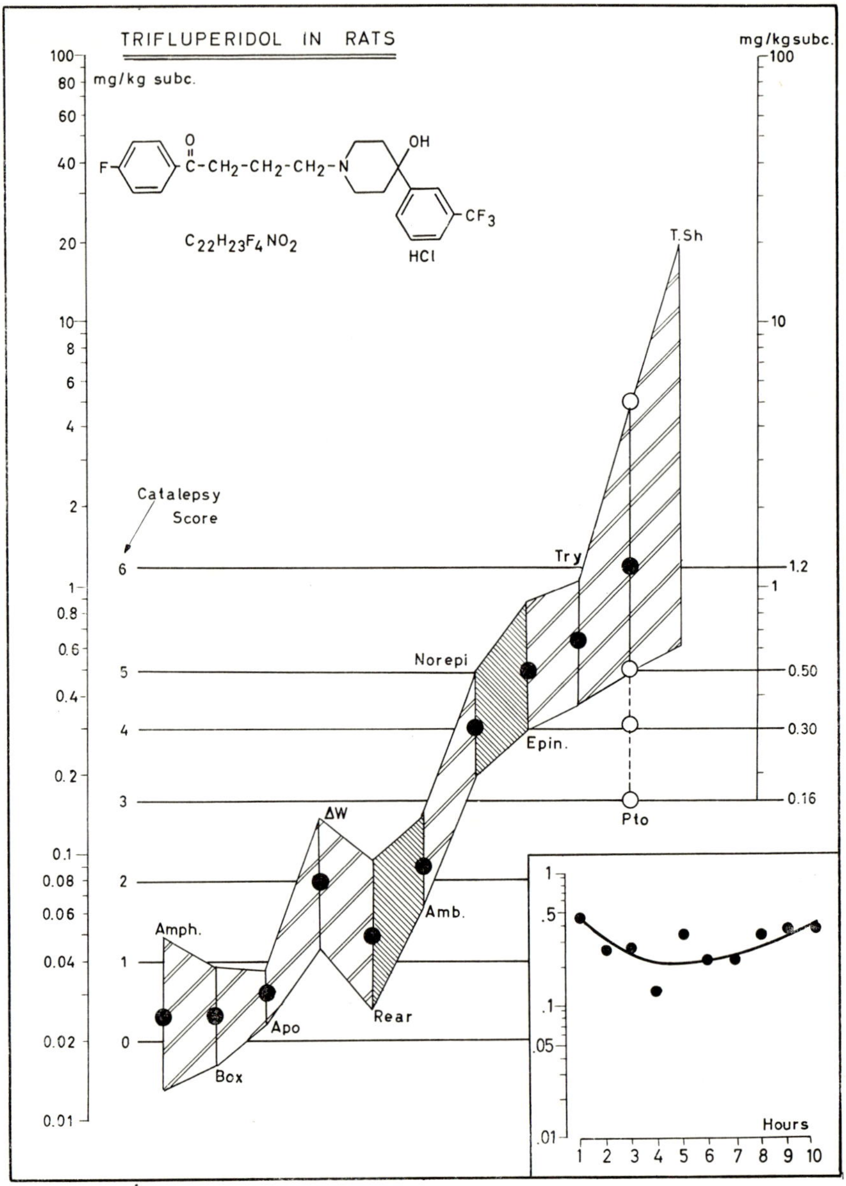

FIG. 1b. Activity spectrum of trifluperidol in rats.

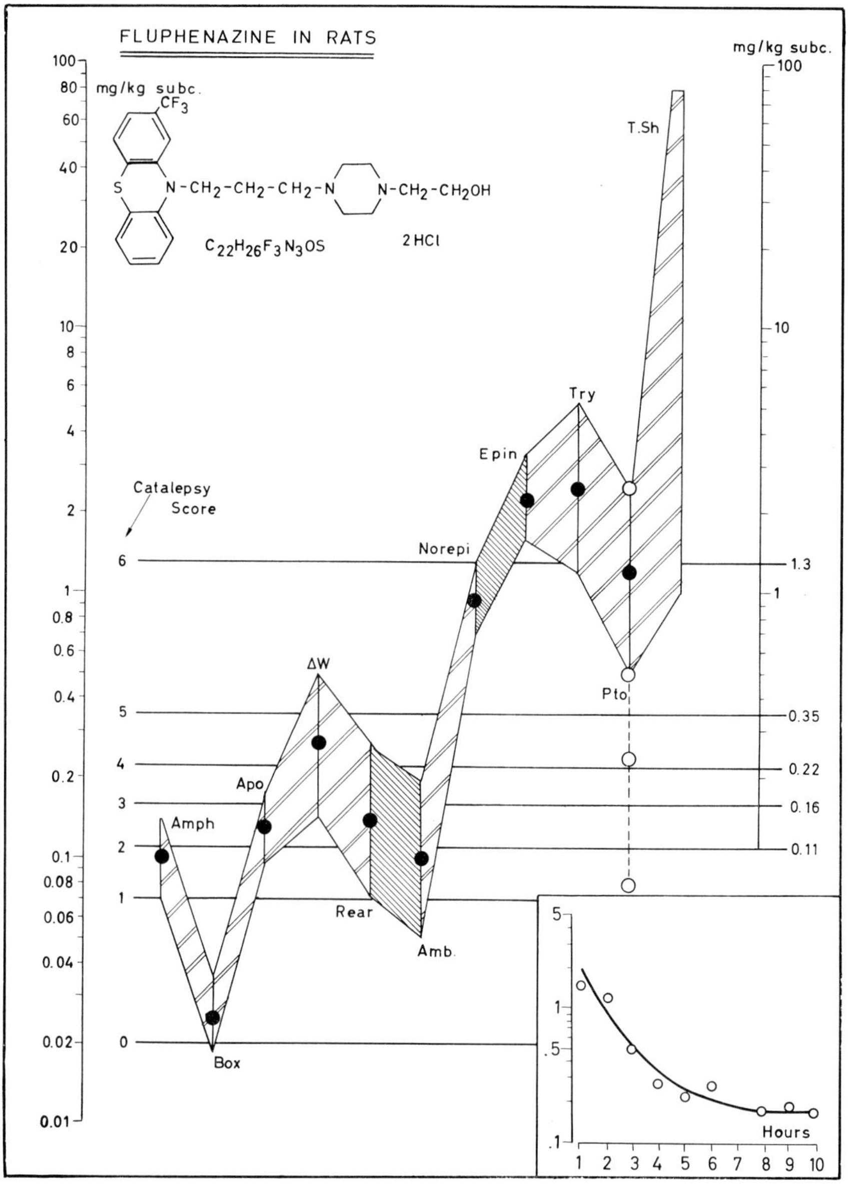

FIG. 1c. Activity spectrum of fluphenazine in rats.

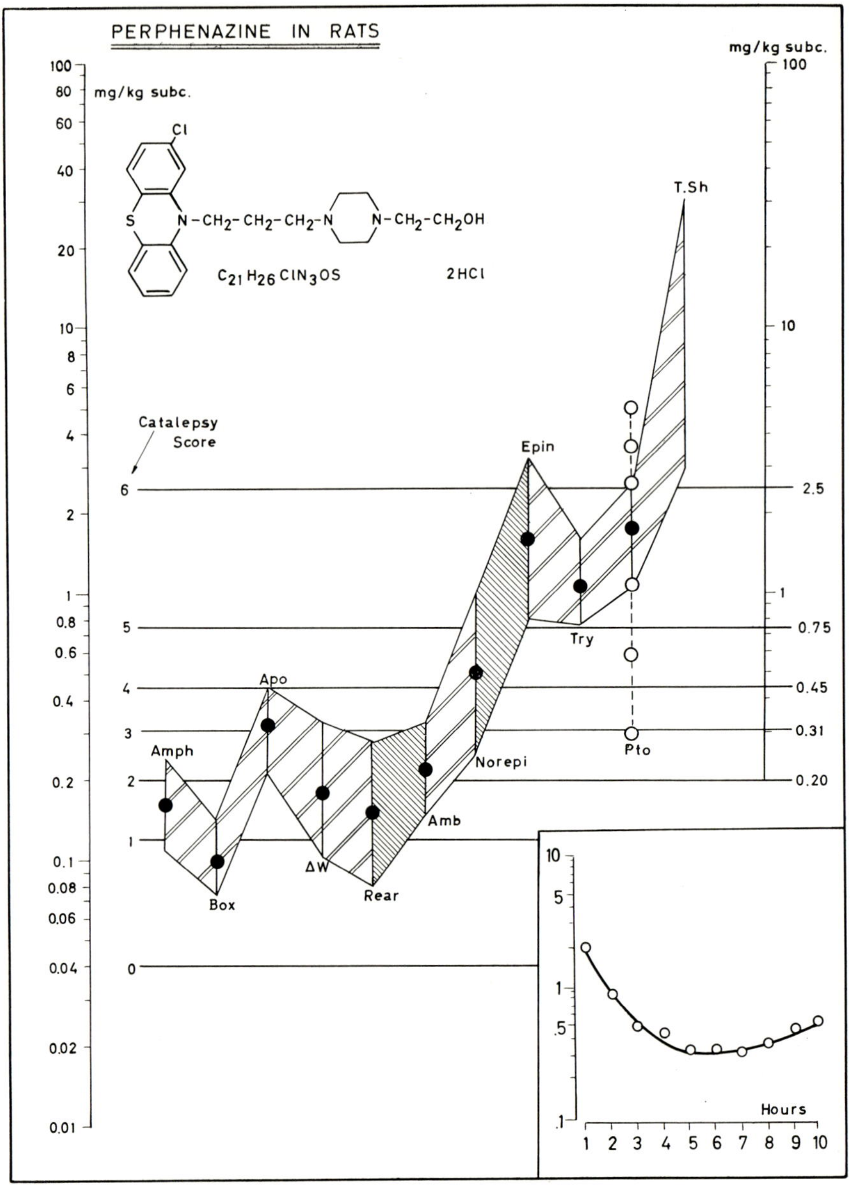

Fig. 1d. Activity spectrum of perphenazine in rats.

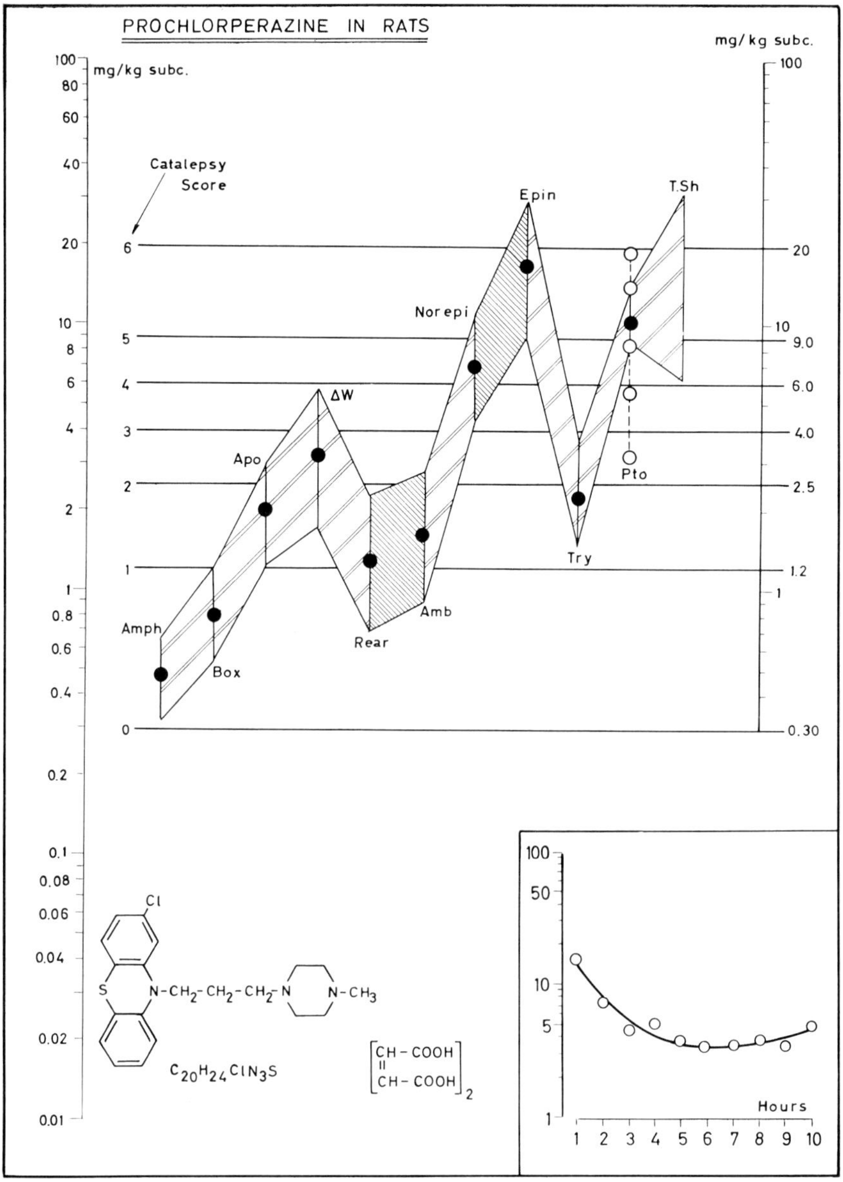

Fig. 1e. Activity spectrum of prochlorperazine in rats.

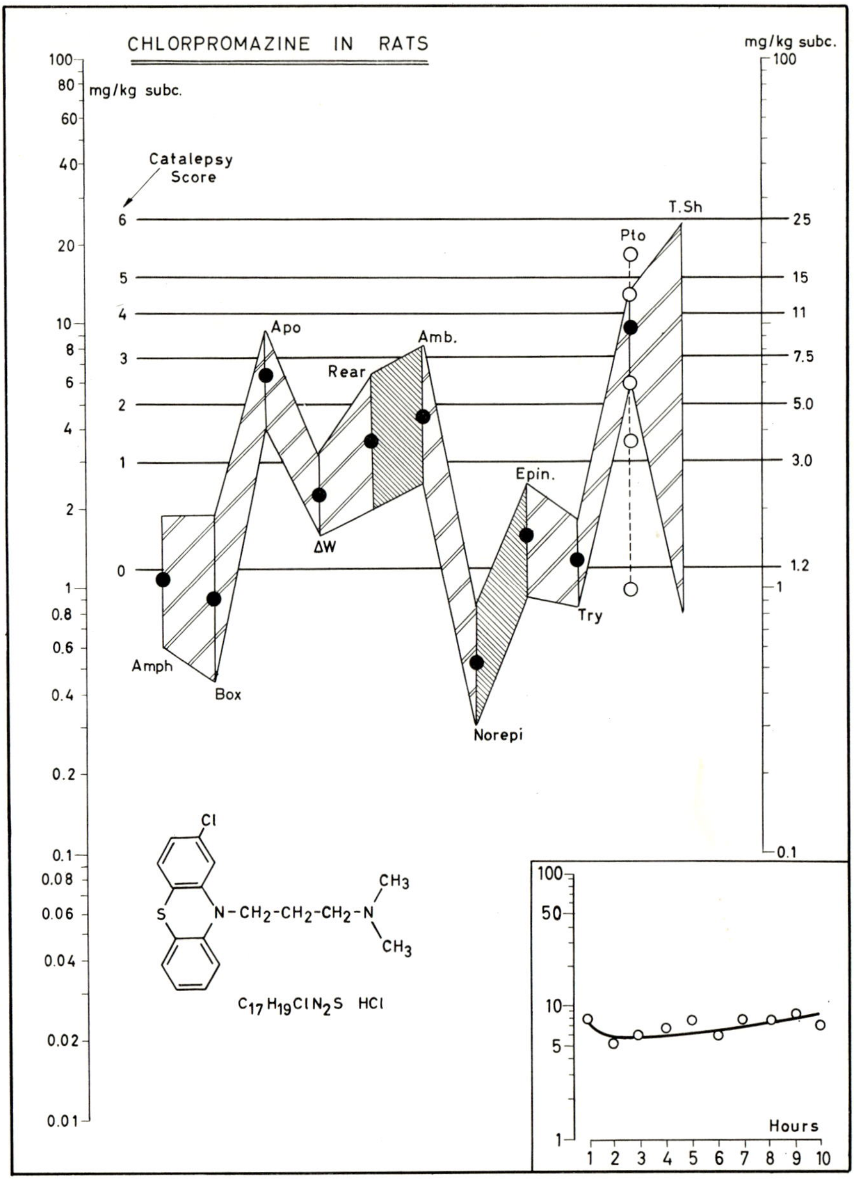

FIG. 1f. Activity spectrum of chlorpromazine in rats.

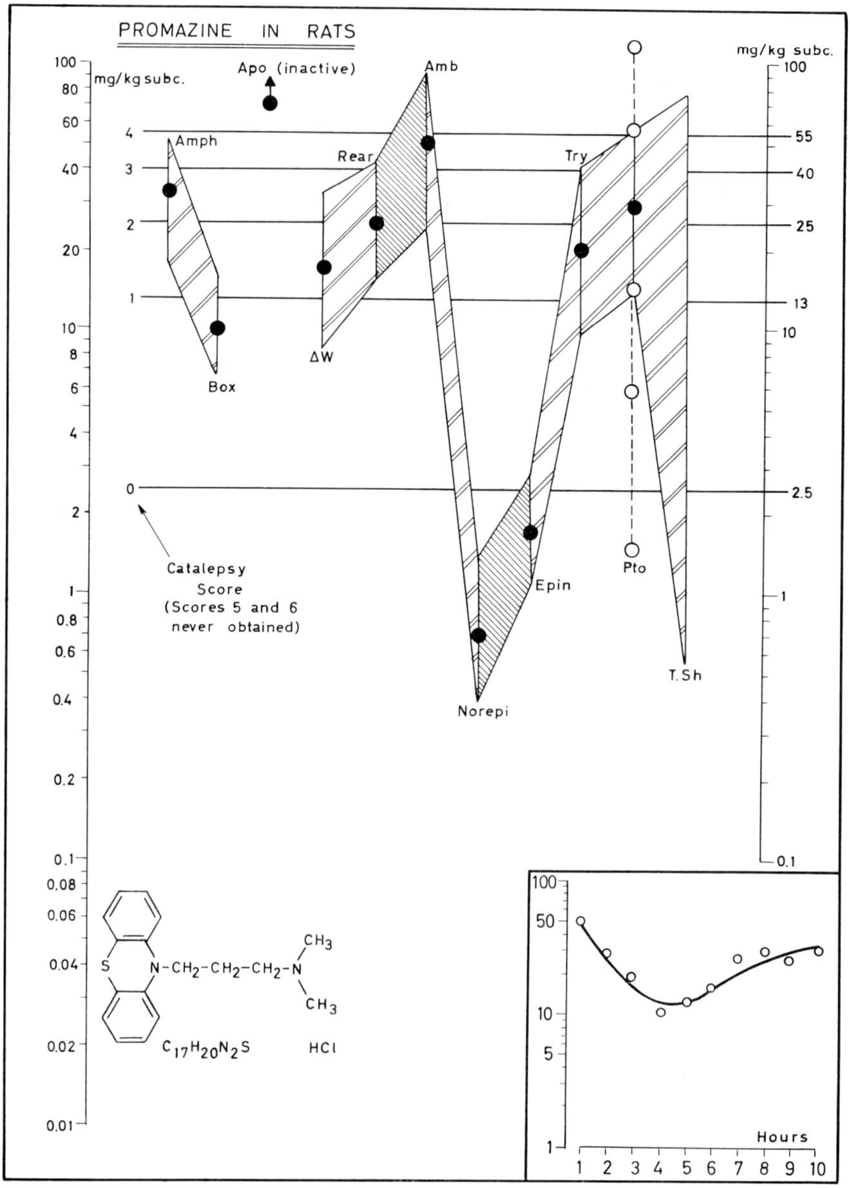

FIG. 1g. Activity spectrum of promazine in rats.

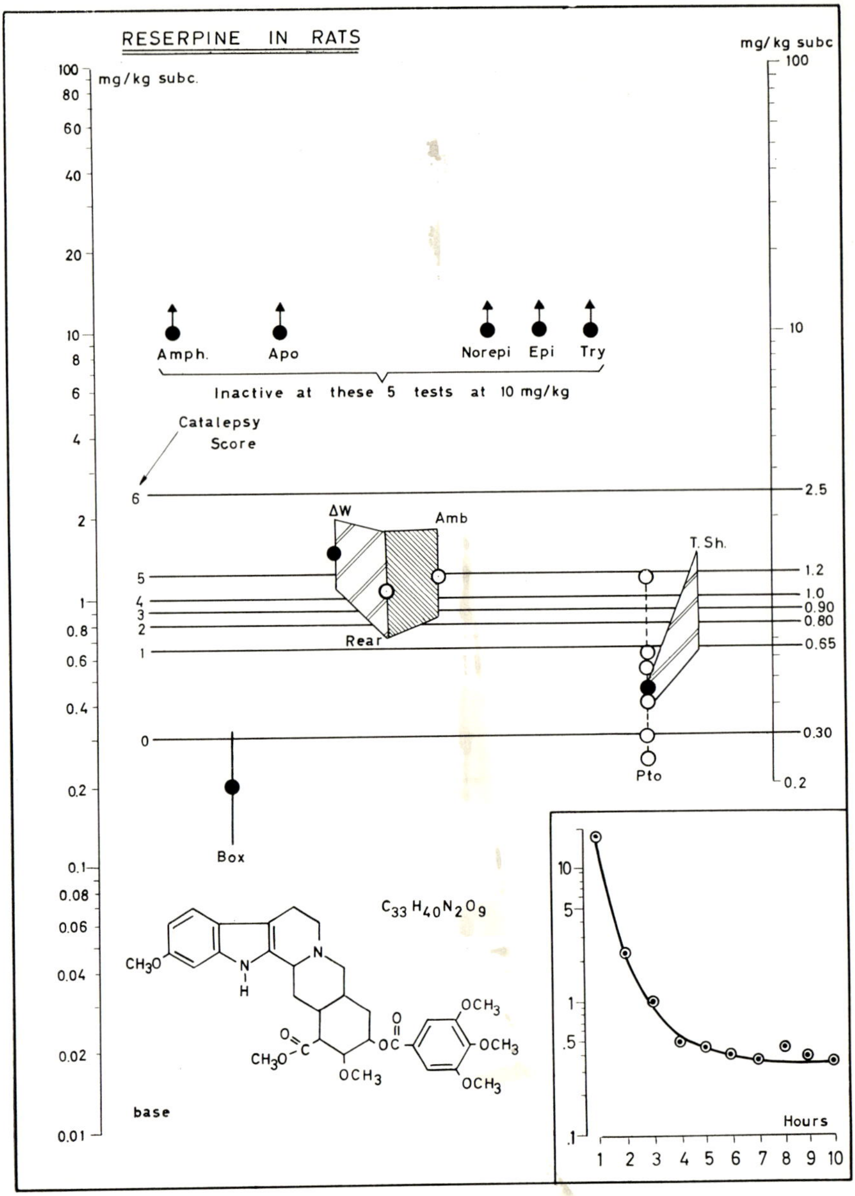

FIG. 1h. Activity spectrum of reserpine in rats.

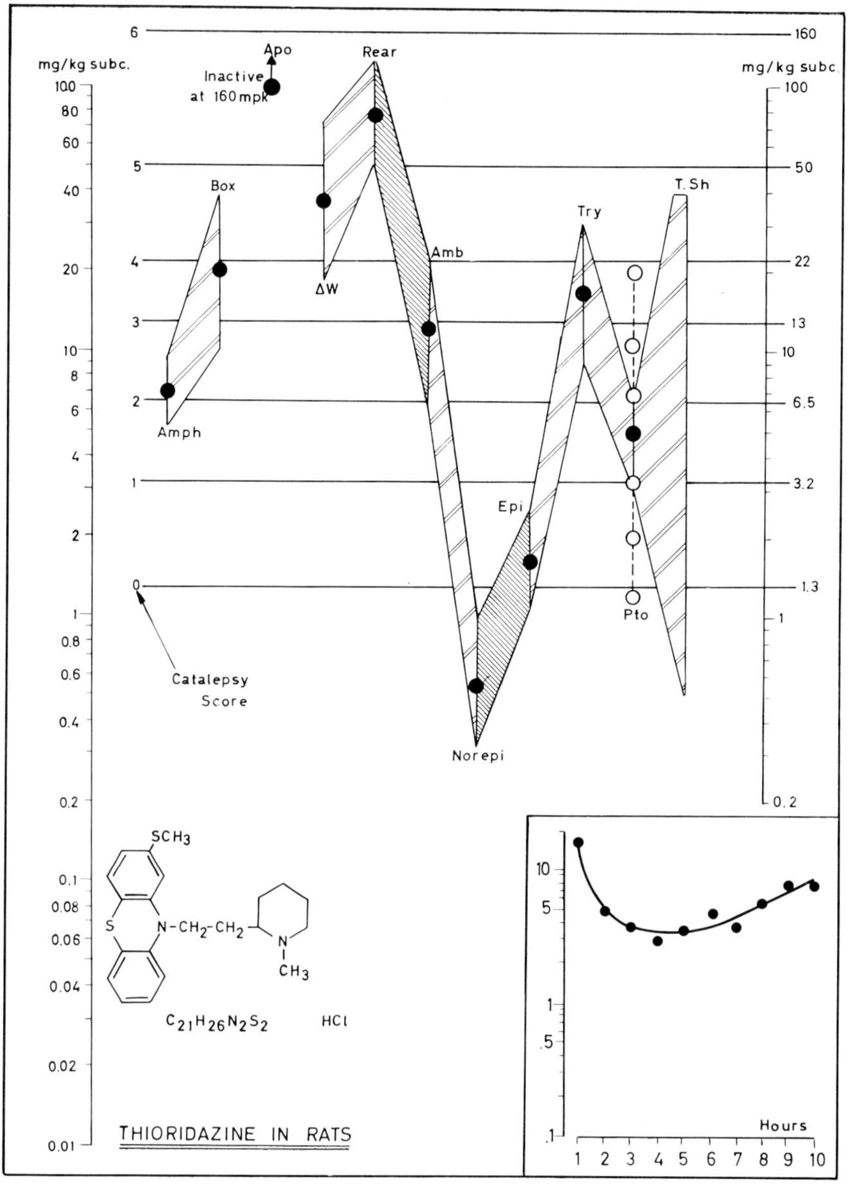

FIG. 1i. Activity spectrum of thioridazine in rats.

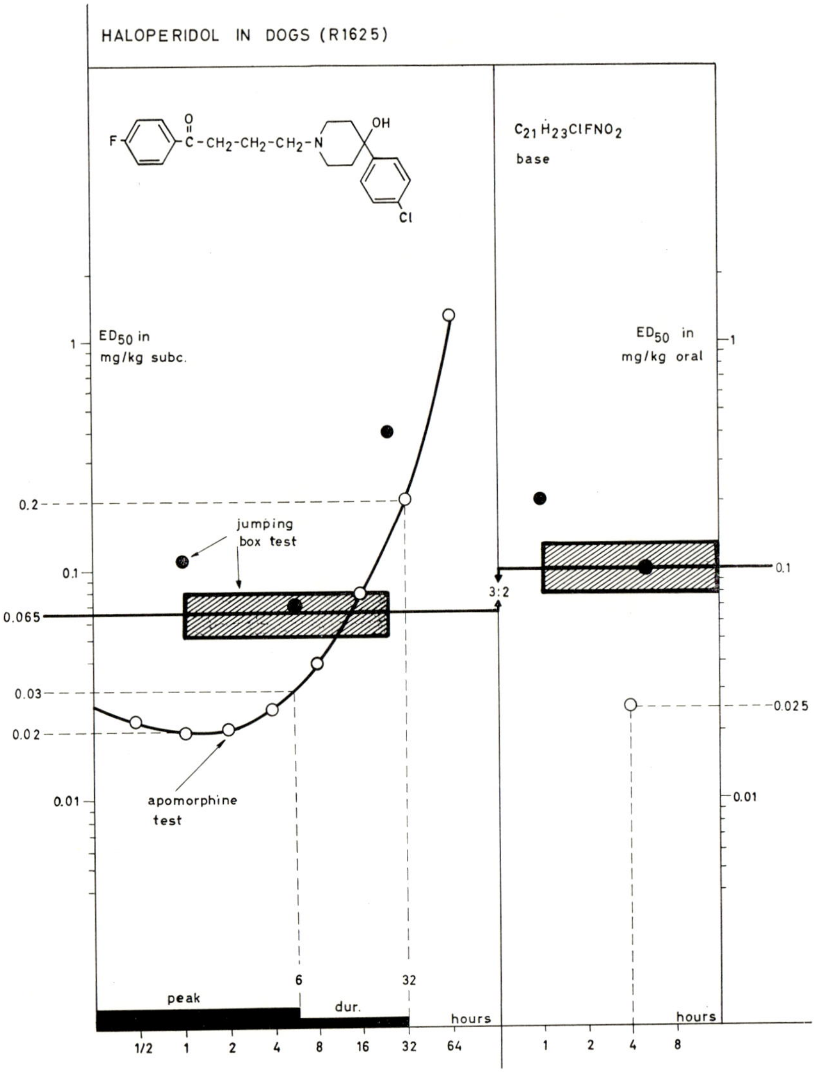

FIG. 2a. Activity spectrum of haloperidol in dogs.

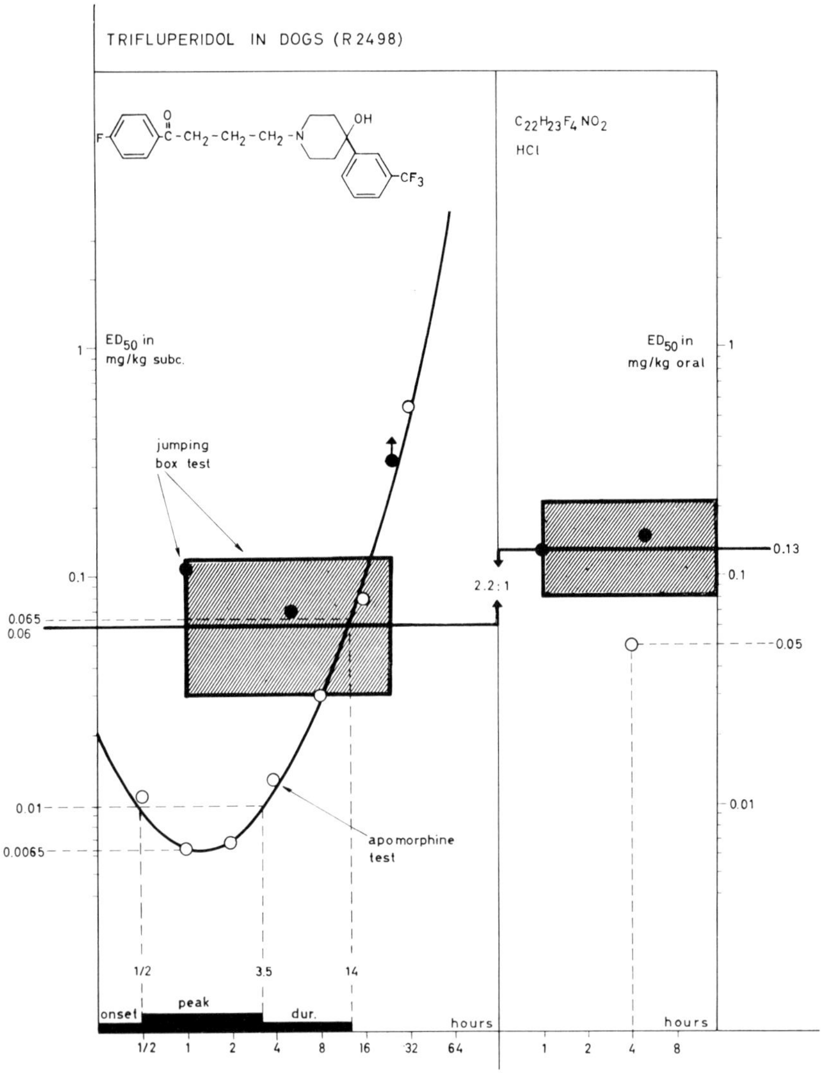

FIG. 2b. Activity spectrum of trifluperidol in dogs.

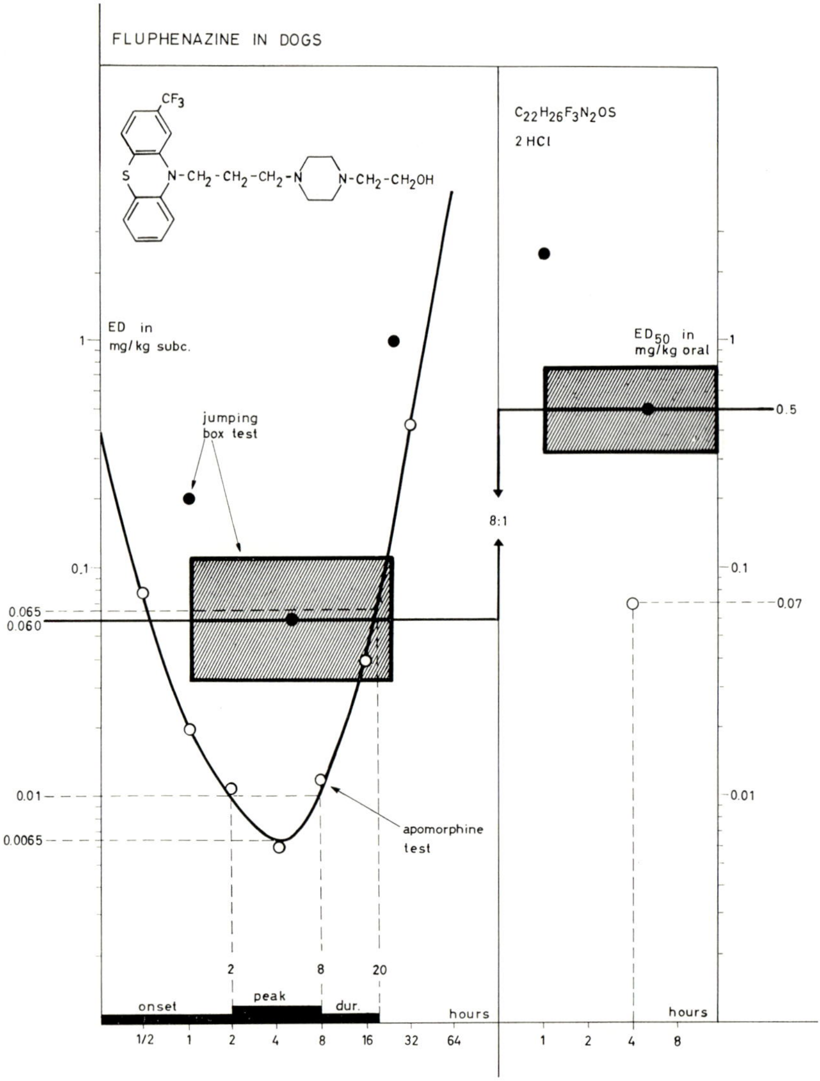

FIG. 2c. Activity spectrum of fluphenazine in dogs.

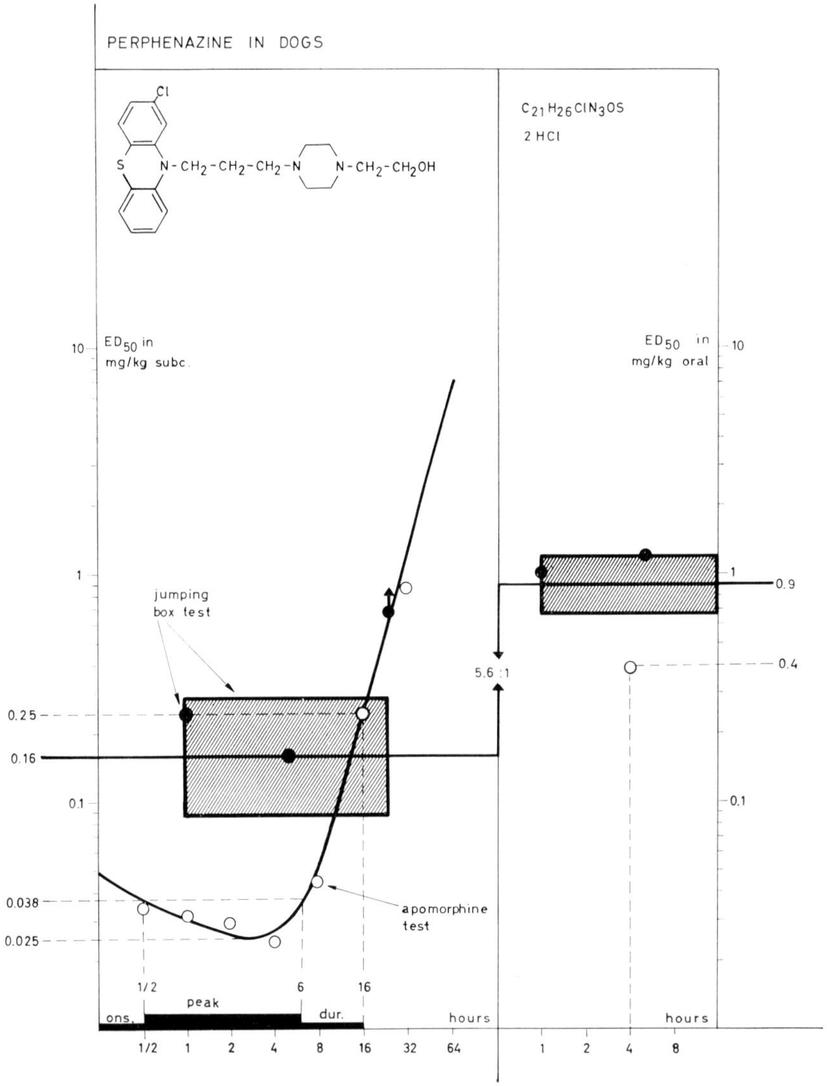

FIG. 2d. Activity spectrum of perphenazine in dogs.

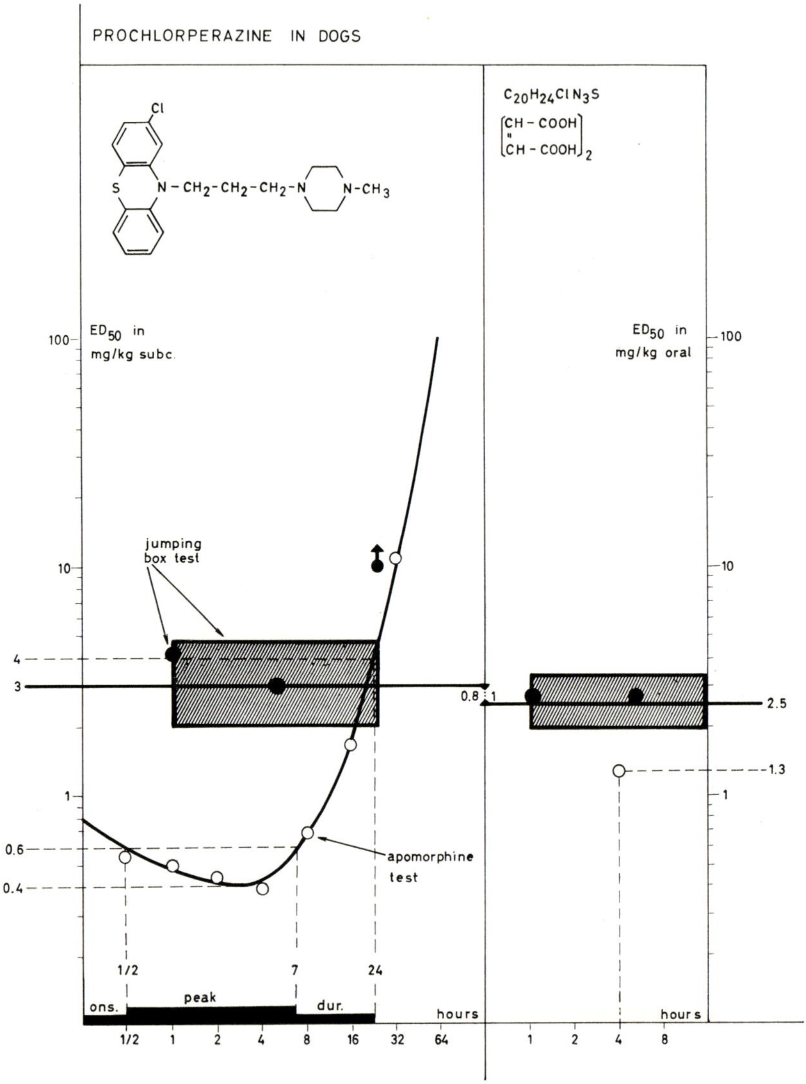

FIG. 2e. Activity spectrum of prochlorperazine in dogs.

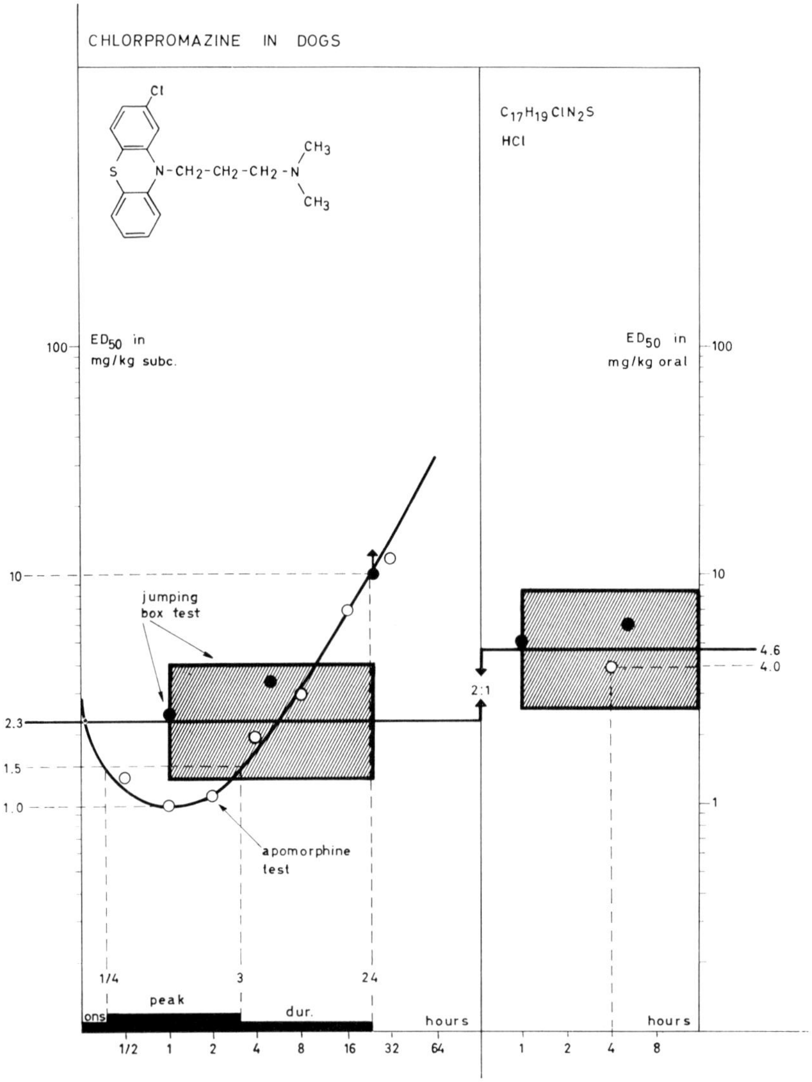

Fig. 2f. Activity spectrum of chlorpromazine in dogs.

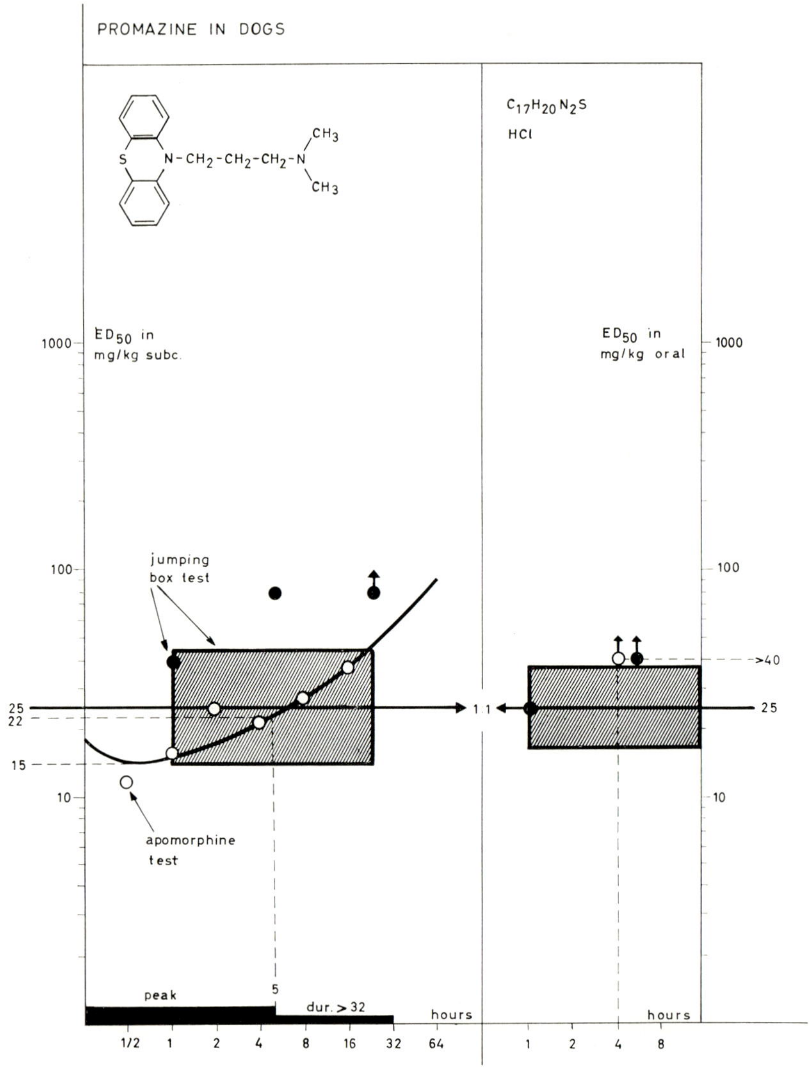

FIG. 2g. Activity spectrum of promazine in dogs.

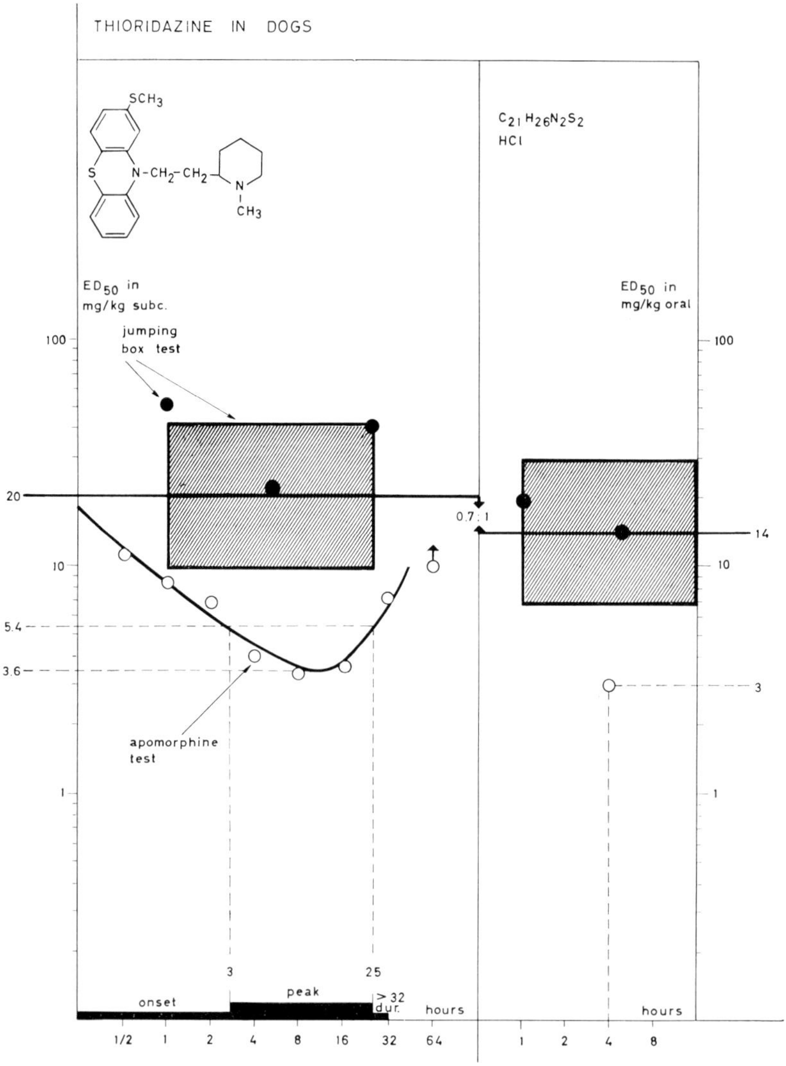

FIG. 2h. Activity spectrum of thioridazine in dogs.

TABLE VI
THE INTENSITY OF CATALEPSY (SCORES 0 TO 6) OBSERVED AT THE VARIOUS ED LEVELS LISTED IN TABLE IV AND FIGS. 1a–i (SUBCUTANEOUS INJECTION IN RATS)[a]

Screening method	Haloperidol	Trifluperidol	Fluphenazine	Perphenazine	Prochlorperazine	Chlorpromazine	Promazine	Reserpine	Thioridazine
Antiamphetamine	0	0	2	1–2	0	0	2–3	∞	2
Jumping box	0	0	0	1	0	0	1	0	4
Antiapomorphine	3	0	2–3	3	2	2–3	∞	∞	∞
ΔW	4	2	4	2	2–3	1	1	5	4–5
Rearing	2	1	3	1–2	1	1	2	4	5
Ambulation	3	2	2	2	1–2	2	4	5	3
Antinorepinephrine	6	4	6	4	4	0	0	∞	0
Antiepinephrine	6	5	6	5–6	6	0	0	∞	0
Antitryptamine	6	5	6	5–6	2	0	2	∞	3–4
Ptosis (ED_4)	6	6	6	5–6	5	3–4	2	0–1	1–2
Antishock	6	5	6	6	4	0	0	1	0

[a] A neuroleptic drug is said to be "specifically active" in a given screening test when the intensity of catalepsy observed at the ED_{50} level is low, i.e., mean catalepsy score 0 to 1. Its action is said to be "aspecific" when the mean score for catalepsy is high, i.e., 5 or 6. The symbol ∞ indicates lack of activity at the highest (subtoxic) dose level tested.

cataleptic immobility in mice, rats, dogs as well as in other laboratory animals. Table V gives the ranking order for cataleptigenic potency (chlorpromazine = 1) in rats.

2. At low dose levels, not significantly affecting gross behavior, a typical neuroleptic drug is a "specific" blocker of learned conditioned avoidance responses, e.g., in the jumping box test (Table VI). In Table VII the potency ratios (chlorpromazine = 1) are given.

3. At dose levels producing a moderate degree of catalepsy, a typical neuroleptic drug inhibits food consumption in the ΔW-test and decreases rearing and ambulation activity in the open

TABLE VII
JUMPING BOX POTENCY

Drug	Rats Subc.	Rats Oral	Dogs Subc.	Dogs Oral
Trifluperidol	35	10	40	35
Haloperidol	15	50	35	45
Fluphenazine	35	15	40	9
Perphenazine	9.5	4.5	15	5
Reserpine	4.5	1	Toxic	Toxic
Prochlorperazine	1	2	$\frac{3}{4}$	2
Chlorpromazine	①	①	①	①
Thioridazine	$\frac{1}{20}$	$\frac{1}{5}$	$\frac{1}{12}$	$\frac{1}{3}$
Promazine	$\frac{1}{10}$	$\frac{1}{6}$	$\frac{1}{10}$	$\frac{1}{5}$

TABLE VIII

Drug	ΔW-Test	Open field test: Rearing	Open field test: Ambulation
Trifluperidol	30	75	50
Haloperidol	10	30	20
Fluphenazine	8.5	25	45
Perphenazine	15	25	20
Reserpine	1.5	3.5	4
Prochlorperazine	$\frac{3}{4}$	3	3
Chlorpromazine	①	①	①
Thioridazine	$\frac{1}{15}$	$\frac{1}{8}$	$\frac{1}{3}$
Promazine	$\frac{1}{7}$	$\frac{1}{7}$	$\frac{1}{10}$

TABLE IX

Drug	ED_{50} (mg/kg) a Jumping box	b Norepinephrine	c Epinephrine	ED_{50} ratios b/a	c/a	Catalepsy score at dose level (0 to 6) b	c	Degree of specificity as catecholamine blockers
Fluphenazine	0.025	0.93	2.3	37/1	92/1	6	6	Very low
Haloperidol	0.058	2.1	14	35/1	233/1	6	6	
Trifluperidol	0.025	0.30	0.5	12/1	20/1	4	5	Low
Prochlorperazine	0.80	7.0	17	9/1	21/1	4	5/6	
Perphenazine	0.10	0.50	1.6	5/1	16/1	4	5/6	
Chlorpromazine	0.93	0.52	1.6	1/2	3/2	0	0/1	Moderate
Promazine	10	0.70	1.7	1/14	1/6	0	0	High
Thioridazine	20	0.55	1.6	1/36	1/13	0	0	
Reserpine	0.20	∞	∞	∞/1	∞/1	—	—	Nil

field test. Table VIII compares potency ratios (chlorpromazine = 1; rats; subc.) obtained from these two tests.

4. In all these tests in rats and in dogs, trifluperidol and haloperidol are about 10 to 75 times more potent than chlorpromazine; fluphenazine is about equally active; perphenazine and reserpine are less potent than the butyrophenones, but more potent than prochlorperazine and chlorpromazine; thioridazine and promazine are less active in all these tests than the other seven neuroleptics.

5. A major difference between the nine neuroleptics listed in Tables IV and VI lies in their relative degree of specificity as epinephrine and as norepinephrine blockers (Table IX).

These results are in good agreement with other pharmacological data in the sense that these drugs, except reserpine, have adrenolytic properties (alpha receptor blockade *in vitro*, epinephrine reversal *in vivo*), promazine, thioridazine, and chlorpromazine being significantly more specific in this respect than the other phenothiazines and the butyrophenones. Reserpine is furthermore the only drug of this series with brain-catecholamine- and brain-serotonin-depleting properties.

Another difference among these drugs can be studied by listing the degree of palpebral ptosis (scores 0 to 8) most frequently observed in drug-treated rats with catalepsy score 0 to 6 (Table X). Haloperidol, trifluperidol, fluphenazine, and perphenazine are relatively weak and aspecific palpebral-ptosis-inducing neuroleptics in handled rats, whereas promazine, thioridazine, and particularly

TABLE X

DEGREE OF PALPEBRAL PTOSIS IN RATS WITH DIFFERENT CATALEPSY SCORES

	Mean catalepsy score:						
Drug	0	1	2	3	4	5	6
Haloperidol	0	0	0	1	1.5	3	4
Trifluperidol	0	0	0	1	2	3	4
Fluphenazine	0	0	1	1	2	2.5	4
Perphenazine	0	0	0	1	1.5	2.5	5
Prochlorperazine	0	0	0	1.5	2	3	7
Chlorpromazine	1	2	2.5	3.5	4.5	5.5	6.5
Promazine	1.5	3	4	4	5	—	—
Thioridazine	1	3	5	6	7	7	—
Reserpine	2	6	6	6	6	7	8

reserpine are relative strong and specifically active in this respect. Prochlorperazine and chlorpromazine are in-between.

Amphetamine, apomorphine, and tryptamine blockade is also observed (ED_{50}) in rats showing a variable degree of catalepsy (Table XI).

TABLE XI

Mean Catalepsy Score at ED_{50} in Three Tests in Rats[a]

Drug	Antiamphetamine		Antiapomorphine		Antitryptamine	
Trifluperidol	0	++	0/1	++	5	--
Haloperidol	0	++	3	+	6	--
Fluphenazine	½	++	⅔	+	6	--
Perphenazine	½	++	3	+	5/6	--
Prochlorperazine	0	++	2	+	2	+
Chlorpromazine	0	++	⅔	+	0	++
Promazine	⅔	+	∞	0	½	+
Thioridazine	2	+	∞	0	¾	-
Reserpine	∞	0	∞	0	∞	0

[a] ++, High specificity of action; +, moderate specificity of action; -, low specificity of action; --, very low specificity of action; 0, no activity.

Comparison of the various "neuroleptic activity spectra" for dogs (Fig. 2a–h) leads to the classification in Table XII.

From all the foregoing analyses it is concluded that trifluperidol and haloperidol are more closely related to fluphenazine, both quantitatively and qualitatively, than to the other phenothiazines. These three drugs have therefore probably a similar mode of action. Haloperidol and trifluperidol are, however, faster acting and better absorbed orally than fluphenazine. Haloperidol is longer acting and trifluperidol shorter acting than fluphenazine. Trifluperidol is from 1.5 to 3 times more potent than haloperidol. Reasoning by analogy one would, of course, predict clinical similarity between these three drugs (Janssen, 1964a).

III. Clinical Results

Most of the clinical results obtained with both butyrophenones are predictable from animal data. Haloperidol and trifluperidol are

TABLE XII

Activity	Triflupe-ridol	Fluphe-nazine	Halope-ridol	Perphe-nazine	Prochlor-perazine	Chlorpro-mazine	Proma-zine	Thiori-dazine
Potency (subc.)								
Jumping box	40	40	35	15	1.5	①	1/10	1/10
Antiemetic (max)	150	150	50	40	2.5	①	1/15	1/4
Duration (hours)								
Peak effect	3.5	8	6	6	7	3	5	25
Total effect	14	20	32	16	24	24	Long	Long
Onset (hours)								
Peak effect	Fast	Slow	Moderate	Moderate	Moderate	Moderate	Fast	Slow
Relative oral vs. subc. effectiveness	Good	Poor	Excellent	Poor	Excellent	Good	Excellent	Excellent

indeed powerful neuroleptic drugs (major tranquilizers) in man. Both drugs are about equally active orally as parenterally. Haloperidol, longer acting than trifluperidol, is being used at daily dose levels of 0.5 to 30 mg and trifluperidol at daily doses of 0.25 to 15 mg. Both butyrophenones are being extensively used in the treatment of psychotic patients, of patients with psychomotor agitation of various etiology (e.g., mania, alcoholic delirium, tic nerveux, and aggressive personality), in anesthesiology, and as antiemetic drugs. The most important undesirable features associated with high dose therapy are reversible neurological effects (e.g., muscular rigidity, tremor, akathisia, and dyskinesia). Fluphenazine and related phenothiazines are known to produce similar side effects. With haloperidol and trifluperidol the incidence of chronic toxicity reactions (e.g., jaundice, blood dyscrasias, and allergic reactions) is extremely low. For detailed clinical information the reader is referred to the extensive clinical literature on haloperidol, trifluperidol, and methylperidol, which now numbers more than five hundred published articles, including Danik and Goverdhan (1963), Delay and Deniker (1961a,b), Delay *et al.* (1960), Divry *et al.* (1958, 1959, 1960), Gallant *et al.* (1965), and Lehman and Bann (1964).

IV. Structure–Activity Considerations

The most potent neuroleptic drugs known are all derivatives of the following basic propylamine structure:

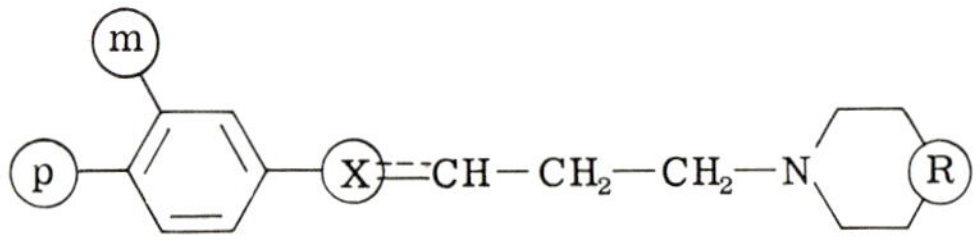

where p is preferably F or H; m is preferably CF_3, SO_2NMe_2, Cl, or H; X is nitrogen, carbon, or oxygen; and R is carbon or nitrogen. This statement is illustrated in Table XIII (Janssen, 1964b).

V. Ideas and Suggestions for Further Research

Further research in this field will probably tend to further elucidate a number of problems related to the mechanism of action of neuroleptic and morphine-like drugs, the correlation between chemical structure, physical properties, and neuroleptic or morphine-like potency, and the metabolic pathways of these drugs. The

TABLE XIII

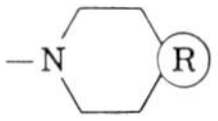	X=CH	I/II[a]	m/p	Generic name
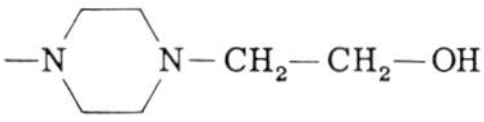	$>N-CH_2-$	I	CF_3	Fluphenazine[b]
		I	Cl	Perphenazine
		I	$COCH_3$	Acetophenazine
	$>C=CH-$	I	Cl	Chlopenthixol
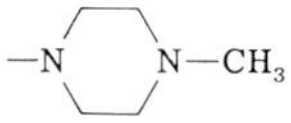	$>N-CH_2-$	I	CF_3	Trifluoperazine[b]
		I	Cl	Prochlorperazine
		I	SO_2NMe_2	Thioperazine[b]
		I	COC_3H_7	Butyrylperazine
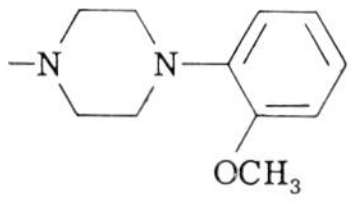	$-C(=O)-CH_2-$	II	F	Fluanisone, R 2028[b] (Janssen, 1961a)
	$-CH(OH)-CH_2-$	II	F	Anisopirol, R 2159
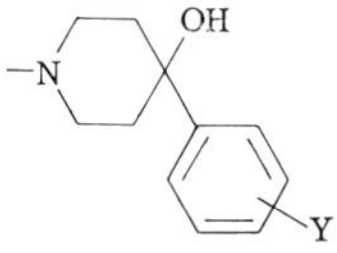 Y = 3 CF_3	$-C(=O)-CH_2-$	II	F	Trifluperidol, R 2498[b]
Y = 4 Cl		II	F	Haloperidol, R 1625[b]
Y = 4 CH_3		II	F	Methylperidol, R 1658, (moperone) (Janssen *et al.*, 1959c)
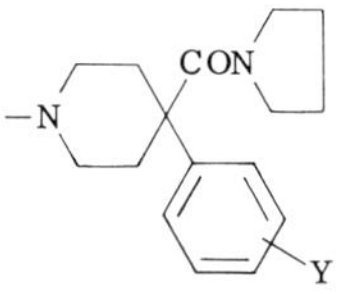 Y = 3 Cl	$-C(=O)-CH_2-$	II	F	Haloperidide, R 3201[b], (Niemegeers and Janssen, 1960a; Schaper *et al.*, 1960; Janssen, 1961a)
Y = 3 CH_3		II	F	Methylperidide, R 2963[b], (Janssen, 1961a)
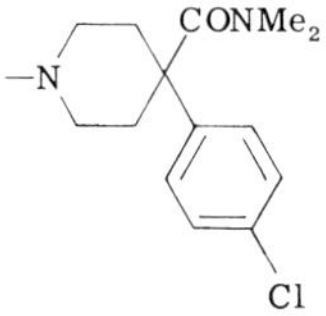	$-C(=O)-CH_2-$	II	F	Paraperidide, R 2962, (amiperone)

TABLE XIII (Continued)

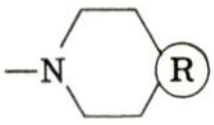	X⩵CH	I/II[a]	m/p	Generic name
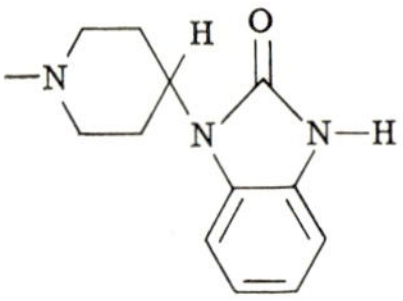	$-\overset{O}{\overset{\|}{C}}-CH_2-$	II	F	Benperidol, R 4584
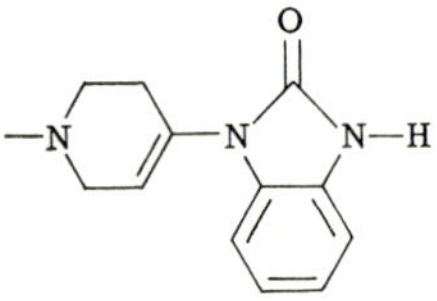	$-\overset{O}{\overset{\|}{C}}-CH_2-$	II	F	Droperidol, dehydrobenzperidol, R 4749 (Janssen *et al.*, 1963b)
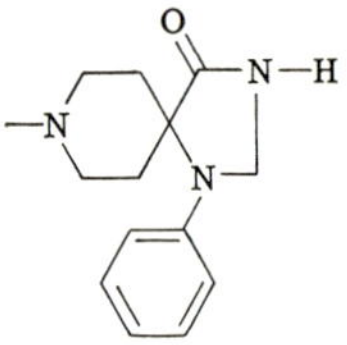	$-\overset{O}{\overset{\|}{C}}-CH_2-$	II	F	Spiroperidol, R 5147[b]
	$-O-CH_2-$	II	F	Spiramide, R 5808
	$-\overset{CH_3}{\overset{\mid}{C}}=CH-$	II	F	Spirilene, R 6109[b]

a

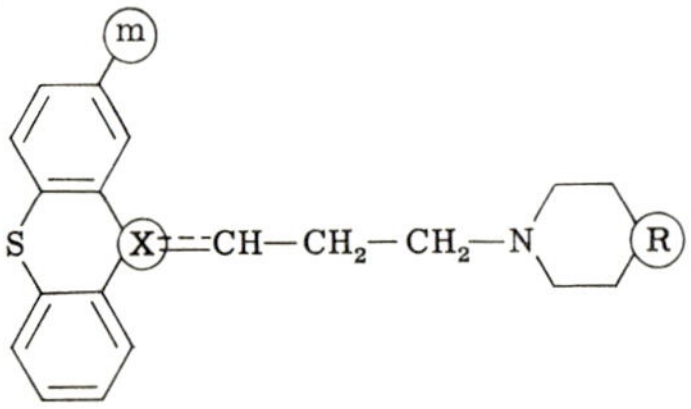

I

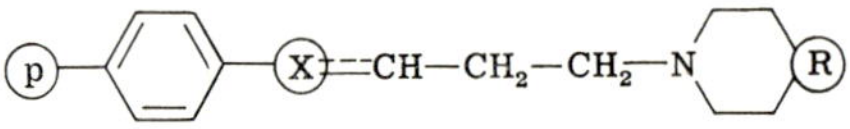

II

[b] Most potent of series.

general formula (III), where X, Y, and R represent carbon, nitrogen, or oxygen, is offered as a source of inspiration for medicinal chemists interested in preparing new and potent neuroleptics.

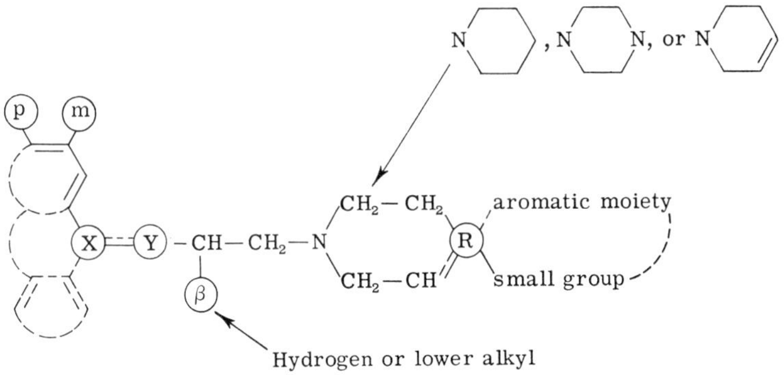

(III)

As pointed out above all known potent and specific neuroleptic drugs are derivatives of this general structure.

Even reserpine is essentially a substituted propylamine. The absolute configuration of this alkaloid is shown in IV (Janssen, 1964b).

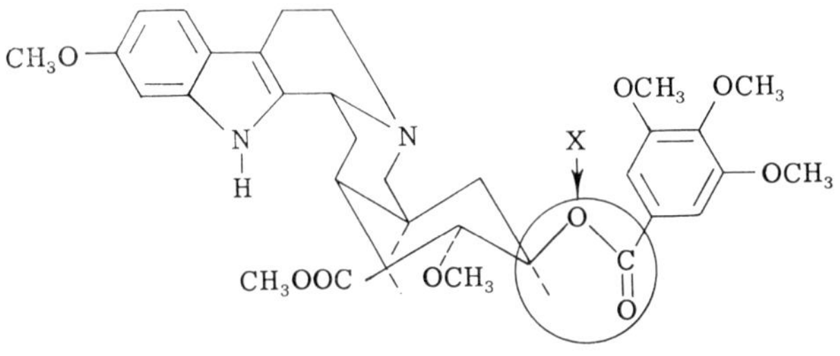

(IV)

$p = m = OCH_3$
$X = CHOCO$; $Y = CH_2$
R = carbon
β = alkyl

The mode of action of neuroleptic drugs is, of course, largely unknown. There are, however, a few striking facts that seem to be relevant:

1. As pointed out before, all potent and specific neuroleptic drugs have a strikingly similar chemical structure. This would of

course suggest a common basic mechanism of action and almost forces us to bring in the receptor concept.

2. There is striking similarity between the chemical features associated with strong neuroleptic potency, on the one hand, and the chemical features associated with strong γ-aminobutyric-acid-like (GABA) depressant activity, on the other hand. In both series the 3-substituted propylamine structure is associated with highest activity. If it is true that GABA and glutamic acid are in competition for the same receptor site on neuronal transmitter receptor membranes, that glutamic acid excites certain neurons by a membrane polarization effect, that GABA depresses these cells and antagonizes glutamic acid without altering membrane potential, the action of both amino acids being mediated by cellular and subcellular membrane permeability changes (Buniatian, 1963; Curtis and Watkins, 1960) and unrelated to a transmitter function (Ryall, 1964), and if it is, furthermore, true that the glutamic acid–GABA system is particularly important in areas of the brain belonging to the extrapyramidal motor system (Mueller and Langemann, 1962), then it appears reasonable to advance the working hypothesis that potent neuroleptics would decrease cellular and subcellular membrane permeability processes, particularly in neurons belonging to the extrapyramidal motor system, e.g., by occupying GABA receptors and making them inaccessible to glutamic acid.

3. Direct evidence for this theory is completely lacking, but there is convincing evidence to show that chlorpromazine-like neuroleptics do, in fact, decrease the permeability of a variety of biological membranes for a great many different types of molecules (Seeman and Bialy, 1963).

4. Seeman and Bialy (1963) have found that potent neuroleptics, including reserpine, reduce surface tension in extremely small concentrations of the order of $10^{-7}\,M$ by adsorbing onto the air–water interface and that surface activity is strikingly correlated with neuroleptic potency.

It was calculated that the surface film is virtually a monomolecular layer of neuroleptic molecules, the surface concentration being from 100,000 to 1,000,000 times the concentration in the bulk solution. We have confirmed these findings and extended them to a large series of potent neuroleptics of various structures without finding an exception to the rule that for some reason neuroleptic drugs lower surface tension in proportion to their neuroleptic potency in rat, dog, and man.

Neuroleptic drugs therefore apparently reduce membrane permeability to practically all solutes by formation of a diffusion-limited monomolecular subfilm on the outer aspect of the cell membrane, thus adding another 15–20 A to its thickness.

5. In view of all these considerations, one is tempted to assume that potent neuroleptics have a much greater tendency to form a monomolecular film on, e.g., GABA-receptor-containing membranes than on others. The oil-soluble aromatic portion of the molecule, i.e., the phenothiazine ring or the benzoyl moiety of the butyrophenones, could adsorb onto the lipophylic portion of the receptor area, the basic six-membered and 4-substituted piperidine or piperazine ring could possibly fit into a partly charged or ionized hydrophylic portion of the receptor area and the propylene side chain could form an adequate bridge between these two portions.

6. If this were all true, then we would expect low doses of potent neuroleptics to interfere specifically with transport mechanisms through certain cellular and subcellular membranes of the extrapyramidal system where permeability is largely regulated by the GABA–glutamic acid system. At much higher dose levels we would expect these drugs to decrease permeability and interfere with transport mechanisms through other membranes.

7. There is no direct evidence to demonstrate the exact nature or the physiological significance of the GABA-containing membranes in the extrapyramidal system that are hypothetically more readily influenced by neuroleptic drugs than other membranes. Indirect evidence, however, suggests that certain membranes of central adrenergic neurons might be involved.

8. The fact that many if not all potent neuroleptics are specific blockers of tranylcypromine-induced elevation of norepinephrine concentration in the rat brain, but have little or no specific effect on reserpine-induced depletion of central catecholamines, is best explained by the assumption that neuroleptics inhibit the transport mechanism of catecholamines into vesicles of central sympathetic nerve endings and axons containing bound reserpine-depletable norepinephrine, but not the mechanism releasing these catecholamine pools into the surrounding monoamine-oxidase-containing (MAO) cell fluids (Dresse and De Meyer, 1965; Kopin, 1964).

9. Carlsson and Lindqvist (1963) reported that the accumulation of methoxytyramine and normetanephrine in brain after treatment with a MAO inhibitor is enhanced by chlorpromazine and haloperidol. Low doses of these two drugs and also of reserpine

furthermore produce a transient increase of 3,4-dihydroxyphenylacetic acid and a somewhat slower, more prolonged increase of homovanillic acid in the rabbit corpus striatum. This and similar indirect evidence (Dresse, *loc. cit.*) would indicate that neuroleptics may produce their typical central nervous system effects by inhibiting the transport mechanism of norepinephrine, dopamine, and similar hypothetical central nervous transmitters through the cellular membrane into the cytoplasm of the nerve ending or back into the small transmitter pool releasing transmitter molecules by nerve stimulation, through the subcellular membrane into intracellular storage granules, through the membranes surrounding the receptor site into the receptor area, and also through the membranes surrounding the whole synaptic area through which *o*-methylated and other metabolites are probably eliminated. A similar permeability block would explain how chlorpromazine-like neuroleptics decrease peripheral uptake of exogenous catecholamines and act as adrenolytics or so-called alpha-receptor blocking agents *in vitro.*

10. In order to test these theories experimentally, the easiest approach seems to be to investigate the mechanism of the anti-emetic action of neuroleptics in detail. In the dog extremely small, behaviorally inactive doses of potent and specific neuroleptics, such as haloperidol or fluphenazine, will prevent the emetic effect of large doses of apomorphine and similar stimulants of the emetic chemoreceptor trigger zone of Borison and Wang, which is located in the area cinerea at the floor of the fourth ventricle (Fig. 3). In this area circulating apomorphine probably penetrates into the trigger zone through the vascular foot of a small astrocyte containing a reddish fluorescent substance (Dresse, 1964). Here, conceivably, apomorphine could depolarize the astrocytic membrane and electrically stimulate an adrenergic neuron of the chemoreceptor trigger zone, which in turn could stimulate non-adrenergic, possibly cholinergic neurons of the vomiting center, hereby triggering the emetic process. Circulating neuroleptics probably also penetrate the area cinerea through the vascular feet of the same or similar astrocytes, which they probably use for transport to the membranes of the first adrenergic synapse. Here they would prevent released transmitter from reaching the receptors by forming a permeability-decreasing monolayer on the surface of the membranes surrounding the receptors. We would consequently

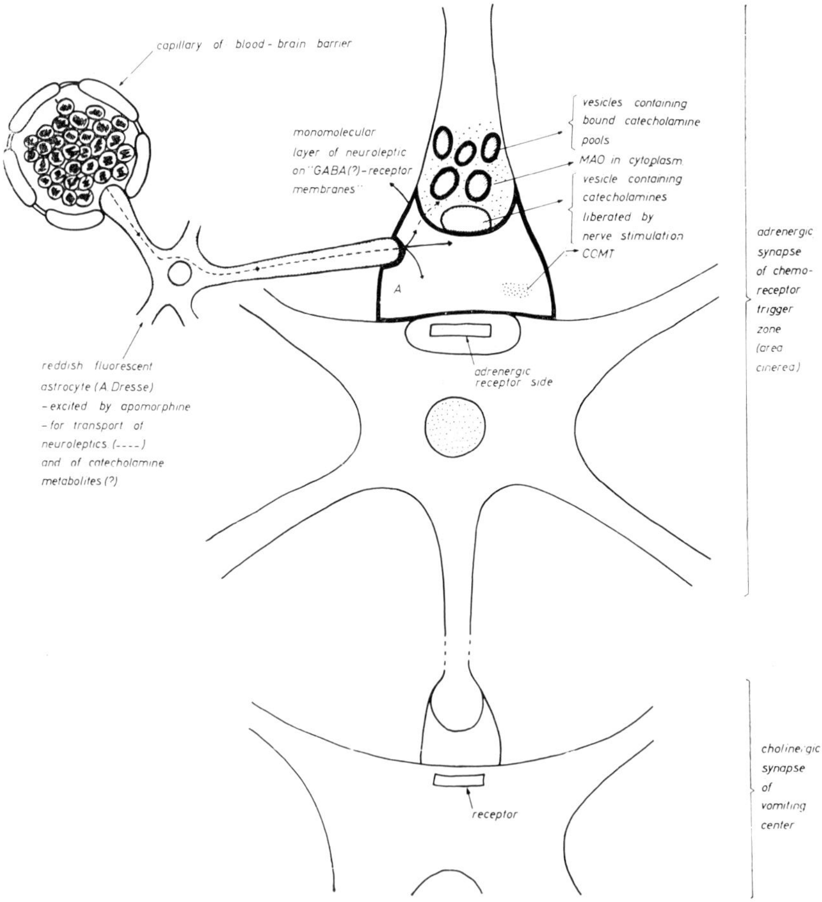

FIG. 3. Specific neuroleptics are potent blockers of apomorphine-induced emesis in dogs. The site of this action is the trigger zone of Borison and Wang (no direct effect on the vomiting center). Graphical representation of the working hypothesis: neuroleptic molecules are picked up from serum by special astrocytes and transported through these astrocytes into the lumen of an adrenergic synapse in the trigger zone where they form a permeability-blocking monolayer on GABA-receptor-containing (?) membranes by occupying these receptors. Apomorphine depolarizes the red astrocytes, whereafter catecholamines are released from a small vesicle pool in the adrenergic synapse but fail to penetrate through the membrane surrounding the receptor side. Adrenergic transmission is blocked, the vomiting center remains inactivated, hence no emesis MAO- and COMT-catecholamine metabolites accumulate in area A as another consequence of reduced membrane permeability.

suspect the GABA–glutamic acid system to play an important role in regulating the normal permeability of this membrane.

To what extent a basically similar mechanism of action would suffice to explain the other typical properties of neuroleptic drugs is not clear. How are most of the behavioral effects of amphetamine-like drugs antagonized by extremely small doses of most neuroleptics and why is reserpine relatively inactive in this respect? How do small doses of all neuroleptics inhibit operant behavior in general, increase the reaction time of conditioned operant responses in trained animals following a conditioning auditory or visual stimulus, decrease exploratory behavior and produce a state of cataleptic immobility at higher dose levels? Why are all neuroleptics potent inhibitors of lever-pressing activity in self-stimulating rats with electrodes implanted in Olds' positive reward centers? How do central anticholinergic drugs antagonize certain neuroleptic effects? How can one explain the typical effects of neuroleptics on muscular tone? Why is it that behaviorally equivalent doses of moderately active neuroleptics reduce autonomic reactivity more readily, produce much more soporific effects, are more potent adrenolytics, induce more hypothermia, possess a much greater barbiturate-potentiating effect, etc. than most potent neuroleptics? What is the significance of the fact that a neuroleptic such as reserpine depletes brain catecholamines and brain serotonin, whereas most other neuroleptics do not have this effect? How can one correlate all these pharmacological properties with antipsychotic activity in man? I would like to suggest that the answer to this question lies in specific areas of the extrapyramidal midbrain system, in the fact that all potent neuroleptics are substituted propylamines with other common specific chemical features similar to the γ-amino acids of the GABA type, in the fact that neuroleptic potency is correlated with surface-tension-lowering or monolayer-forming ability, in membrane-permeability-lowering phenomena, in the fact that neuroleptics are blockers of inflow into cells and vesicles more than of outflow (outflow can even be increased), in the transport function of specialized astrocytes of the blood–brain barrier around the ventricles and in the inhibition of adrenergic neurons in these same areas, and in the concept that in a given situation typical psychological changes are the predictable consequence of the basic biophysical, biochemical, and neurological effects of drugs. These are the pieces of the puzzle—how they fit together remains to be seen.

REFERENCES

Boissier, J. R., and Pagny, J. (1960). *Thérapie* **15,** 479.

Boissier, J. R., and Simon, P. (1963). *Thérapie* **28,** 1257.

Boissier, J. R., and Simon, P. (1964a). *Arch. Intern. Pharmacodyn.* **147,** 372.

Boissier, J. R., and Simon, P. (1964b). *Encéphale* **53,** 109.

Boissier, J. R., Pagny, J., Mouillé, P., and Forest, J. (1960). *Acta Neurol. Psychiat. Belg.* **60,** 39.

Boissier, J. R., Pagny, J., and Font di Picart, Y. (1961). *Thérapie* **16,** 279.

Boissier, J. R., Simon, P., and Lwoff, J. M. (1964). *Thérapie* **19,** 571.

Buniatian, H. C. (1963). *J. Neurochem.* **10,** 461.

Carlsson, A., and Lindqvist, M. (1963). *Acta Pharmacol. Toxicol.* **20,** 145.

Curtis, D. R., and Watkins, J. C. (1960). *J. Neurochem.* **6,** 117.

Danik, J. J., and Goverdham, M. (1963). *Am. J. Psychiat.* **120,** 389.

Delay, J., and Deniker, P. (1961a). *In* "Système extrapyramidal et neuroleptiques" (Jean-Marc Bordeleau, ed.), p. 301. Editions Psychiatriques, Montreal.

Delay, J., and Deniker, P. (1961b). *In* "Méthodes Chimiothérapiques en Psychiatrie," pp. 150, 211, 383, 385, 401. Masson, Paris.

Delay, J., Pichot, P., Lempérière, T., Elissalde, B., and Peigne, F. (1960). *Ann. Méd.-Psychol.* **118,** 145.

Divry, P., Bobon, J., and Collard, J. (1958). *Acta Neurol. Psychiat. Belg.* **58,** 878.

Divry, P., Bobon, J., Collard, J., Pinchard, A., and Nols, E. (1959). *Acta Neurol. Psychiat. Belg.* **59,** 337.

Divry, P., Bobon, J., and Collard, J. (1960). *Acta Neurol. Psychiat. Belg.* **60,** 7.

Dresse, A. (1964). *Compt. Rend. Soc. Biol.* **158,** 1741.

Dresse, A., and De Meyer, R. (1965). *Biochem. Pharmacol.,* in press.

Frommel, E., and Chmouliovsky, M. (1964). *Compt. Rend. Soc. Biol.* **158,** 48.

Frommel, E., and Joye, E. (1963). *Méd. Hyg.* **21,** 675.

Frommel, E., Fleury, C., Schmidt-Cinzkey, J., and Béguin, M. (1960). *Thérapie* **15,** 1175.

Gallant, D. M., Bishop, M. P., Nesselhof, W., Jr., and Sprehe, D. J. (1965). *Psychopharmacologia* **7,** 37.

Gözsy, B., and Kato, L. (1962). *Compt. Rend. Soc. Biol.* **156,** 556.

Jageneau, A. H. M., and Janssen, P. A. J. (1956). *Arch. Intern. Pharmacodyn.* **106,** 199.

Janssen, P. A. J. (1960). *In* "Synthetic Analgesics. Part I: Diphenylpropylamines" (D. H. R. Barton and W. Doering, eds.), Vol. 3, International Series of Monographs on Organic Chemistry. Macmillan (Pergamon), New York.

Janssen, P. A. J. (1961a). *Arzneimittel-Forsch.* **11,** 819, 932.

Janssen, P. A. J. (1961b). *Psychopharmacologia* **2,** 141.

Janssen, P. A. J. (1962a). *Anaesthesist* **11,** 1.

Janssen, P. A. J. (1962b). *Brit. J. Anaesthesia* **34,** 260.

Janssen, P. A. J. (1962c). *Encéphale* **51,** 582.

Janssen, P. A. J. (1964a). *Ciba Foundation Symp.,* p. 264. Churchill, London.

Janssen, P. A. J. (1964b). *4th Intern. C.I.N.P. (Collegium Intern. Neuro-Psychopharmacol.) Meeting, Birmingham, August, 1964.*

Janssen, P. A. J., and Eddy, N. B. (1960). *J. Med. Pharm. Chem.* **2**, 31.
Janssen, P. A. J., and Jageneau, A. H. M. (1956). *Experientia* **12**, 293.
Janssen, P. A. J., and Jageneau, A. H. M. (1957). *J. Pharm. Pharmacol.* **9**, 381.
Janssen, P. A. J., and Jageneau, A. H. M. (1958). *J. Pharm. Pharmacol.* **10**, 14.
Janssen, P. A. J., and Niemegeers, C. (1959). *Arzneimittel-Forsch.* **9**, 765.
Janssen, P. A. J., and Niemegeers, C. J. E. (1961a). *Arzneimmittel-Forsch.* **11**, 1037.
Janssen, P. A. J., and Niemegeers, C. J. E. (1961b). *Nature* **190**, 911.
Janssen, P. A. J., Jageneau, A. H. M., van Proosdij-Hartzema, E. G., and de Jongh, D. K. (1958). *Acta Physiol. Pharmacol. Neerl.* **7**, 373.
Janssen, P. A. J., Jageneau, A. H. M., Demoen, P., van de Westeringh, C., de Cannière, J., Raeymaekers, A., Wouters, M., Sanczuk, St., and Hermans, B. (1959a). *J. Med. Pharm. Chem.* **1**, 309.
Janssen, P. A. J., Jageneau, A. H. M., Demoen, P., van de Westeringh, C., Raeymaekers, A., Wouters, M., Sanczuk, St., Hermans, B., and Loomans, J. (1959b). *J. Med. Pharm. Chem.* **1**, 105.
Janssen, P. A. J., van de Westeringh, C., Jageneau, A. H. M., Demoen, P. J. A., Hermans, B. K. F., Van Daele, G. H. P., Schellekens, K. H. L., Van der Eycken, C. A. M., and Niemegeers, C. J. E. (1959c). *J. Med. Pharm. Chem.* **1**, 281.
Janssen, P. A. J., Jageneau, A. H. M., Demoen, P., van de Westeringh, C., de Cannière, J., Raeymaekers, A., Wouters, M., Sanczuk, St., and Hermans, B. (1960a). *J. Med. Pharm. Chem.* **2**, 271.
Janssen, P. A. J., Jageneau, A. H. M., and Niemegeers, C. J. E. (1960b). *J. Pharmacol. Exptl. Therap.* **129**, 471.
Janssen, P. A. J., Niemegeers, C. J. E., and Jageneau, A. H. M. (1960c). *Arzneimittel-Forsch.* **10**, 1003.
Janssen, P. A. J., Jageneau, A. H. M., and Schellekens, K. H. L. (1960d). *Psychopharmacologia* **1**, 389.
Janssen, P. A. J., Niemegeers, C. J. E., and Schellekens, K. H. L. (1960e). *Arzneimittel-Forsch.* **10**, 955.
Janssen, P. A. J., Niemegeers, C. J. E., and Dony, J. G. H. (1963a). *Arzneimittel-Forsch.* **13**, 401.
Janssen, P. A. J., Niemegeers, C. J. E., Schellekens, K. H. L., Verbruggen, F. J., and Van Nueten, J. M. (1963b). *Arzneimittel-Forsch.* 13, 205.
Janssen, P. A. J., Niemegeers, C. J. E., and Schellekens, K. H. L. (1965). *Arzneimittel-Forsch.* **15**, 104.
Kopin, I. J. (1964). *Pharmacol. Rev.* **16**, 179.
Lehmann, H. E., and Bann, T. E. (1964). *1st N. Am. Symp., Quebec, January, 1964. Quebec Psychopharmacol. Res. Assoc. Rept.*
Mueller, P. B., and Langemann, H. (1962). *J. Neurochem.* **9**, 399.
Niemegeers, C. (1960). Thesis, University of Paris, Paris, France.
Niemegeers, C. J. E., and Janssen, P. A. J. (1960a). *J. Pharm. Pharmacol.* **12**, 744.
Randrup, A., Munkvad, I., and Udsen, P. (1963). *Acta Pharmacol. Toxicol.* **20**, 145.
Raynaud, G., and Valette, G. (1963). *Arch. Intern. Pharmacodyn.* **142**, 425.
Revol, M. L. (1961). *Bull. Trav. Soc. Pharm. Lyon* **5**, 69.
Ryall, R. W. (1964). *J. Neurochem.* **11**, 131.

Schaper, W. K. A., Jageneau, A. H. M., Huygens, J., and Janssen, P. A. J. (1960). *Med. Exptl.* **3**, 169.

Seeman, P. M., and Bialy, H. S. (1963). *Biochem. Pharmacol.* **12,** 1181.

Van Nueten, J. M. (1962). Thesis, University of Paris, Paris, France.

Weaver, L. C., Rahdert, E., Richards, A. B., and Abreu, B. E. (1964). *J. Pharm. Sci.* **53**, 417.

AMPLITUDE ANALYSIS OF THE ELECTROENCEPHALOGRAM

Review of the Information Obtained with the Integrative Method

By Leonide Goldstein and Raymond A. Beck

Section on Neuropharmacology, Bureau of Research in Neurology and Psychiatry, Princeton, New Jersey

"Here hills and vales, the woodland and the plain,
Here earth and water seem to strive again,
Not chaos-like together crush'd and bruis'd
But, as the world harmoniously confus'd:
Where order in variety we see,
And where, tho' all things differ, all agree."

Alexander Pope

I. Introduction

Almost four decades have elapsed since Hans Berger (1929) described to an incredulous world of neurologists and physiologists the curious electrical phenomena occurring ceaselessly in the brain of man. Since then, Berger's finding has not only been confirmed but so largely extended that an entire new branch of science has developed, that of electroencephalography.

During the first 10 to 15 years of EEG research, impressive correlations were found between the morphology of brain waves and physiologico-behavioral conditions (sleep, wakefulness) as well as in relation to pathological states (epilepsy, brain tumor). From the former, one could predict the latter, and even, within limits, define a "normal" tracing, i.e., a tracing not containing any visible suggestions of association with known or suspected manifestations of brain dysfunction (Gibbs and Gibbs, 1952). Of special interest to the medical profession was the fact that no complex measurements were needed to analyze EEG records. The main qualifications were a prolonged training, a well-developed gift of observation, and an ability to recognize artifacts.

However, as the years passed and more and more recordings were obtained not only on man but on numerous animal species (including such unlikely candidates as the alligator and the elephant), exceptions to originally established criteria were reported. These exceptions were especially prominent in regard to relationships between EEG and behavioral characteristics, so that eventually the expression "dissociation of EEG and behavior" appeared more and more frequently in the literature (Wikler, 1952; Bradley and Elkes, 1955; Longo, 1956; Domino and Hudson, 1959). Furthermore, despite the use of almost entirely distortion- and artifact-free amplifiers and recorders, no correlation was found respecting the extremes of the intelligence quotient, nor, for example, did neurotics display "abnormal" brain waves. Even in chronic schizophrenics, with brains obviously functioning in a markedly different manner from that of nonpsychotic subjects, the EEG most often appeared "normal."

Paralleling qualitative studies, work on the quantitative analysis of brain waves also progressed from the early days of electroencephalography, although at a pace less rapid and intense. For a few "mechanistically" minded physiologists, the failures of the EEG method appeared to be due not to an absolute obstacle, but rather to the limitations of the human eye to distinguish the trees in an amazingly complex forest. They maintained that if a more intensive method of analysis were applied to EEG signals, other and perhaps entirely new information would emerge, resolving at least some of the contradictions between brain wave morphology and the physiological state. Was such a claim justified? This review attempts to answer the question with a presentation of data obtained from one of the currently available methods of quantification, that involving the amplitudes of brain waves.

II. Methodological Basis for Amplitude Measurements

The EEG is essentially the manifestation of spontaneously occurring potential differences of 0 to 300 μv and with frequencies ranging from 1 to 300 or more per second. It is most important to understand clearly the implications of this fundamental concept.

In a system involving a potential difference between two discrete points, the characteristics of the intervening or constituent potential differences cannot be specifically deduced from the end points alone. That is, an increase or decrease in over-all potential difference does not necessarily indicate the direction of the changes of the individual potentials; an *increase* in the value of this total difference may actually reflect *decreases* in the constituent values and vice versa. Furthermore, the degree of homogeneity implied by the end point (output) potentials does not reflect directly the state of distribution prevailing among the constituent potentials. For example, the term "hypersynchronization" is often used to refer to an EEG record comprising successive identical events; at the other extreme, "desynchronization" refers to the absence of such homogeneity. However, a hypersynchronous over-all output does not necessarily mean hypersynchronization "within and between" constituent parts. On the contrary, as shown in Table I, one can easily construct a model to demonstrate that if the variability in the output is brought to zero, i.e., the output is continuously held constant,

TABLE I
MODEL OF A SYSTEM IN WHICH THE OUTPUT REPRESENTS THE DIFFERENCE BETWEEN THE VALUES OF TWO COMPONENT PARTS (1 AND 2)[a]

	Initial state			Condition A			Condition B		
	1	2	Output	1	2	Output	1	2	Output
	50	26	24	50	25	25	60	35	25
	46	19	27	46	21	25	39	14	25
	56	33	23	56	31	25	28	3	25
	64	36	28	64	39	25	51	26	25
	51	34	17	51	26	25	70	45	25
	42	20	22	42	17	25	64	39	25
	58	32	26	58	33	25	53	28	25
	58	30	28	58	33	25	68	43	25
	67	43	24	67	42	25	56	31	25
	61	32	29	61	36	25	32	7	25
Mean	55.3	30.5	24.8	55.3	30.3	25.0	52.1	27.1	25.0
SD	8.0	7.2	3.6	8.0	8.0	0	18.1	14.7	0
CV[b]	14.4	23.8	14.6	14.4	26.3	0	34.7	54.3	0

[a] Under conditions A and B the output is made to be constant although in A, component 1 is not changed, and in B, both components are made to be more variable.

[b] Coefficient of variation.

the constituent parts may be manipulated toward increased or decreased variability without affecting the variability level of the over-all output.

These factors are of extreme importance in that they illustrate the difficulties involved in such a system when *only* the over-all output is considered.

The kind of problem encountered here reminds one of that which confronted naturalists throughout the eighteenth and nineteenth centuries when they tried, unsuccessfully, to design a theory of evolution from observations of the morphological characteristics of randomly selected individual animals or plants. Even if such work had extended through ten or more centuries, even if it had been done by scientists with infinite patience and extraordinary acuteness of observation, failure to build a sound theory accounting for the changes in the morphology, physiology, and biochemistry of living creatures throughout the ages would still have resulted. It was only when analyses of changes were extended from individuals to populations, and even further to the dynamics of population changes, that such concepts as mutation pressure, selection pressure, and migration patterns were developed, and an over-all widely accepted statistical theory of evolution formulated (Fisher, 1930; Haldane, 1932; Wright, 1940).

The analogy between the characteristics of populations and that of brain waves is perhaps more than fortuitous. In both cases, analysis is hindered by a lack of knowledge of the fundamental state of the units involved. For instance, we do not know the absolute potential values whose difference is described by x-μv in wave w; similarly not knowing the genotypes of the progenitors of organism o, the latter can be described only by its phenotype. However, in both cases, we encounter the prominent feature of variability (so prominent, in fact, that it is most often ignored). No two organisms of the same species, subspecies, or even of the same variety are exactly alike; no two brain waves, except in very special cases, are exactly alike. Since information on evolutionary factors in related organisms is obtained through what amounts to a statistical analysis of variability in time, it is tempting to use the same approach in dealing with populations of related brain waves. In view of the impossibility of determining directly the behavior of constituent parts of brain electrical potentials, an indirect approach is used by analyzing their relationships. In other words, instead of describing or analyzing states as separate entities, information is obtained through the study of their relationships.

The idea of statistical analysis of brain waves, with its implication of a series of means computed from periods of varying duration, can appear totally artificial. Yet, the often used notion of "EEG pattern" is, in fact, a form of averaging. Since brain waves are extremely variable, one can argue that a single arbitrarily chosen sample can be highly *mis*representative of the condition of the brain at that time. Over-all expressions, covering as wide a range of events as possible, could be more informative, provided one specifies the limiting characteristics of that range.

This suggests considering brain waves as populations of electrical events, amenable to statistical analysis as applied to any other type of population. It precludes, unfortunately, the use of the well-established and highly useful classification of brain waves in terms of amplitude/frequency characteristics (alpha, beta, delta, theta, etc.) since these then become merely components of the global population. However, as will be shown later, when the presence of such rhythms appears to be statistically significant, their significance is emphasized by the quantitative approach, perhaps even more effectively than by qualitative observation alone.

III. Measurement of Amplitudes

The first attempt to quantify the EEG, presented by Kornmuller in 1937, consisted primarily of amplitude measurements. It is of interest to describe his work as an illustration of the problems involved in such a procedure. Kornmuller determined the amplitude of successive waves, peak positive to peak negative, for periods of 1-minute duration. To perform such measurements, an ordinary desk ruler was used, the measured values summed up, and the over-all cumulative amplitude calculated. Then, Kornmuller divided this global value by 60, expressing *a mean amplitude per second* (rather than dividing by the number of waves to express a mean amplitude per wave). A further refinement was the transformation of such data into actual microvolts per second by means of the calibration characteristics, specifically, the height of the wave evoked by feeding into the oscillograph the standard 50 μv signal.

Although this early attempt at quantification yielded some interesting facts, it was far from satisfactory from the physical point of view. For instance, no mention is made in this work of a base line or zero line, and yet it is obvious that in peak positive to peak negative determinations, the position of the base line is most important. In fact, if this position is not constant, comparisons of different recordings become meaningless. Since, as previously mentioned, brain waves are potential differences between variables, the absolute values of which one cannot know, it follows that the only correct reference, or zero line, is that corresponding to potential differences equal to zero. Needless to say, this value has only a derived, theoretical position, and cannot be measured on the recorded EEG tracing. Therefore, such peak-to-peak measurements have little or no validity.

An even more important reason for rejecting this simplified approach to quantification concerns the recording of only one of the values of a potential difference *varying in time,* thus neglecting most of the informational content. That is, one would be treating as static an essentially dynamic phenomenon whose assumed relationships with brain function can be established only through kinetic studies. For example, in the EEG, dome-shaped and spiky waves, frequently occurring adjacent to each other, may also have identical peak amplitudes. The former may well represent a slowly developing phenomenon with regularly spaced small increments, followed beyond a certain point, by identically spaced, slowly developing decrements. On the other hand, a spiky wave may correspond to a rapidly occurring, rapidly disappearing event, involving geometric-type progressions in the extrusion and contraction of the electrical gradient. Hence, in spite of their identical peak amplitudes, the treatment of both waveforms as identical in other parameters would obviously be wrong.

The solution to such a problem is to measure not the maximal heights of successive waves, but rather the entire linear course pursued in the evolution of each individual wave tracing with concomitant measurement of the area subtended. This was first attempted by Drohocki (1937) by means of a planimeter, a relatively simple, but very precise device which determines the surface of the plane area subtended by any curve form. With brain waves, this type of measurement obtains the integral of varying potential differences between successive points which most often serve as time references. Such integrals may be considered direct representations of the electrical energy displayed in either a single wave or in many waves. The base line, established directly by the planimeter, is that straight line connecting the starting and end points of the measured areas.

The planimetric method was used for a few years by Drohocki (1937), Berger (1938), and André (1945); later by Goldstein and Minz (1955) and by Bruck (1960). Owing to the fact that this procedure was exceedingly tedious and time consuming, only very short intervals of a recording were submitted to measurement. Hence, in these early analyses, it was not unusual to define states or conditions of the brain from a single 10-second sample. Again stressing the extreme variability of the EEG, it is readily apparent that such restricted measurements could be misleading. Therefore, an automatic device that would perform measurements directly on the EEG signals, i.e., one that would integrate the brain waves continuously, was much to be desired, if not required.

IV. The Electronic Integrator

By 1948, Drohocki was able to design an automatic integrator for electroencephalography which overcame some technical difficulties in unique ways. The classical electronic integrator is simply a capacitor which is charged by the incoming signal through a resistor. The size of the capacitor determines the maximum energy (charge) that can be stored, and this, together with the size of the resistor, determines the rate at which the energy can be stored. This simple circuit becomes nonlinear (logarithmic rise) as its maximal charge is approached; the smaller the proportion of maximum charge, the more linear the circuit. This places a practical limit on the response range of the device. Also, when the maximum value is reached, there must be some way of shorting the capacitor momentarily, so that it again has zero charge, and integration can be resumed. The Drohocki circuit meets these problems by charging the capacitor through a high-gain, sharp cut-off pentode. The large plate resistance of this tube plus the effective amplification of the value of the capacitor (Miller effect) results in an integrator of very large time constant with the linear portion of its range being extended enough to be of practical value. The discharge of the capacitor is effected by means of a gas-discharge (thyratron) tube. This tube has the characteristic of being virtually nonconductive (having a very large plate resistance) until a fixed value of grid voltage is reached, at which time, the gas (argon) in the tube becomes ionized (average time, 0.5 μsec). The plate resistance then drops to a very low value, and the tube conducts off the charge which has accumulated on the capacitor. Deionization occurs in about 75 μsec, and the circuit is then ready to resume storing charge. The thyratron is also in the plate circuit of the pentode, so that its firing occurs at a time which is entirely synchronous with the accumulation of the desired charge on the capacitor. The time constant of the entire circuit can easily be changed by modifying the value of the capacitor. This is done by means of a front panel selector switch.

The circuit is also arranged so that the firing of the thyratron and the discharge of the capacitor trigger a monostable multivibrator, which then gives an approximately 10-volt pulse as the output signal of the device. This pulse can be viewed on an oscilloscope or recorded on paper or magnetic tape.

The Drohocki integrator is by no means the only device available for integration, although it was the first one designed to give an output in the form of pulses which can be treated as numbers and submitted to the statistical analytical procedures discussed in this paper (Drohocki, 1957c). It has remained until recently the only one which did not need a relay for resetting, a highly useful feature in view of the well-known difficulties encountered with such devices.

Of course, with the integrator, as with all such circuits for analysis of harmonic functions, the incoming signal must first be rectified, so that the average value will not be zero.

Since each pulse from the integrator represents a fixed increment of electrical energy, the number of pulses in a given period of time will be a direct reflection of the amount of electrical energy (joules) in the input signal during that time. As illustrated in Fig. 1, this is frequency-independent for the frequency range under study, because of the very large time constant of the entire integrator circuit.

As can also be seen in Fig. 1, the output from the integrator is fed into the oscillograph so that a direct waveform tracing and its quantitated counterpart appear on the record simultaneously. An advantage of this graphic arrangement is that elimination of any portion of the EEG presenting an artifact necessarily includes removal of its quantitated counterpart. Also, one may arbitrarily select a specific portion of the EEG tracing, possessing pattern characteristics of qualitative interest, and obtain, at the same time, its corresponding quantitative measurements.

However, perhaps the main attribute of this method is that it permits not only instant characterization of any change, however fast or slow, but further permits statistical evaluation of its possible significance. This is of particular value when dealing with a system,

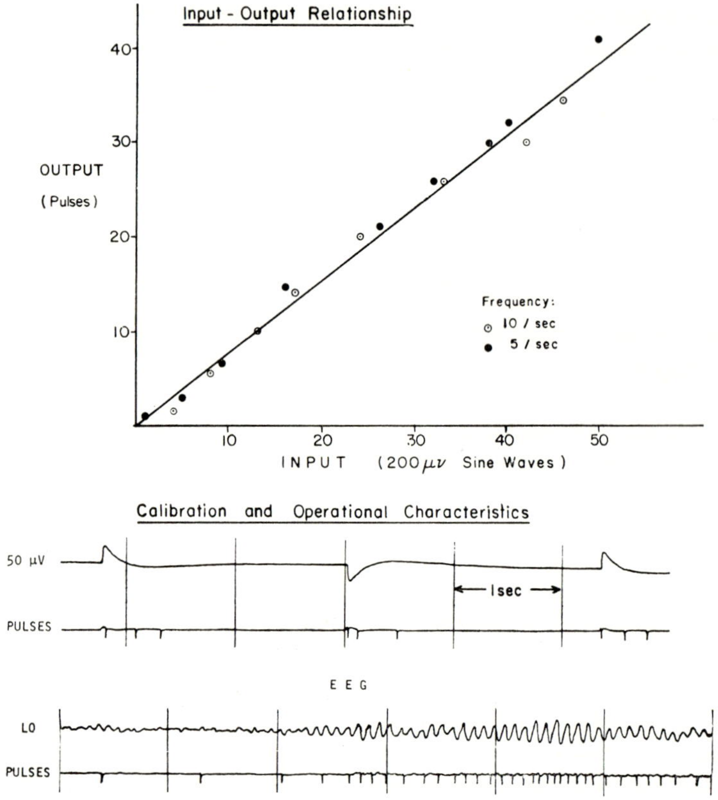

FIG. 1. Mode of operation of the Drohocki integrator. Upper graph: relationships between energy input (number of 200 μv sine waves) and integrator output (number of pulses delivered). As seen, direct proportionality is maintained despite variation of the frequency of sine waves fed into the analyzer (i.e., 5 or 10 cps). Lower graphs: calibration characteristics and actual integration of a 6-second strip of EEG recording (monopolar derivation from the left occipital in a normal human subject). The standard 50-μv calibration signal corresponds to 3 pulses regardless of polarity (since the integrator performs full-wave rectification). In the 6-second EEG sample, 34 pulses were cumulated and may be expressed as 34/6 or an average of 5.7 pulses per second. The average value may further be transformed in relation to calibration characteristics, and expressed as the mean energy content (MEC).

such as the EEG, in which a "pure" or homogeneous state, per se, does not seem to exist. Finally, direct data obtained from different subjects (animals or human) exposed to identical conditions may not unreasonably be simply averaged, provided such data has been initially submitted to some simple and preferably straightforward transformations in order to bring it all to the same initial level. The most often used transformation has been, until now, the indicial one (by which any set of values is equated to a mean of 100). In many cases, however, use was made of the "calibration transformation" since the selection of the time constant of integration was to be adjusted in relation to the relative level of "EEG abundance" of the subjects or animals. In this case, measurements are expressed, following transformation, in terms of the calibration characteristics established immediately before any one of the recording runs. (See Fig. 1 for an example of such manipulation of the data.)

It should be well understood, however, that data obtained through the integrator have value only if treated with statistical methods; this is an averaging method, and perhaps nothing more than an averaging method. Hence, the detection of unique, isolated waveforms from integrator data is hardly possible since no averaging method is sufficiently sensitive to single out events of rare or infrequent occurrence in a highly variable population of events.

As previously mentioned, it is primarily because of the wide variability of the EEG that the integration method is uniquely useful. In fact, it distinguishes the significant from the aleatory, as can be demonstrated by well-known procedures for examining the relationships between samples. In the EEG, e.g., this specifically entails the statistical comparison of a large number of successive periods of the electrical activity in respect to their numerical pulse content. From such treatment, values are obtained for the average *amplitude* (henceforth designated as mean energy content or MEC) and for the *variability* of the population which it represents, the latter statistic being determined from periods involved in the calculation of the MEC and most often expressed as the coefficient of variation (CV).

V. Analysis of the Resting EEG

The resting EEG has been extensively studied in animals and man to provide a "base line" in relation to which all changes can be expressed. Interestingly enough, it has yielded surprisingly consistent data characterized by two apparently opposite features: (1) a wide variability in the successive periods of integration enumerated during short time intervals (1–10 seconds) and, (2) a remarkable constancy between such successive levels of cumulated pulses during more prolonged time intervals. Figure 2 illustrates these facts with actual data taken from a representative recording of a normal human subject and a rabbit. As can be seen, with increasing length of time, the number of pulses counted and successive points plotted produce a progressively flattening curve to the ultimate level of a straight line. This corresponds to 250 seconds both in man and in rabbits. This finding shows that if a sufficiently large group of electrical energy levels is considered, a normal distribution results so that values above and below the mean cancel out each other.

A direct demonstration of this property of brain electrical activity was provided by Drohocki (1947, 1956, 1957b, 1962c) and Drohocki *et al.* (1955, 1956a) who studied a large number of distributions of integration pulses obtained for various time intervals in transcranial recordings in rabbits. Statistical tests showed that they were always within the range of expectation for a Gaussian curve. By recording from various cortical areas, the same authors found that in spite of differences in the mean level of electrical energy, symmetrical spreads of the individual values around the different means always existed.

In man, in recordings obtained from the parietal area of 60 normal adult volunteers during five successive sessions of 20 minutes to 1 hour each, Drohocki (1954a) found that a characteristic value (or "constant") could be determined for each subject. Although this value was fairly constant from recording to recording for each subject, large differences were noted between subjects. Plotting the successive values of either a single session or of all sessions globally for each volunteer produced almost perfect distributions.

From integration of monopolar recordings of the left occipital areas of 30 normal volunteers, Goldstein *et al.* (1963a) carried the study a step further. Instead of using direct data (the values for each of 30 successive 20-second intervals), such data was initially related to the MEC for the individual by indicial transformation, whereby the mean for each 10-minute "run" per subject was always

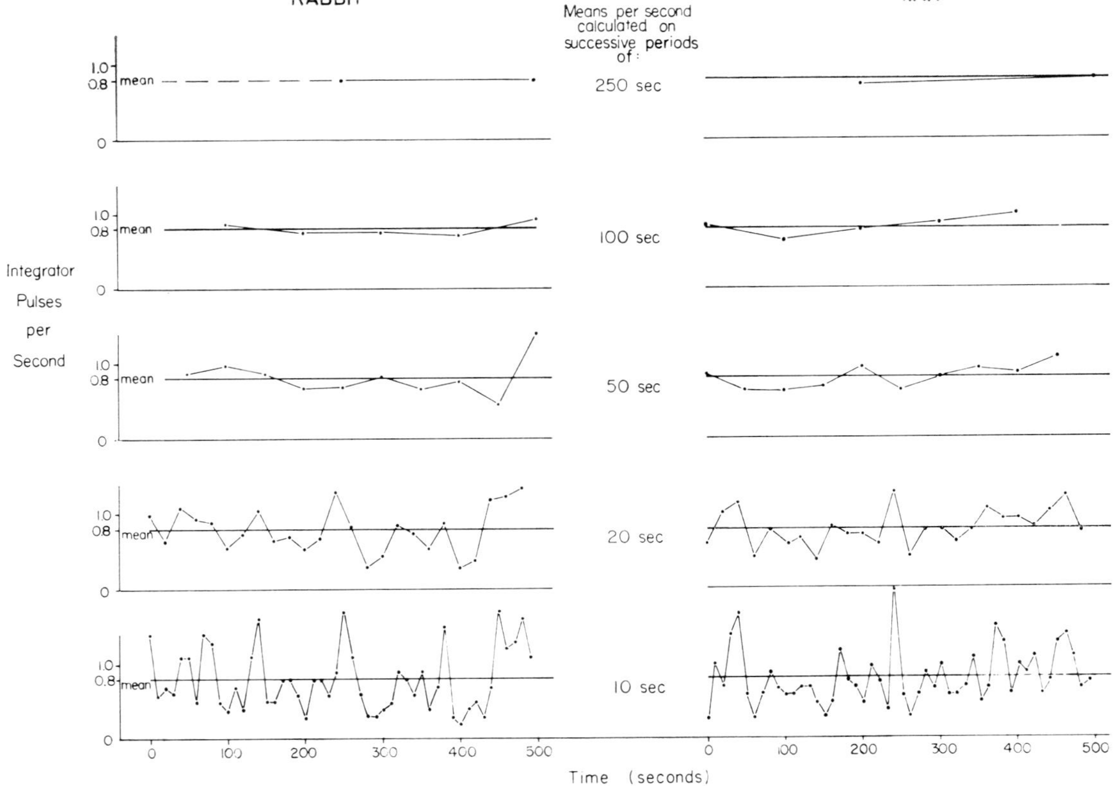

FIG. 2. The increasing variability in the mean number of pulses per second (MEC) is shown as progressively smaller samples of a 500-second strip of the EEG are considered. The straight horizontal line in each graph represents the mean number of pulses per second for the entire 500-second sample. The plotted points represent the means of the number of pulses for the time intervals listed in the center column.

equated to 100. Under such conditions, data between subjects could then be grouped and compared, providing close to 3000 values. The histogram of frequency distribution was typically Gaussian, with an over-all CV equal to 14.5 (standard deviation, 14.5% of the mean).

In further studies (Goldstein *et al.*, 1964a) the time basis for measurement was varied to include 5 periods ranging from 1 second to 1 minute. The relationships between the time unit of measurement and the value of the CV are listed in Table II. No exceptions

TABLE II
RELATIONSHIPS BETWEEN TIME BASIS OF MEASUREMENT OF THE QUANTITATED EEG AND CORRESPONDING STANDARD DEVIATIONS OF THE DISTRIBUTION OF THE VALUES[a]

Time basis (sec)	Normal subjects			Chronic schizophrenics		
	No. of measurements	Mean	SD	No. of measurements	Mean	SD
1	12,000	2.64	1.25	12,000	2.61	0.80
5	2,400	13.20	4.37	2,400	13.06	2.16
10	1,200	26.40	7.49	1,200	26.12	3.12
20	600	52.80	13.30	600	52.24	5.15
60	200	158.40	33.15	200	156.72	11.01

[a] Data obtained from 20 records of normal volunteers and 20 records of male chronic schizophrenics matched for similar individual and over-all energy contents (Goldstein *et al.*, 1964a).

to the rule mentioned above were found; it is obvious that they represent normal distributions in every case.

Aside from its theoretical implications, which will be discussed later, the outstanding advantage of this type of data is that it permits the use of parametrical statistical procedures which are notably simpler than nonparametrical. In addition, it provides justification for the definition of the resting EEG in terms of its MEC and CV. Drohocki (1954a), in fact, suggested the possibility of using the lower and higher limits of the MEC values of a large, homogeneous population to define normalcy within such a population, at least in relation to the level of electrical energy. Goldstein *et al.* (1963a), Pfeiffer *et al.* (1964a), and Sugerman *et al.* (1964), on the other hand, consider the CV to be a more sensitive indicator of this type of characterization.

VI. Analysis of the Resting EEG in Brain Disorders

The first attempt to analyze EEG's in brain disorders was by Drohocki (1954b) who studied the quantitated records of 33 newly admitted epileptic patients, age from 17 to 26, not yet exposed to anticonvulsant therapy. He found that the MEC's in these records were as much as four times higher than those of the 60 normal volunteers analyzed by the same author (as previously mentioned). Furthermore, in the integrator-processed data, the distribution of the successive measurements around their respective means yielded, instead of a one-peak plot, bimodal and even plurimodal curves.

This disruption in the distribution of measurements was interpreted as a change in the bioelectrical manifestations of cortical function as influenced by the presence of an epileptic focus. Of interest was the fact that this change in the distribution shape was evident in recordings of the parietal cortex regardless of the location of the foci—an indication that widespread changes in cortical function can be brought about by apparently small, well-delineated areas of pathology.

Goldstein *et al.* (1963a, 1964a) focused their attention on male chronic schizophrenics. Monopolar EEG's were recorded from the left occipital area on 101 patients in sessions lasting at least 10 minutes each. From the great wealth of data obtained, a very striking fact emerged, namely, that the coefficient of variation for the schizophrenic group was one-half that calculated for a group of 104 normal volunteers. On the other hand, no significant difference could be detected between male patients and male nonpsychotics in regard to the over-all MEC. In other words, although the means of the distribution curves of EEG measurements in normal and schizophrenic subjects occupied the same position, the spread of values around the mean was markedly wider in the case of the normals. Further EEG recordings established the fact that the difference in variability existing between normal and psychotic groups was not an artifact due to a chance selection of the time period for measurement, but, as shown in Table II, could be demonstrated in measurements from different time-intervals varying in duration from 1 second to 1 minute. It also appeared that this difference in variability was independent of the levels of the MEC as well as independent of alpha indices.

VII. Analysis of Changes Produced by Modification of Physiological Conditions

A. Hyperventilation

Investigations of hyperventilatory effects were performed by Drohocki (1954c, 1960b, 1962a), Drohocki and Duflo (1958, 1959), Drohocki and Soussen (1959), and Soussen and Chassaing (1960), on both children and adults in apparent good health. The quantitated bipolar EEG was recorded from the parieto-occipital areas during a 5-minute control period, 3 minutes of hyperventilation, and finally a 1-minute posttreatment period. Of 37 children studied (age from 9 to 13 years), 28 showed a one- to fourfold increase in MEC during hyperventilation. It appeared that the lower the energy content of the control period, the larger the increase produced by forced breathing. In the remaining 9 subjects, no change of any kind was detected.

In adults (mean age 23), 102 experiments were performed. The inverse relationship between the initial control level and the extent of increase during hyperventilation was again found. Quantitative studies showed no relationships between the increased amount of exhaled air or increased respiratory rate during hyperventilation and the over-all change in electrical energy. The spread of the distribution of integration pulse frequencies was not modified during the phase of increased energy; however, the entire distribution was shifted to a higher range.

B. Flicker Stimulation

In each of 40 normal adults, Drohocki (1954c, 1960a, 1960c) found that flicker-light stimulation resulted in an increase in the MEC. There also existed a certain subject-specific frequency, located between 3 and 19 cps, at which a further increase in energy occurred. This specific frequency of stimulation appeared to be independent of the individual alpha rhythm.

C. Sound Stimulation

Forty subjects, studied by Drohocki (1962b), on exposure to sound stimulation (400 cps for 3 seconds) manifested two successive phases in the evolution of the EEG: first, a decrease of the MEC; second, a "rebound" increase, elevating the energy content above the control level. During the decrease, variability was lowered, returning to control levels or higher during the second phase.

D. Visual Field Stimulation

A number of normal subjects and male chronic schizophrenics were recorded in a dimly lit room before and immediately following opening of the eyes. The procedure was done in both the supine and sitting positions (Goldstein *et al.*, 1964a). In normals, eye opening was followed by an abrupt fall in MEC and a decrease in EEG variability. These changes occurred in both the supine and the sitting positions, although the decreases in MEC and CV were more pronounced in the sitting position. In male chronic schizophrenics only minimal, nonsignificant changes, in either MEC or CV, were observed during or following eye opening; a shift to the sitting position had no effect on the typical low level of EEG reactivity in these patients.

E. Blood Pressure and Hematocrit

In unanesthetized rabbits, Muñoz and Goldstein (1961a) induced hypovolemic hypotension by bleeding while recording the parieto-cortical EEG from transcranial electrodes. Removal of a volume of blood amounting to 1% body weight resulted in a large increase in the MEC as is characteristic of sedation ("hypersynchronization"). Replacement of the depleted volume with an equivalent volume of dextran restored the EEG to the control level. This procedure could be repeated as many as five times, to the extent of decreasing the hematocrit to one-third of its original level while maintaining the original fluid volume without significant alteration of the EEG. To explore physiological mechanisms possibly influencing the effect of hypotension on the EEG, such operations as section of the spinal cord at C2, denervation of the carotid sinuses, or section of both vagi at the level of the neck were performed. However, the inverse relationship of MEC and blood pressure levels was not affected by these procedures.

F. Blood Circulation and Oxygenation

Studies were performed on 22 dogs submitted to long-term partial cardiopulmonary bypass using a disposable bubble oxygenator or a "Kay-Cross disc oxygenator." The extracorporeal blood flow was kept constant, mostly at a rate of 600 ml/minute, corresponding to about 40% of the control cardiac output. The results of these experiments have been described in detail by Hopf *et al.* (1961).

A few minutes after initiation of the heart-lung bypass, a pronounced decrease (up to 40%) of the MEC was observed in bipolar recordings of the frontoparietal cortex. This decrease, persisting throughout the experiments (up to 10 hours), was not affected by varying either the extracorporeal flow from 0 to 900 ml/minute or the carotid blood flow from 83 to 143 ml/minute. The lowered MEC could only be returned to, and maintained at, control levels for periods of up to 3 hours following the introduction into the perfusing blood of 100 mg of hydrocortisone. This finding suggests that under the conditions of cardiopulmonary bypass there occurs an inhibition or a depletion of cortical adrenal hormones.

VIII. Analysis of Changes Produced by CNS Stimulants and Antidepressant Drugs

The study of CNS stimulant and antidepressant drugs may transcend the limits of therapeutics in that such agents can induce a state of brain function of unspecific clinical significance but of utmost importance to the homeostatic economy of the organism, namely, arousal. For one, widespread searches have revealed the existence of numerous naturally occurring stimulants. Further, as will be shown, there are many indications that certain psychotic states are essentially states of hyperarousal or hyperstimulation. It is not surprising, therefore, that there has been extensive research in the analysis of the quantitated EEG of animal and man exposed to naturally occurring or synthetic CNS stimulants.

One problem encountered in the study of such compounds is that when administered to awake, unsedated subjects in small doses, their effects are generally rather mild and short-lasting; hence it is difficult if not impossible to ascertain by mere visual inspection of the EEG the significance of the changes induced. The quantitative method, however, obviates these difficulties by permitting appraisal of drug-induced EEG changes in relation to the predrug control period, whatever its variability. Also, as will be seen, quantitation describes the stimulant effect (desynchronization) simply and directly by a decrease in both the MEC and the CV.

A. Naturally Occurring Compounds with Stimulant Properties

Studies of these compounds were conducted mostly on rabbits, although some cats and dogs were included.

1. *Catecholamines*

It was found by Goldstein and Muñoz (1960, 1961b) that epinephrine and norepinephrine at dose levels of 1 to 5 μg/kg, iv, produced significant, short-lasting changes in the EEG toward stimulation, or what is usually referred to as "desynchronization"; this occurred, however, in only 20% of the animals tested (45 rabbits, 7 cats, 2 dogs). As will be described, further studies involving pretreatment of the animals with other specific drugs prior to administration of these neurohormones resulted in significant stimulation in 100% of the cases.

2. *Histamine*

This compound was tested by Goldstein *et al.* (1963c, 1964b) in rabbits prepared with chronic indwelling electrodes and protected against peripheral vascular effects with promethazine methosulfate or diphenhydramine trimethylammonium chloride. Potent and long-lasting stimulant effects of histamine were demonstrated with intravenous doses of 1 mg/kg. Of interest is the fact that *N*,*N*-dimethyl histamine, a naturally occurring metabolite of histamine (Fram and Green, 1963), proved to be more effective than histamine, in that a smaller dose produced an identical shift in the EEG toward a lowered level of the MEC. Other metabolites or congeners, such as imidazole methyl histamine, imidazole acetic acid, and histidine, showed no stimulant effects.

3. *Choline*

In a large range of oral doses, choline exerted no apparent effect on the EEG of man. An intravenous injection of 5 mg/kg was without effect on the EEG of rabbits; but 1 mg/kg, iv, produced a short-lasting decrease in the MEC of the parietal cortex of normal human volunteers (Pfeiffer *et al.*, 1960).

B. Congeners, Derivatives, or Precursors of Naturally Occurring Compounds

1. *Isoproterenol*

Muñoz and Goldstein (1961b) and Goldstein and Muñoz (1960, 1961b) found that this compound, at doses of 1 to 5 μg/kg, iv, produced short-lasting stimulant effects in most of the animals tested (rabbits, cats, dogs). The effect coincided with the maximal hypotension and tachycardia induced by isoproterenol, but disappeared before return to normotension. Denervation of the carotid sinuses (in rabbits) shifted the effect from that of stimulation to one of sedation.

2. *Dichloroisoproterenol* (*DCI*)

The same authors found in rabbits that 4 mg/kg of this structural analog of isoproterenol (which characteristically effects beta-adrenergic blockade) produced marked and long-lasting arousal effects, as measured by reversal of pentobarbital-induced sedation. Smaller doses had only a partial reversing effect.

3. *Amphetamine*

Muñoz and Goldstein (1960, 1961a) and Beck *et al.* (1963) performed extensive experiments with amphetamine administered to rabbits equipped with chronically implanted electrodes and methodically trained to withstand intravenous injections under minimal stress and unrestrained conditions. To ensure the delineation and precise measurement of drug effect, the rabbits were initially lightly sedated with 3 mg/kg, iv, of sodium pentobarbital, thus inducing an acceptably constant level of hypersynchronization. Varied doses of amphetamine were given intravenously immediately thereafter—one dose level per group of 5 to 10 animals.

The degree of stimulation was determined by the reversal of the level of the MEC of the barbiturate-induced sedation toward the MEC level existing during the control period prior to sedation. Applying such an experimental procedure, linear log-dose-effect relationships could be demonstrated on appropriately plotted curves; from the latter, in turn, 50% reversal doses (of pentobarbital sedation) could be determined to serve as relative indications of test-drug activity. Thus, the average dose of *d*-amphetamine required to produce a 50% reversal was found to be 0.01 ± 0.005 mg/kg.

The aforementioned relationships enable the evaluation of the stimulant effect to a more precise degree than possible with qualitative observation alone in which only extensive change can convincingly carry significance.

The effects of *d*-amphetamine in normal human subjects were studied by Pfeiffer *et al.* (1960) and Murphree *et al.* (1962b). The EEG was recorded from the parietal area; measurements for analysis were obtained by "sampling" the record for 5 minutes at 30-minute intervals for a period of 3 hours. In 7 subjects, 0.1 mg/kg, iv, produced a significant decrease in the parietal EEG after a short latent period.

With 15 mg *per os* (8 subjects) a significant change was also detected, this time in the occipital area; the stimulant effect was not, however, consistently present and acquired significance only when the total data obtained from all 8 subjects were averaged. The measured EEG changes amounted to a 20% decrease in the MEC and a 20% decrease in the CV. This effect first appeared in the recorded electrical activity in a 10-minute "sample" obtained 30 minutes after drug administration, attained a peak at 60 minutes, and returned to the control level after 2 hours.

4. *Deanol (2-Dimethylaminoethanol)*

Primarily, deanol is a precursor of choline (trimethylaminoethanol) which has been shown by Groth *et al.* (1958) to penetrate the blood–brain barrier freely. Choline, in turn, is known to be a precursor of acetylcholine, a neurochemical mediator important for maintenance of the vigilant state of the organism.

Goldstein (1960b), Pfeiffer *et al.* (1963), and Beck *et al.* (1964) studied the effects of this compound on the rabbit EEG. The action of deanol appears to depend on the behavioral state of the animal at the time of drug administration. A dose of 5 mg/kg, injected intravenously, into awake, spontaneously alert rabbits, produces within 20 to 30 minutes, an EEG consisting of sporadic "hypersynchronus" patterns corresponding to increases in both MEC and CV. Administered to animals, either spontaneously sedated or pretreated with minimal doses of pentobarbital, the same intravenous dose of deanol produced, after a 15 to 20 minutes latent period, a distinct and sudden shift in the EEG pattern toward stimulation. Dose–effect curves, established by the experimental design described previously for amphetamine, revealed that the dose of deanol exerting a 50% reversal of sedation was 1.8 ± 0.5

mg/kg. Of interest is the fact that monomethylaminoethanol produced the identical reversal at the much higher dose level of 13.2 mg/kg. This tends to indicate, for certain compounds, a relationship between the degree of methylation and their stimulant potency. Other examples of this type of structure–activity relationships are to be mentioned later.

In man, the effects of single-dose administration of deanol were studied by Pfeiffer *et al.* (1960, 1964b) and by Goldstein *et al.* (1963b). The dose most frequently employed orally was 200 mg, although in several cases the effects of 1-gm doses were studied; also, on a group of 7 subjects, an intravenous dose of 1 mg/kg was administered. In regards to the MEC, the EEG changes observed were very similar to those produced by *d*-amphetamine, i.e., a decrease attaining its peak (20%) 1 hour after drug treatment. However, exactly contrary to the pronounced decrease in CV occurring with amphetamine, deanol increased the variability of the EEG energy levels to 120%; this altered variability still existed 2 hours after drug administration, although the MEC had since returned to the control level.

Chronic administration of deanol was effected only in male chronic schizophrenic patients, as part of a year-long study involving different drug treatments, to be described in detail later. Sixteen patients, not exposed to any acute or chronic drug treatment for at least 3 months were involved in that study. Their base-line recordings had the typical characteristics of a very small CV, of the order of 7%. Deanol was administered daily at the oral dose of 1 gm. Recordings, performed at the end of 1 month of such treatment, revealed a 30% increase in the CV of the group. There was, however, no significant change in the over-all MEC and no changes in behavioral ratings (Sugerman *et al.*, 1964).

C. Other Types of CNS Stimulant Drugs

A number of compounds were studied in rabbits for possible stimulant properties by Goldstein (1960b) and Beck *et al.* (1964; Beck and Goldstein, 1964). In most cases, dose–effect curves were established by the procedure applied to the study of amphetamine.

1. *Tropines*

Of this group of compounds, atropine and scopolamine are of special interest in that they are known to produce behavioral stimulant effects (in many species) along with a seemingly contradictory hypersynchronized pattern in the EEG. As a matter of fact, it is in reference to these specific compounds that the expression "dissociation between EEG and behavior" was originally used (Wikler, 1952). Atropine, 1 mg/kg, iv, did indeed shift the normal pattern of the EEG toward a type resembling either sedation or light sleep. However, statistical analysis of the *quantitated* EEG revealed an important difference between the two types of hypersynchronization, inapparent to observation with the naked eye. Under true sedation, the distribution of successively measured periods of electrical energy (periods of 1-second duration) was markedly widened in comparison to its spread during normal wakefulness. Under atropine, however, the limits of the distribution remained unchanged from that before drug administration; rather, the "sedation" effect consisted in a shift of the entire system toward higher values of electrical energy.

Furthermore, if the dose of atropine administered is decreased to 5–10 μg/kg, the behavioral stimulant effect of higher doses again appears; but now, in contradistinction to high-dose effect, the EEG pattern is that of a long-lasting desynchronization. Thus it was established that in the parameter of the EEG, atropine produced two opposite effects dependent on dose level: at 1 to 50 μg/kg, a progressively increasing stimulant effect prevailed (as evidenced by the per cent reversal of pentobarbital-induced sedation); whereas, doses above 50 μg/kg produced, in place of the low-dose arousal, a deepening of the sedated state. The same relationships were found to occur with scopolamine except that the dose level thresholds for arousal and sedation were one-twelfth–to one-twentieth that defined for atropine.

2. *Physostigmine*

This cholinesterase inhibitor exerted a distinct stimulant effect at a threshold dose level of 20 μg/kg, iv; the effect lasted 30 minutes. From preliminary unpublished observations, it appears that unlike all the chemical compounds discussed in this review, physostigmine studies do not yield dose–effect curves, thus implying the existence of an "all-or-none" phenomenon.

3. *Nicotine*

The dose of nicotine producing a 50% reversal of sedation was found to be 19 μg/kg. It is to be emphasized that contrary to the action of most stimulants, the effects of this alkaloid were found to be extremely short-lasting, appearing 2 minutes after intravenous administration, and disappearing completely within 6 to 8 minutes (Beck, 1965).

4. *Caffeine*

Only preliminary data are at present available concerning the effects of caffeine on animals. It appears that the 50% reversal dose is approximately 1 mg/kg, administered intravenously. A significant effect becomes evident after a latent period of 3 to 5 minutes and persists for a relatively long period of time (30 minutes or more).

In normal human subjects, the effects of a single oral dose of 250 mg of caffeine were studied by Goldstein *et al.* (1963b). The EEG stimulant effect appeared very rapidly, attained an approximate maximal point 30 minutes after drug administration, and persisted for at least 3 hours. The observed changes resembled those produced by amphetamine except that they were comparatively more accentuated; that is, caffeine induced a 30% decrease in the MEC, and a 35% decrease in the CV. Unlike their response to amphetamine, all subjects reacted to caffeine essentially in the same fashion and with little variation.

5. *Ethylenediamine Compounds*

Beck *et al.* (1964) studied a series of methylated derivatives of ethylenediamine to ascertain the degree to which progressive methylation may promote simulant properties of the ethylenediamine moiety. As in the investigations of drugs already described, the effective potency of each substituted compound was evaluated in terms of the dose level producing a 50% reversal of pentobarbital-induced sedation. The results demonstrated a direct relationship between the degree of methylation of the amino groups and the stimulant effect evoked. For example, the 50% reversal dose of the *N*-monomethyl derivative was 36.0 mg/kg, iv, as compared to 5.7 mg/kg for the trimethyl compound, implying increasing stimulant potency with progressive methylation.

6. *Ibogaine*

This alkaloid extracted from the shrub *Tabernanthe iboga* was tested by Drohocki (1954d) in man. Monopolar EEG recordings were obtained from the vertex; the integrator pulses were measured in units of 1-second time intervals. Significant changes were reflected in the spread of the distributions, in the position of the mean, or in both parameters, and occurred chiefly at the time the subjects reported "psychic excitation."

D. Antidepressant Agents

At the present time, antidepressant drugs investigated in man include only the monoamine oxidase inhibitors, tranylcypramine (20 mg total dose, orally), and the experimental compound, 2-methyl-3-piperidinopyrazine or W3207 B (50 and 120 mg total doses, orally). The results of these studies were essentially negative (Goldstein *et al.*, 1963b), as shown by no significant change in MEC or CV over a 6-hour period, other than a transient increase in the MEC 2 hours after the larger 120-mg dose of W3207 B.

However, clinically, these antidepressant drugs are well known to be slow in onset of action, necessitating relatively prolonged administration to evoke the desired behavioral effects. Hence, it is not surprising that, in the above study, quantitated EEG changes were undetectable following a single-dose administration and a relatively short period of EEG recording.

IX. Analysis of Changes Produced by Hallucinogenic Drugs

Ever since the discovery of the remarkable capacity of lysergic acid diethylamide (LSD) to induce hallucinatory states in man, there has been considerable interest in this specific compound, and others with similar activity. Although prominent changes were demonstrated in the EEG's of animals under the influence of LSD, mescaline, and psilocybin, distinctive features in the electrical activity of the human brain could not be detected by visual inspection of records alone even during the occurrence of drug-induced hallucinations. Hence, the quantitative method of EEG analysis was applied in an attempt to uncover the apparently subtle effects of hallucinogenic drug action.

A. Experimentation in Man

Goldstein *et al.* (1963a,b) administered LSD orally to normal volunteers at the two dose levels of 0.3 and 1.0 μg/kg. Ten-minute recordings were obtained from the left occipital area every 30 minutes for a period of 3 hours. As in all quantitative EEG studies, electrical energy levels and the variabilities therein were expressed in relation to their control levels in a fixed period to drug administration. After the lower dose of 0.3 μg/kg, the 6 subjects tested reported no behavioral effects other than a slight restlessness. Further, no significant change in the MEC of the quantitated EEG was detected during any of the sampling periods. However, a significant decrease in the CV (from the control value of 17.6 to 11.7%) occurred 90 minutes after drug ingestion. This lowered variability was still detectible after 2 hours. At the higher dose of 1 μg/kg, producing visual hallucinations and other LSD effects in most of the 13 subjects studied, the decrease in EEG variability was even more pronounced (from the control value of 14.7 to 7.9%). Moreover, along with this change, the level of the MEC decreased by 23%. Maximal decrease in electrical activity occurred in 90 minutes; that of the CV, in 150 minutes.

Thus, in the quantitated EEG's of normal volunteer subjects, LSD does, indeed, induce prominent changes. The latter are similar to those observed with amphetamine and caffeine: a decrease in MEC and variability; the decreases, however, were relatively pronounced and longer lasting with LSD.

Of interest at this point are the experimental reports that overdosage with amphetamine may produce visual hallucinations. Also to be considered is the fact that the decreased EEG variability typical of drug-induced hallucinations is very similar to that found in the resting EEG of the chronic schizophrenic. In both cases, the variability is approximately one-half that found in normal, untreated subjects.

Goldstein *et al.* (1963a) administered LSD (1 μg/kg orally) to each of 10 male chronic schizophrenics. There was no change in the MEC during 2 hours following drug administration. On the other hand, the CV increased rather than decreased, as occurred in the nonpsychotic subject. This could be interpreted as a "rebound" phenomenon, although no striking behavioral changes were observed in the patients throughout the period of action of LSD.

B. Experimentation in Animals

The effect of hallucinogenic drugs on rabbits was studied by Pierre (1957), Goldstein *et al.* (1962), and Beck *et al.* (1963). As anticipated from the findings in normal human volunteers, these drugs proved to be equally powerful CNS stimulants in rabbits.

Using the previously described technique, and determining the dose necessary to reduce the energy levels attained during pentobarbital-induced sedation by 50%, the following values were obtained: LSD—0.23 μg/kg; bufotenine—0.08 mg/kg; psilocybin—0.27 mg/kg; mescaline—1.7 mg/kg. In all cases, the stimulant effect was long-lasting.

Goldstein *et al.* (1965) and Pfeiffer *et al.* (1965) compared in rabbits the changes induced by LSD at cortical and rhombencephalic levels to changes occurring during "paradoxical" or "fast" sleep. This study was prompted by the observation that in both cases the cortex exhibited an identical pattern of "hyperarousal" and that an unquestionable resemblance existed between dreaming and hallucinations. As shown by the work of Dement and Kleitman (1957) there are numerous indications that dreaming takes place during the stages of paradoxical sleep. Quantitative integration of the EEG recorded during paradoxical sleep revealed that the energy content and variability are quite low at cortical levels and very high in the subcortical, caudal, pontine nucleus. Following LSD (5 μg/kg, iv), similar effects were seen at cortical levels, but in the rhombencephalic area, no significant difference from wakefulness was found in either energy content or CV. This could mean that different mechanisms (or perhaps different neuronal pathways) are involved in dreaming and drug-induced hallucinogenesis.

X. Analysis of Changes Produced by Antianxiety Drugs

A. Animal Studies

Drohocki and Goldstein (1957) studied the effects of benactyzine, meprobamate, and the experimental compound, phenylparachlorophenyl morpholinoethoxymethane (LD 2630) on the cortical EEG of rabbits. All three drugs produced a shift of the EEG toward sedation, corresponding to increases in the MEC and CV. The doses doubling the control energy level (within a period of 20 minutes) were: benactyzine—0.8 mg/kg; LD 2630—3.0 mg/kg; and meprobamate—1.0 mg/kg. The duration of effect was longest with LD 2630 and shortest with benactyzine.

The data in these studies were analyzed in a somewhat different manner, yielding, as a result, additional and unanticipated information; that is, successive 10-second intervals of the EEG were measured, the time-unit values cumulated, and then plotted to obtain linear regression lines, for the period of drug action (the first 20 minutes following drug administration). The slopes of the regression lines were found to be directly dose-related, suggesting a one-step relationship between the dose of the drug and the number of time units involved.

B. Studies on Normal Volunteers

A number of antianxiety agents were studied by Goldstein *et al.* (1963d), Pfeiffer and Schultz (1964), Pfeiffer and Goldstein (1964), and Pfeiffer *et al.* (1964a). The EEG was evaluated from successive 10-minute units, sampled from the recording every hour for a period of 6 hours. As with most of the previous studies, measurements were expressed in relation to a 10-minute, predrug, control recording.

1. *Meprobamate*

A total oral dose of 800 mg was administered to 10 normal volunteers. Two hours after drug administration, the MEC was decreased by 30%; after 6 hours, it had returned to the control level. The CV, on the other hand, increased progressively and markedly, attaining a peak in the fifth hour postdrug sampling. and still 25% above normal at the conclusion of the experiment.

2. *Chlordiazepoxide*

Similar changes, i.e., decrease in MEC and increase in CV, were observed in the 9 subjects studied (20 mg total oral dose). However, the appearance of effects in relation to time differed from that of meprobamate. With chlordiazepoxide, the MEC was not significantly decreased until 4 hours after drug administration, nor did it return to control level at the conclusion of the 6-hour duration of the experiment. Further, the CV did, indeed, tend to increase, but significantly so only in the second and sixth hour samples of the EEG record.

3. *Diphenhydramine*

This antihistaminic agent was tested at two dose-levels, 20 and 50 mg (total oral dose), on 10 and 13 subjects, respectively. Similar, though more pronounced, inverse relationships between the MEC and CV were observed as with meprobamate and chlordiazepoxide. For example, with 50 mg, the MEC decreased, 6 hours after drug administration, to 28% of its control value; at the same time, the CV almost doubled in value. In both EEG parameters, the degree of change was shown to be dose-related.

4. *Orphenadrine*

The EEG changes produced by this drug resembled those described for diphenhydramine. Total doses of 20 and 50 mg, administered to each of 10 and 13 subjects, respectively, produced a similar decrease in the MEC and increase in the CV. However, compared to aforementioned drugs, orphenadrine effects were both more accentuated in nature and differently spaced in time.

5. *Atropine*

One milligram total oral dose (the sole dose level studied), effected no change in the MEC measured throughout a 6-hour period. However, a significant trend toward increase in the CV was observed.

6. *Ethanol*

Each of 10 subjects received an oral dose of ethanol amounting to 0.25 ml/kg (95% solution). Within 60 minutes, the MEC of the quantitated EEG decreased by 17%; at the same time, a slight, nonsignificant, increase in the CV occurred. The maximal drop in MEC appeared 90 minutes after drug administration.

7. *Phenobarbital*

Total oral doses of 20 and 40 mg were given to each of 2 groups of 10 subjects, respectively. The EEG changes again included a decreased MEC and increased CV, but unlike the compounds discussed above, these trends were not uniform but presented, instead, a variable course of events: 1 hour after drug administration, the MEC decreased; in the second- and third-hour EEG samples, the energy content returned to normal levels; in the fourth hour, a second more pronounced decrease in MEC occurred (as compared to the first sampling), and persisted to the conclusion of the 6-hour experimental period.

Since sampling errors are always possible despite the averaging of data on as many as 10 subjects, Pfeiffer (1965) repeated the same study on an entirely new group of 10 subjects. The results obtained were strikingly similar to those obtained for the first groups. It would appear, therefore, that the biphasic drop in MEC under phenobarbital reflects a characteristic feature of the action of this drug. It is tentatively suggested that the second (fourth-hour) decrease in MEC may be due to the effect of a metabolite of phenobarbital, exerting stronger effects than the barbiturate itself.

8. *Pentobarbital*

Twenty and 40 mg total oral dose produced no significant change in either MEC or CV throughout experimental sessions lasting 6 hours. As will be discussed, higher doses did exert significant effects, but of a nature more characteristic of hypnotic rather than antianxiety activity.

The decreased MEC induced by antianxiety agents might, indeed, seem puzzling (if not paradoxical) when considered in relation to the CNS stimulant drugs which similarly effect a diminution in electrical activity. However, in contrast to the decreased CV observed with stimulant drugs (amphetamine, caffeine, LSD), variability in the EEG is increased with the antianxiety agents. Following administration of the latter, EEG recording examined by visual inspection alone, reveal a pattern resembling that of drowsiness, namely, juxtaposited intervals of alpha rhythm, nonrhythmic beta activity, and even sporadic slow waves of sleep. In comparison, the state of arousal or stimulation is characterized by a fairly constant reduction in brain-wave amplitude persisting for a relatively long period of time. It is precisely this difference in the variability of the quantitated EEG which distinguishes the action of antianxiety agents (increased CV) from that of stimulant agents (decreased CV).

XI. Analysis of Changes Produced by Hypnotic and Anesthetic Agents

A. Pentobarbital

This familiar compound is of special importance in animal brain investigations in that it provides an effective base line of mild sedation to which stimulant activity of varied agents can be more precisely referred.

In unrestrained rabbits equipped with chronically implanted intracranial electrodes (parietal cortex) and carefully trained to experimental procedures, Muñoz and Goldstein (1961b), Pfeiffer *et al.* (1963), Beck *et al.* (1963, 1964), and Beck and Goldstein (1964) found that pentobarbital in doses of 3 to 6 mg/kg, iv, increased the MEC of the EEG to 200% or more above control levels. This effect required approximately 5 minutes to reach a fairly constant level which then persisted for 20 to 30 minutes or more. The CV was most often doubled. At higher doses, such as 30 mg/kg, iv (administered over a period of 1 minute), Drohocki *et al.* (1956b) distinguished three phases in the evolution of the MEC: an initial phase (lasting approximately 200 seconds after injection) showing a decrease in MEC; a second phase of rapid increase of MEC (lasting from 300 to 400 seconds); and finally, the appearance of a plateau of more or less constant activity. Plotting of the logarithmic values of successive 1-second intervals of the second phase of rapid increase in MEC yielded a linear regression, which, in turn, indicated a geometric progression of the measured values per time unit in the development of the hypnotic effect.

In man, pentobarbital effects were studied by Drohocki (1957a), Jenney *et al.* (1962), Murphree *et al.* (1962a), and Pfeiffer *et al.* (1965).

1. *Normal Subjects* ($N = 13$)

A total oral dose of 200 mg produced a phase division of the MEC levels as observed in rabbits, namely, an initial decrease (duration—12 minutes), a geometric-type increase (duration—19 minutes), and a slow arithmetic increase requiring 6 minutes to reach the maximal level of a plateau. An additional, primary stage (duration—7 minutes), not seen in rabbits, corresponded to a latency period between administration of drug and beginning of effect; this difference is, however, most likely due to the difference in routes of administration, namely, intravenous in the rabbit, oral in man. The maximal level of electrical energy at plateau level averaged 80% above that of the control period. The CV increased both during the period of latency and during the first phase of the rise in MEC; it was further augmented during the phase of arithmetical growth, remaining considerably elevated thereafter.

2. *Male Chronic Schizophrenics*

In this group, response to pentobarbital was characterized by a relatively prolonged latent period (22 minutes), and absence of initial decrease of the MEC. The geometric-type increase was replaced by an arithmetic progression of 17 minutes duration, leading up to a plateau of constant activity, but only 25% above control level. Variability was unchanged during the latent period and only slightly higher during the two last phases.

B. Thiopental

This drug was studied only in human subjects.

1. *Normal Subjects (N = 10)*

A dose of 1.5 mg/kg, iv, rapidly administered, produced an immediate, short-lasting but very marked increase in energy content. After 2 minutes, the MEC temporarily returned to the control level after which it decreased over the next 10 minutes by as much as 90% of its control value; the behavioral correlate of the reduced energy period was that usually referred to as "activation." As expected, it corresponded to a reduction in EEG variability.

2. *Male Chronic Schizophrenics*

Somewhat similar changes were found in the averaged EEG data obtained from 10 patients. However, recordings of the latter displayed a greater and more prolonged reduction in electrical energy and variability than did normal subjects, a finding confirming Goldman's report (1962) of the existence of a difference between normals and schizophrenics.

C. Butyric Acid Derivatives

The two closely related compounds studied in man were butyrolactone (2.5 gm) and γ-hydroxybutyrate (1.5 to 4.0 gm). After a latent period of 12 minutes, butyrolactone induced behavioral sleep with a concomitant increase in MEC to levels of 100 to 120% above control level. The attained plateau persisted for 25 minutes or more. γ-Hydroxybutyrate exhibited no behavioral or EEG effects up to 1.5 gm; larger doses produced an irregular CNS depression starting 15 minutes after dosage and lasting up to 2 hours. Despite increases in the MEC almost as pronounced as with butyrolactone, only light anesthesia resulted in a certain number of the subjects. Interestingly, as the subjects roused from the γ-hydroxybutyrate effects, they verbalized spontaneously and coherently despite a coexistent EEG picture of high-voltage humps and sleep spindles, features corresponding to a high level of electrical energy and an increased variability.

D. Ethyl Carbamate

This anesthetic was studied in rabbits by Drohocki *et al.* (1956b). Administration of 1 g/kg of the drug was followed by deep sleep within 15 minutes. Although the mean energy content of the EEG (parietal leads) increased markedly, a plateau of constant activity was not attained; that is, electrogenic levels shifted unpredictably from values of 3 to 300% above control level to values equal to or even below those observed before drug administration. The statistical distribution of integrator pulses, examined at different stages of sleep development or with different time units of measurement, failed to reveal any trend or organization whatsoever.

XII. Analysis of Changes Produced by Antipsychotic Medication

A. Chlorpromazine and Perphenazine in Chronic Schizophrenics

Quantitative EEG analyses were performed on a group of 16 male chronic schizophrenics for a period of 1 year; 10-minute EEG recordings on each patient were taken monthly. The treatment routine was as follows: chlorpromazine (CPZ) (300 mg daily) for 1 month; placebo for 3 months; finally, perphenazine (16–32 mg daily), administered either alone or in combination with deanol (previously described), for the remainder of the study. The results of this investigation, performed in a double-blind design, have been reported by Sugerman *et al.* (1964) and Murphree *et al.* (1963).

It is to be emphasized that the control, pretreatment level of the coefficient of variability of the EEG of the these patients was relatively low. (See section on the resting EEG in schizophrenic patients.) The action of *chlorpromazine,* evaluated from recordings at cessation of drug treatment, reflected a slight increase in the over-all MEC of the group, and a nonsignificant increase in the CV. Replacement of the phenothiazine by placebo maintained the trend toward increasing MEC and CV for the following 2 months. At the end of this time, the MEC was 27% above predrug level, whereas the CV had doubled its original value. However, at the conclusion of 3 months of placebo treatment, the trends of increasing MEC and CV reversed; both parameters now returned to approximately control values.

Perphenazine alone, but especially in combination with deanol (1 g daily), produced a striking change in the CV to the extent of a threefold increase. In contrast to the increased MEC due to CPZ, these drugs effected a decrease in MEC to a plateau level 40% below initial value. Also unlike CPZ action, replacement of perphenazine with placebo resulted in markedly decreased EEG variability within 1 month. In other words, after 2 months of placebo treatment which concluded the entire experimental study, the CV approached the low variability level characteristic of male chronic schizophrenics not exposed to drug therapy.

Perhaps the chief finding of this investigation was the demonstration of the direct correlation of clinical improvement in schizophrenic behavior (as measured by the Psychotic Reaction Profile and Inpatient Multidimensional Psychiatric Scale) and the increase in the CV of the quantitated EEG; similarly this direct correlation applies to the association of exacerbated schizophrenic symptoms with decrease in the CV.

B. Chlorpromazine in Rabbits

Goldstein and Muñoz (1961b) and Muñoz and Goldstein (1960, 1961b) administered CPZ to rabbits in doses of 0.5 to 2.0 mg/kg, iv. In the quantitated, parietal EEG, the drug increased the MEC to 75–82% above control level. However, in contrast to the action of other agents producing a similar rise in the MEC (such as barbiturates), the CV was not significantly affected. Further studies (to be discussed later) were conducted to evaluate possible alpha-adrenergic blocking activity of CPZ in relation to the EEG behavior of catecholamines, amphetamines, and other CNS stimulants.

XIII. Analysis of Drug Interactions in Rabbits

A. Morphine–Nalorphine

Interest in the interaction on the CNS of these two agents centers on their individual abilities to induce identical shifts in the EEG pattern to that of hypersynchronization. Nalorphine, however, administered at the peak of the sedating action of morphine, institutes an immediate and complete reversal of the latter sedation, as seen by the shift of EEG hypersynchronization to distinct arousal. The animal remains in this alerted state for 10–20 minutes, after which the EEG gradually resumes the initial morphine-induced pattern. The reciprocal of this phenomenon does not occur; nor does nalorphine antagonize its own hypersynchronous effect. The unique features of this interaction prompted Seevers and Woods (1953) to postulate the possible existence of competitive antagonism between two drugs having similar effects but different affinities for the same receptor—thus, a resultant displacement of morphine by nalorphine.

Goldstein and Aldunate (1960) studied the quantitative EEG changes induced in rabbits by morphine and nalorphine, either separately or consecutively. A slow continuous injection of morphine, effecting measureable dose levels of 0.1 to 20 μmoles/kg, yields a linear log-dose-effect relationship between 0.5 and 5.0 μmoles/kg. (The effect measured was the MEC in successive time-unit intervals throughout drug administration.) Below 0.5 μmole/kg changes were not significant; above 5.0 μmoles/kg, the MEC did not increase beyond 325% above the pretreatment, control level. With nalorphine injected under similar conditions, a log-dose related increase in MEC was also obtained. However, the lowest effective dose was 10 times smaller than that of morphine, the plateau level reached with 0.5 μmole/kg, and the plotted data revealed a sigmoid, rather than linear, curve. These facts implied a difference in mechanism of action between the two drugs. Further, the antidoting of morphine action by nalorphine evidently obeys an "all-or-none" law at a variable threshold of 1 part nalorphine to 400 parts of morphine or 1 to 600 parts, respectively. Curiously, nalorphine at the latter, the lower dose level, produces morphine antagonism proportionately longer in duration than that obtained at the higher dose level.

B. Morphine–Quaternary Ammonium Compounds

Knoll and Komlos (1951) and Szerb (1957) reported potentiation of the analgesic effects of morphine by compounds such as choline and neostigmine. It seemed of interest to examine the statistical significance of this phenomenon, and further, to explore other compounds for possibly similar action. Thus, Goldstein (1960a) designed appropriate experiments on rabbits equipped with chronically implanted electrodes and carefully trained for their consistently steady responses to sedative and stimulant agents.

The first step in this work was to determine a dose level of morphine which would have absolutely no effect on the EEG whether administered once or two or three times throughout a 12-hour period, thus precluding cumulative action. Such a level, which provided a "base line" for measurement of morphine potentiation, appeared to be 0.05 mg/kg, iv. Similarly, potential potentiating agents were necessarily screened to establish threshold doses which of themselves also had no effect on the cortical electrical activity. Finally, interaction studies were performed to determine the most effective time spacing of test drug and morphine injections, this interval being obviously dependent upon the mechanism of action of the chemical compounds involved.

By such methods, a large series of quaternary ammonium compounds of widely differing pharmacological properties, were shown to potentiate or enhance the central action of morphine. These include: atropine methyl bromide, scopolamine methyl bromide, homatropine methyl bromide, methantheline, *d*-tubocurarine, decamethonium, succinylcholine, neostigmine, choline, and methacholine. On the other hand, tertiary ammonium analogs of some of these drugs (atropine, scopolamine, homatropine, physostigmine) and other unrelated tertiary compounds (hexamethonium, mecamylamine, β-erythroidine, phentolamine, ergotamine, and dibenzyline) were entirely devoid of potentiating properties. This study offers an unbiased confirmation of the Knoll and Komlos hypothesis which views such potentiation as an occupation of morphine receptors by nonspecific, quaternary ammonium compounds in addition to morphine itself, resulting in an additive analgesic effect.

C. Adrenergic Blockers–Catecholamines and Related Compounds

As previously mentioned, Goldstein and Muñoz (1961b) and Muñoz and Goldstein (1961b) performed numerous electroencephalographic experiments on rabbits to determine effects of adrenergic antagonist agents in relation to the reactivity of the adrenergic system of the brain. (Either curarized rabbits or waking, unrestrained animals with chronically implanted electrodes were used.) These studies were extended to include an investigation of adrenergic antagonists and are summarized as follows:

1. Epinephrine and norepinephrine produced significant arousal reactions in only 20% of the animals.

2. Following pretreatment with dichloroisoproterenol (DCI), a

beta-adrenergic blocker, epinephrine and norepinephrine not only produced arousal in *all* the animals, but an arousal of prolonged duration.

3. The alpha-adrenergic blockers, chlorpromazine, phenoxybenzamine, and dibenzyline, suppressed the stimulant action of catecholamines, whether in the 20% spontaneous group or following treatment with DCI. However, other blocking agents, such as azapetine, dihydroergotamine, and phentolamine, failed to inhibit the central effects of catecholamines, even at doses that did inhibit the peripheral effects of catecholamines.

4. Isoproterenol exerted an EEG stimulant effect which could be blocked by DCI and by all the alpha-adrenergic blockers. Following such a block of either alpha- or beta-adrenergic receptors, the effect of isoproterenol was now one of sedation. A later study (Goldstein, 1962), showed that LSD (5 to 100 μg/kg, iv) also blocked the EEG effects of isoproterenol, in a manner similar to the action of DCI. On the other hand, its nonhallucinogenic analog, 2-brom LSD, produced no blocking effect even at very high doses.

5. Epinephrine, but not norepinephrine, evoked an EEG pattern of hypersynchronization when administered after injection of alpha-blocking agents (characterized by their ability to suppress the stimulant activity of catecholamines). Another condition under which epinephrine displays a sedative rather than stimulant effect was described by Drohocki *et al.* (1956c). The degree of sedation in rabbits anesthetized with ethyl carbamate was increased following administration of epinephrine.

6. DCI reversed and/or prevented the EEG sedative effects of a variety of agents apparently unrelated to the adrenergic system, such as pentobarbital, morphine, and meprobamate. It was ineffective against EEG hypersynchronization induced by chlorpromazine or phenoxybenzamine (Goldstein *et al.*, 1961).

7. The universal stimulant effects of amphetamine were suppressed by the same agents which were found to be effective against catecholamines.

8. The specificity of the aforementioned reactions was emphasized by the inability of either alpha- or beta-blocking agents (or the simultaneous injection of both) to affect the EEG stimulant properties of caffeine or pentylenetetrazole.

These studies, based on statistical criteria of significance in relation to changing MEC levels (corresponding to changing sedation–arousal states), may be interpreted as evidence for the existence of two adrenergic pathways in the central nervous system: one related to the alpha receptors and involved in arousal phenomena, and the other related to the beta receptors, intervening in sedation phenomena.

D. Alpha–Adrenergic Blockers and Histamine

As mentioned in the section on histamine, this naturally occurring amine typically exerts an EEG stimulant effect. An indirect mechanism of action, involving release of stimulant catecholamines by histamine, has been frequently considered. However, such a mechanism has been refuted by Goldstein *et al.* (1964b) in a study of animals pretreated with chlorpromazine; the latter drug had no effect on the EEG stimulant properties of histamine. On the other hand, pretreatment with promethazine, a centrally acting antihistaminic agent, did abolish the stimulant effect of histamine.

E. Atropine–Cholinergic and Adrenergic Drugs

In rabbits, Goldstein (1960b) studied the effect of atropine on the central action of deanol, a choline precursor which (as previously mentioned) does influence brain activity.

In animals displaying EEG hypersynchronization following pretreatment with deanol, atropine (1 mg/kg, iv) caused an immediate reversal of the latter sedation pattern to one of alertness; the effect was quantitatively indicated in the integrated recording by a return to control MEC levels. This alert state persisted for 12 to 15 minutes, after which hypersynchronization resumed. Atropine (1 mg/kg) *alone* induces a hypersynchronized pattern characterized by a shift in the statistical distribution of energy measurements to a higher level without change in the fiducial limits; in contrast, deanol-induced hypersynchronization produces a marked widening of the distribution curve.

It seemed of interest to determine whether the EEG sedation following atropine reversal (arousal) of the deanol hypersynchronization was due to resumption of deanol activity or due to an additional atropine effect delayed by the presence of deanol. The problem was resolved by identifying the nature of the distribution curve of measurements for the sedation period in question. It proved to be a deanol-type distribution, implying resumption of deanol activity.

An interaction of choline and deanol was also reported in this study. Pretreatment of rabbits with choline more than doubled the time (latent period) necessary for deanol to reach the peak of its hypersynchronization effect.

Another example of atropine interaction concerned its tendency at very low doses (5–10 μg/kg) to induce EEG arousal in comparison to the hypersynchronization typically effected by larger doses (1 mg/kg). Pretreatment of the rabbits with chlorpromazine (1 mg/kg, iv) completely abolished the arousal effect (Beck and Goldstein, 1964). This was viewed as a possible indication that the EEG arousal of very low doses of atropine was due to an indirect release of catecholamine.

F. Ethanol–CNS Stimulants

Greenberg *et al.* (1964) studied the effect of various stimulant agents on rabbits treated with ethanol at a dose maintaining a blood level of 300 mg %. This concentration of ethanol produced an EEG pattern of deep sedation with a concomitant high increase in the MEC. Amphetamine (5 mg/kg, iv), deanol (100 mg/kg, iv), carnitine (100 mg/kg, iv), and LSD (5 μg/kg, iv) reverted the hypersynchronous activity to approximately pre-ethanol levels. Under these conditions, EEG arousal did not necessarily correspond to behavioral arousal, although the apparent dissociation was difficult to evaluate in the relatively constrained animals.

G. Hypovolemic Hypotension–Adrenergic and Ganglionic Blockers

As mentioned previously, hypovolemic hypotension, induced in rabbits by draining a volume of blood corresponding to 1% body weight, effected an EEG pattern of sedation, with a large increase in MEC.

Goldstein and Muñoz (1961a) performed such experiments in animals pretreated with various agents to determine whether the EEG effect was due directly to a change in blood mass, or indirectly due to the physiological effects of bleeding on alternate CNS pathways.

Phenoxybenzamine (1–5 mg/kg, iv), an alpha-adrenergic blocking agent suppressing the arousal effect of catecholamines, did not prevent an increase in MEC following bleeding. Phentolamine (5–10 mg/kg), also an alpha-adrenergic blocker (which does not, however, affect the EEG stimulant action of catecholamines) significantly reduced the sedation due to hypovolemic hypotension. Similar interaction was demonstrated with DCI (a beta-adrenergic blocker) and with amphetamine. Hexamethonium (0.1–1.0 mg/kg, iv) had an inverse effect in deepening the level of postbleeding sedation.

XIV. Miscellaneous Drug and Placebo Effects

A. Curare

Although it is generally believed that *d*-tubocurarine does not cross the blood–brain barrier, and so exerts its apparent central effects indirectly, Drohocki and Goldstein (1956b) analyzed the EEG's of rabbits under subparalytic doses (50–200 μg/kg), which induced relaxation of only the neck and ear muscles. They found that although the MEC did not differ significantly in the pre- and posttreatment recordings, the shape of the statistical distribution of measurements was indeed affected by the drug. In place of a sharply defined peak for the class corresponding to the mean, there occurred at least two adjoining classes with identical frequency of occurrence.

B. Pentylenetetrazole

This convulsant agent was studied by Drohocki and Goldstein (1956a) in that it afforded an opportunity to analyze the shifts in three apparently continuous, overlapping states of the central nervous system, namely, wakefulness, excitation, and convulsions. Following administration of progressively increasing doses of pentylenetetrazole, EEG measurements were made for very short time intervals, most often of 1-second duration. Ten and 20 mg/kg, iv, effected a significant decrease in both the mean number of pulses per unit time and a decrease in the variability. With doses of 40 mg/kg, iv, the decrease in both parameters was still initially evident but then was overshadowed in 20 to 30 seconds by a large increase in energy content associated with the appearance of convulsive activity. In decided contrast to other known states of increased MEC, the variability of the EEG during convulsions was almost zero. A search for possible continuum or developing trend within the MEC levels immediately preceding the convulsive phenomena was inconclusive. That is, the shift was so rapid as to obscure the possible existence of an energy state intermediate between mere excitation and drug convulsion. This turning point, between a sharply delimited pattern of decreased MEC and an abruptly appearing pattern of increased MEC, actually suggested two individual EEG's rather than the EEG of one animal.

C. Placebo

As has been frequently observed, the effects of pharmacologically active drugs (such as stimulants, sedatives, antianxiety agents) may often be convincingly replicated on surreptitious substitution of the active agent by a pharmacologically inert compound or placebo (such as lactose or starch). Therefore, in all quantitated EEG drug studies performed on human subjects (at least in the United States), administration of placebo was included. A "triple-blind" design was routinely applied, so that neither subject nor medical investigator nor the technician analyzing EEG records was informed as to the nature of the agent (drug or placebo) administered in a particular study.

Investigations of placebo effects were conducted by Goldstein *et al.* (1963a), Murphree *et al.* (1964), Pfeiffer *et al.* (1963), and Pfeiffer (1965). In most subjects, placebo produced no significant change in either the MEC or the CV. However, in a few volunteers, the EEG did reveal significant decreases or increases in the MEC (as compared to preplacebo control levels), with or without associated changes in the CV. Such changes were detectable in EEG samples taken at various times during the usual 6-hour period of recording. In contrast to the EEG effects of active drugs, placebo effects on the MEC or CV seem totally unrelated. For example, a decreased MEC and increased CV identified 2 hours after placebo, may well reverse to an increased MEC and decreased CV 1 hour later. Furthermore, the aforementioned EEG changes have been shown to be randomly distributed; that is, in any single group of at least 8 to 10 volunteers, statistical analysis of the total EEG data, including that obtained from placebo-reacting subjects as well as from nonreactors, reveals no significance in the variations of the EEG parameters considered.

XV. Discussion and Conclusions

The value of the data obtained with the integrative method of EEG analysis is perhaps best judged by answering a simple though highly relevant question: Does such quantitated data provide *more* information, or a *different kind* of information, than that derived from visual inspection of EEG records alone? Indeed, this would appear to be the most critical, if not the only, question to be raised in the present stage of development of electroencephalography as applied to neurophysiology and neuropharmacology. That is, in any purportedly quantitative investigation of biological phenomena, popular criteria of scientific soundness, such as "precision" or "accuracy" or "dynamic range response' are poorly applicable if not invalid. As emphasized in this review, the direct, intrinsic source of the electroencephalogram is as yet unknown, so that the precise relationship of EEG measurements to the *true* state of brain function remains undefined. It is for this reason that the most acceptable criteria currently employed in this field are those of reproducibility and statistical validation.

The application of statistical methodology to measurement of bioelectrical phenomena has thus far been restricted to direct "utilitarian" testing of the significance of changes in states; and such tests are indeed applied to the integrative method. In addition, however, statistical analysis of quantitated electrogenesis may well serve to characterize a bioelectrical state in terms of the interrelationship of a population of events comprising this state. For example, such an interrelationship may be estimated by the variability of the EEG, a parameter, though often neglected, potentially suitable as an indicator more sensitive to change in functional states than reflected by actual levels of over-all activity.

Thus, in summary, data obtained from the quantitative integration of the EEG under varied experimental conditions have revealed the following heretofore unknown or even unsuspected findings:

1. A difference in the level of brain wave variability in normal subjects as compared to male chronic schizophrenic patients
2. A correlation between the level of EEG amplitude variability and psychological behavioral ratings of chronic schizophrenics;
3. A decrease in EEG variability, induced by CNS stimulants and hallucinogens in normal subjects, to a level approaching that typical of the untreated schizophrenic
4. A concept, derived from animal studies, that stimulation is a graded rather than an "all-or-none" phenomenon
5. An increase in the EEG variability (despite a decrease in the

over-all EEG amplitude) of normal subjects treated with anti-anxiety agents

6. An arithmetic type progression in the increased level of MEC in animals treated with antianxiety drugs.

7. A geometric type progression in the MEC changes preceding sleep in normal volunteers treated with pentobarbital.

8. A difference in the slope of the evolution of the MEC, as well as in the level of the plateau attained, following administration of pentobarbital to normal subjects and to chronic schizophrenics

9. An indication that patterns such as hypersynchronization can correspond to different specific distributions of the values of the electrical energy levels around their means

10. A practical, reproducible method for evaluating chemical agents in respect to such specific factors as onset, peak, and duration of pharmacological action, as well as determination of their relative potencies

11. More generally, an instrument to define the bioelectrical events corresponding to a given behavioral state, e.g., by the limits of distribution of measurements obtained during its occurrence; from such a definition, the possibility to ascertain statistically not only the significance of a change, but also the characteristics of the state evolved by such change. (See Table III for a summary of EEG data obtained in human subjects.)

On the basis of these observations one may conclude that the integrative method of EEG analysis provides both *more* information and also a *different kind* of information than that derived from visual inspection of EEG records alone.

Assuming that integrated EEG data reflects the action of physiological mechanisms of the brain to a reasonable extent, one could cautiously propose a model of brain function derived from such data. Such a model suggests itself in the symmetrical spread of bioelectrical values around their respective means, and in the change of spread of such a distribution in relation to varying states, such as arousal or sedation. In other words it suggests a homeostatic model.

This model of brain function (at cortical levels) is essentially characterized by the regulating mechanisms maintaining a state of equilibrium in a constantly changing environment. Stimulation, hyperexcitation, and hallucinatory states (spontaneous or drug induced) would correspond to different degrees of *hyper*-regulation.

TABLE III
LEVELS OF THE MEC AND CV IN HUMAN SUBJECTS[a]

Condition	N[b]	MEC[c]	CV
Normals—resting EEG	104	32.68	18.52
Chronic schizophrenics			
Undifferentiated	54	35.05	9.18
Hebephrenic	15	37.30	10.02
Paranoid	20	32.77	9.98
Catatonic	12	36.00	7.39
Normals			
Amphetamine 15 mg	8	26.57	12.17
Caffeine 200 mg	4	19.61	11.01
LSD 1 μg/kg	13	24.22	9.95
Deanol 200 mg	10	26.57	34.93
Normals			
Meprobamate 800 mg	10	23.14	56.20
Chlordiazepoxide 20 mg	9	24.15	32.80
Phenobarbital 20 mg	20	23.49	26.93
Orphenadrine 50 mg	7	9.38	31.90
Chronic schizophrenics			
LSD 1 μg/kg	10	37.33	14.50

[a] The drug values listed correspond to maximal effect.

[b] Number of subjects involved in each study. The number of individual measurements from which the mean energy content (MEC) and coefficient of variation (CV) were estimated was most often 30; for example, 390 measurements were used for the calculation of the levels of the MEC and CV in normals under LSD.

[c] The MEC was determined by transformation of direct integrator data from calibration characteristics existent immediately before the recording of each experiment.

In contrast, drowsiness, sedation, and drug-induced sleep would imply *hypo*-regulation. Normal wakefulness, then, would be considered an optimal level of regulating mechanisms functioning in an intermediate position between mechanisms prevailing during excitation and those prevailing during sedation.

At first sight, such a model might seem to contradict the observation that behavior during excitation or in schizophrenia is decidedly more variable than normal. However, it is to be understood that hyper-regulation corresponds to loss of function. Theoretically, the extent and precision of responsiveness in a homeostat is directly related to the variety of its reactive units (Ashby, 1958). Therefore, the correlation of decreased EEG variability with hyper-regulation of brain mechanisms is not, in effect, contradictory to increased behavioral variability.

It is quite apparent that the aforementioned considerations involve theoretical constructs without much factual basis. It must also be stressed that the integrative method of EEG analysis reveals merely a small chapter of the electrophysiology of brain function. This type of analysis is obviously restricted in that it applies to only one aspect of the EEG, neglecting such parameters as frequencies, phase relationships, and waveform correlations. However, despite its limitations, it does indeed have value as a practical tool for exploring an intriguing feature of what is perhaps nature's most fascinating achievement—the brain.

Acknowledgments

We express a particular debt of gratitude to Dr. Zenon Drohocki, the late Dr. Bruno Minz, Dr. Carl C. Pfeiffer, Dr. Harry L. Williams, Dr. James A. Bain, Dr. Henry B. Murphree, Dr. A. Arthur Sugerman, and Miss Elizabeth H. Jenney. The able assistance of Mmes. Diane Leibach, Jenney Stephan, and Martha Hopkins is gratefully acknowledged.

The work done in the U. S. A. was supported in part by grants from the Geschickter Fund for Medical Research and the American Medical Association Education and Research Foundation.

References

André, J. (1945). "Thesis in Medicine." C. Thomas, Nancy, France.

Ashby, W. R. (1958). *Cybernetica* **1**, 83.

Beck, R. A. (1965). Unpublished observation.

Beck, R. A., and Goldstein, L. (1964). *Federation Proc.* **23**, 561.

Beck, R. A., Goldstein, L., and Pfeiffer, C. C. (1963). *Pharmacologist* **5**, 238.

Beck, R. A., Pfeiffer, C. C., and Goldstein, L. (1964). *Pharmacologist* **6**, 204.

Berger, H. (1929). *Arch. Psychiat. Nervenkrankh.* **87**, 527.

Berger, H. (1938). *Nova Acta Leopoldina* **6**, 6.

Bradley, P. B., and Elkes, J. (1955). *Brain* **80**, 77.

Bruck, M. A. (1960). *Electroencephalog. Clin. Neurophysiol.* **12**, 528.

Dement, W., and Kleitmen, N. (1957). *Electroencephalog. Clin. Neurophysiol.* **9**, 673–690.

Domino, E. F., and Hudson, R. D. (1959). *J. Pharmacol. Exptl. Therap.* **127**, 305.

Drohocki, Z. (1937). *Arch. Ges. Physiol.* **239**, 658.

Drohocki, Z. (1947). *Année Psychol.* **47–48**, 230.

Drohocki, Z. (1948). *Rev. Neurol.* **80**, 619.

Drohocki, Z. (1954a). *Rev. Neurol.* **91**, 304.
Drohocki, Z. (1954b). *Rev. Neurol.* **91**, 305.
Drohocki, Z. (1954c). *Rev. Neurol.* **91**, 305.
Drohocki, Z. (1954d). *Rev. Neurol.* **91**, 306.
Drohocki, Z. (1956). *Rev. Neurol.* **94**, 804.
Drohocki, Z. (1957a). *Rev. Neurol.* **96**, 475.
Drohocki, Z. (1957b). *Rev. Neurol.* **96**, 516.
Drohocki, Z. (1957c). French patent issued to the Centre National de la Recherche Scientifique.
Drohocki, Z. (1960a). *J. Physiol. (Paris)* **52**, 83.
Drohocki, Z. (1960b). *Rev. Neurol.* **102**, 320.
Drohocki, Z. (1960c). *Rev. Neurol.* **103**, 276.
Drohocki, Z. (1962a). *Rev. Neurol.* **107**, 204.
Drohocki, Z. (1962b). *Rev. Neurol.* **107**, 211.
Drohocki, Z. (1962c). *Rev. Neurol.* **107**, 257.
Drohocki, Z., and Duflo, G. (1958). *J. Physiol. (Paris)* **50**, 251.
Drohocki, Z., and Duflo, G. (1959). *Rev. Neurol.* **100**, 330.
Drohocki, Z., and Goldstein, L. (1956a). *Rev. Neurol.* **94**, 901.
Drohocki, Z., and Goldstein, L. (1956b). *Rev. Neurol.* **94**, 904.
Drohocki, Z., and Goldstein, L. (1957). *Arch. Sci. Physiol.* **12**, 59.
Drohocki, Z., and Soussen, G. (1959). *Rev. Neurol.* **100**, 326.
Drohocki, Z., Goldstein, L., and Minz, B. (1955). *Compt. Rend. Soc. Biol.* **149**, 2115.
Drohocki, Z., Goldstein, L., and Minz, B. (1956a). *Rev. Neurol.* **94**, 141.
Drohocki, Z., Goldstein, L., and Minz, B. (1956b). *Rev. Neurol.* **94**, 144.
Drohocki, Z., Goldstein, L., and Minz, B. (1956c). *Rev. Neurol.* **94**, 145.
Fisher, R. A. (1930). "The Genetical Theory of Natural Selection." Oxford Univ. Press, London and New York.
Fram, D. H., and Green, J. P. (1963). *Pharmacologist* **5**, 253.
Gibbs, F. A., and Gibbs, E. L. (1952). "Atlas of Electroencephalography." Addison-Wesley, Reading, Massachusetts.
Goldman, D. (1962). *Ann. N. Y. Acad. Sci.* **96**, 356.
Goldstein, L. (1960a). *Federation Proc.* **19**, 291.
Goldstein, L. (1960b). *J. Pharmacol. Exptl. Therap.* **128**, 392.
Goldstein, L. (1962). *Federation Proc.* **21**, 337.
Goldstein, L., and Aldunate, J. (1960). *J. Pharmacol. Exptl. Therap.* **130**, 204.
Goldstein, L., and Minz, B. (1955). *J. Physiol. (Paris)* **47**, 591.
Goldstein, L., and Muñoz, B. (1960). *Pharmacologist* **2**, 80.
Goldstein, L., and Muñoz, C. (1961a). *Acta Physiol. Latinoam.* **11**, 239.
Goldstein, L., and Muñoz, C. (1961b). *J. Pharmacol. Exptl. Therap.* **132**, 345.
Goldstein, L., Muñoz, C., and Norton, G. (1961). *Electroencephalog. Clin. Neurophysiol.* **13**, 167.
Goldstein, L., Jenney, E. H., Murphree, H. B., and Pfeiffer, C. C. (1962). *Proc. Intern. Union Physiol. Sci.* **2**, 1219.
Goldstein, L., Murphree, H. B., Sugerman, A. A., Pfeiffer, C. C., and Jenney, E. H. (1963a). *Clin. Pharmacol. Therap.* **4**, 10.
Goldstein, L., Murphree, H. B., and Pfeiffer, C. C. (1963b). *Ann. N. Y. Acad. Sci.* **107**, 1045.

Goldstein, L., Pfeiffer, C. C., and Muñoz, C. (1963c). *Federation Proc.* **22,** 424.
Goldstein, L., Pfeiffer, C. C., Murphree, H. B., and Jenney, E. H. (1963d). *Pharmacologist* **5,** 233.
Goldstein, L., Stolberg, H., and Sugerman, A. A. (1964a). *18th Meeting Am. Electroencephalog. Soc., Santa Fe, New Mexico* p. 108.
Goldstein, L., Pfeiffer, C. C., Muñoz, C. (1964b). *Federation Proc.* **23,** 1113.
Goldstein, L., Nelson, S. D., and Henley, K. (1965). *Federation Proc.* **24,** 52.
Greenberg, R. E., Goldstein, L., and Pfeiffer, C. C. (1964). *Pharmacologist* **6,** 170.
Groth, D. P., Bain, J. A., and Pfeiffer, C. C. (1958). *J. Pharmacol. Exptl. Therap.* **124,** 290.
Haldane, J. B. S. (1932). "The Causes of Evolution." Harper, London, England.
Hopf, M. A., Galletti, P., and Goldstein, L. (1961). *Proc. Am. Soc. Artificial Internal Organs* **7,** 231.
Jenney, E. H., Murphree, H. B., Goldstein, L., and Pfeiffer, C. C. (1962). *Pharmacologist* **4,** 166.
Kornmüller, A. E. (1937). "Die bioelektrischen Erscheinungen der Hirnrindfelder." Thieme, Leipzig, Germany.
Knoll, J., and Komlos, E. (1951). *Acta Physiol. Acad. Sci. Hung.* **2,** 57.
Longo, V. G. (1956). *J. Pharmacol. Exptl. Therap.* **116,** 198.
Muñoz, C., and Goldstein, L. (1960). *Pharmacologist* **2,** 80.
Muñoz, C., and Goldstein, L. (1961a). *Acta Physiol. Latinoam.* **11,** 242.
Muñoz, C., and Goldstein, L. (1961b). *J. Pharmacol. Exptl. Therap.* **132,** 354.
Murphree, H. B., Goldstein, L., Pfeiffer, C. C., and Jenney, E. H. (1962a). *Pharmacologist* **4,** 166.
Murphree, H. B., Jenney, E. H., and Pfeiffer, C. C. (1962b). *Federation Proc.* **21,** 337.
Murphree, H. B., Sugerman, A. A., Jenney, E. H., and Schultz, R. E. (1963). *Federation Proc.* **22,** 510.
Murphree, H. B., Goldstein, L., Pfeiffer, C. C., Schramm, L. P., and Jenney, E. H. (1964). *Intern. J. Neuropharmacol.* 3, 97.
Pfeiffer, C. C. (1965). *J. New Drugs* **4,** 299.
Pfeiffer, C. C., and Goldstein, L. (1964). *J. Neuropsychiat.* **5,** 475.
Pfeiffer, C. C., and Schultz, R. E. (1964). *Federation Proc.* **23,** 175.
Pfeiffer, C. C., Goldstein, L., and Jenney, E. H. (1960). *Federation Proc.* **19,** 33.
Pfeiffer, C. C., Goldstein, L., Muñoz, C., Murphree, H. B., and Jenney, E. H. (1963). *Clin. Pharmacol. Therap.* **4,** 461.
Pfeiffer, C. C., Goldstein, L., Murphree, H. B., and Jenney, E. H. (1964a). *Arch. Gen. Psychiat.* **10,** 446.
Pfeiffer, C. C., Goldstein, L., Murphree, H. B., and Jenney, E. H. (1964b). *Neuropsychopharmacol.* **3,** 466.
Pfeiffer, C. C., Goldstein, L., Nelson, S. D., Beck, R. A., and Murphree, H. B. (1965). *Proc. 13th Intern. Congr. Physiol. Tokyo, Japan.*
Pierre, R. (1957). *Compt. Rend. Soc. Biol.* **151,** 698.
Seevers, M. H., and Woods, L. A. (1953). *Am. J. Med.* **14,** 456.

Soussen, G., and Chassaing, H. (1960). Cerebral Anoxia and the Electroencephalogram, *Colloq. Reunion Européenne Inform. Electroencephalog.*, pp. 209–213. (Thomas, Springfield, Illinois.)

Sugerman, A. A., Goldstein, L., Murphree, H. B., Pfeiffer, C. C., and Jenney, E. H. (1964). *Arch. Gen. Psychiat.* **10**, 340.

Szerb, J. C. (1957). *Arch. Intern. Pharmocodyn.* **61**, 314.

Wikler, A. (1952). *Proc. Soc. Exptl. Biol.* **79**, 261.

Wright, S. (1940). *In* "The New Systematics" (J. Huxley, ed.), pp. 161–183. Oxford Univ. Press, London and New York.

AUTHOR INDEX

Numbers in italics refer to pages on which the complete references are listed.

C

D

I

J

Q

R

T

SUBJECT INDEX

F

G

H

I

K

L

U

W